D0810170

TOXIC TERROR

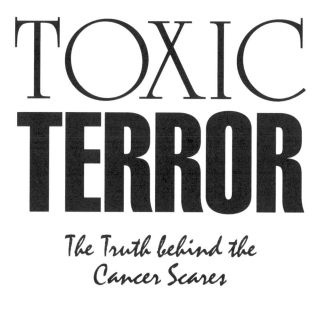

TOXIC TERROR

The Truth behind the Cancer Scares

Elizabeth M. Whelan, Sc.D., M.P.H.

Prometheus Books • Buffalo, New York

Published 1993 by Prometheus Books

97 96 95 94 93   5 4 3 2 1

Library of Congress Cataloging-in-Publication Data

Whelan, Elizabeth M.
     Toxic terror / Elizabeth M. Whelan.—2nd ed.
     Includes bibliographical references.
     ISBN 0-87975-788-4
     1. Environmental health—United States. 2. Pollution—United States—
Environmental aspects. I. Title.
RA565.W47   1993
363.7′00973—dc20   92-34154
                                                                           CIP

Printed in the United States of America on acid-free paper.

Contents

Foreword

A few years ago when I returned home to reside in the United States of America after living and working abroad in a low-income, food-deficit developing nation with limited food production, I experienced a severe cultural shock in reverse.

It appeared to me that our nation was experiencing a curious case of schizophrenia, as it relates to the contributions of science and technology toward the improvement of health, agriculture, food, energy, clothing, housing, transportation, communications, recreation, and industrial development—all of which contribute to the high standards of living enjoyed by Americans today.

On one side, well-organized, noisy consumer-activist groups, aided by a few self-serving Cassandra-type scientists, reinforced by extremists in the environmentalist movement, appeared to be surprisingly effective at preaching "toxic terrorism" and gloom and doom. Through fear they were convincing many people and some political leaders that America is on the verge of being poisoned out of existence. Our predicament, according to these activists, is the direct result of the reckless production and distribution of thousands of new, unnecessary, toxic, carcinogenic, mutagenic, and teratogenic chemical compounds that are being synthesized, manufactured, and sold each year by an irresponsible chemical industry solely for economic profit without regard for public health. According to these alarmists, our water, food, and air are being poisoned, thereby endangering our health.

The promoters of toxic terrorism seem to imply that we must go back to methods of the good old days of the early 1930s, before the use of chemical fertilizers, pesticides, synthetic fibers, and plastics, etc., came into being. At that time world population was 2 billion, whereas today it is 5.4 billion, and growing at the rate of 94 million more per year. One hears little or nothing constructive from these groups about what is to be done to provide for the

7

basic needs of the 3.4 billion additional people who have been added to the world population since 1930. Nor are they very helpful or constructive in taming the family-planning programs. It should be obvious to all Americans that the U.S.A. is today, like it or not, but one of about 165 independent but increasingly interdependent nations of the planet earth. What happens economically, socially, and politically in other countries will have repercussions within the U.S.A., for our economics are ever more intertwined.

Now let us look at the other side of these issues. It appears to me that most Americans are relatively well-satisfied with the substantial—if not truly impressive—improvement in the standard of living that has occurred in the U.S.A. in the past three to four decades, which is in large part attributed to the use of applied science and improved technology.

Most Americans are horrified by the tragic scenes they see on their television screens and read about in newspapers and magazines, depicting hunger, epidemics, poverty, human misery, and famine in Ethiopia and many other African countries. Many Americans, and a few governments, have been generous in providing food and medicine to alleviate the suffering of those who are fortunate enough to receive this assistance. Unfortunately, the magnitude and complexity of the agricultural, food, poverty, and population problem are such that they cannot be solved with food gifts alone. Science and appropriately improved agriculture production technology must be developed and married to enlightened economic and political policy, which will permit its widespread use to increase food production and alleviate human misery in the developing nations.

The U.S.A. today is largely an industrial, commercial, financial, and professional society with only about 2 percent of the active labor force engaged in agricultural production. Consequently most Americans have lost contact with the soil and hence fail to realize the important role that science and technology played in transforming and increasing food and fiber production in the U.S.A. over the last fifty-five years. If they fail to understand what has made American agriculture the most productive in the world it is little wonder that they are bewildered by the reasons for the lack of agricultural productivity and economic progress in the food-deprived nations in Africa at present. Although the present African situation is worsened by drought, it has much deeper underlying causes.

A brief glance at what has happened in American agriculture in the last five decades and in a number of food-deficit nations such as Mexico, India, Pakistan, China, Indonesia, and the Philippines over the past two decades, is relevant to the issue of hunger, poverty, famines—and toxic terrorism. The development and widespread use of improved production technology in the United States—including the use of high-yielding crop varieties, chemical fertilizers, herbicides, insecticides, and fungicides—combined with stimulatory economic policy that encourages the widespread adoption of the new technology, has revolutionized agricultural yields and production in America and other developed countries. For example, as a result of the widespread use of improved production technology and good management, the combined output of the seventeen most important food, feed, and fiber crops, which averaged 252 million metric tons in the 1938–40 period, reached 610 million metric tons in 1978–80, with an increase of only 3 percent in cultivated area. Had our country tried to achieve the 1980 production employing the yield and technology of 1940 it would have required the cultivation of an additional 437 million acres of land. This additional area corresponds to the land area of all of the states east of the Mississippi plus the state of Michigan. It becomes clear from this data that improved technology resulting in higher yields is a substitute for land area.

Agricultural chemicals played the dominant role in increasing yield and production. Had the yields of 1938–40 persisted, to have produced the 1978–80 harvest, it would have been necessary either to have plowed up approximately 73 percent of America's permanent pasture and grazing lands or to have converted 61 percent of the forest and woodland to cropland. In actuality, since many of these lands have much lower productive potential than the land now under cultivation—and are also more vulnerable to erosion—it really would have been necessary to convert a much larger percentage of the pasture land, or forest and woodlands, to crop land than is indicated. Were this to have happened, land for many other uses—including recreation, wildlife habitat, forestry, and urbanization—would have been lost.

These data serve as a clear rebuttal to those who are antiscience, antichemical, and antitechnology, but who nevertheless want to enjoy the good life—including vast areas for recreation, wilderness areas, and areas for wildlife habitat. As a result of the development and widespread use of high-yield production technology the United States has become the largest producer and largest exporter of food in the world. Domestically, as a result of the combined effort of farmers, ranchers, food processors, and the entire food system, American consumers have at their disposal the most diverse, best quality, most inexpensive food supply the world has ever known.

As an agricultural scientist I know that this abundance is in large part the result of skillful management involving the proper use of chemical fertilizers, pesticides, high-yield crop varieties, and sound agronomic practices. Without the availability and proper use of chemical fertilizers, herbicides, insecticides, and fungicides, the worldwide growing demands for food cannot be met, and devastating social, economic, and political chaos are inevitable.

For the past two decades, Americans have been in the grip of a virulent strain of "chemical-phobia." Most people seem convinced that an array of sinister industry-produced chemicals has invaded their air, water, homes, and even their fruit and vegetable bin. The news media regularly carry anxiety-provoking stories about pesticides such as Alar; environmental contaminants like dioxin; industrial chemicals like PCBs; and alleged chemical nightmares at sites such as Love Canal and Times Beach.

Self-appointed representatives of the public interest have demanded bans or severe restrictions on agricultural and industrial chemicals. In 1989, Americans were in a severe state of panic over Alar residues on their apples. Despite the fact that there wasn't one bit of credible scientific evidence that Alar was threatening human health, the Natural Resources Defense Council successfully orchestrated an unprecedented media blitz that resulted in the banning of Alar. Apple growers faced losses of at least $250 million, and taxpayers bought at least $15 million worth of leftover apples.

In her book *Toxic Terror,* Dr. Elizabeth Whelan, president of the American Council on Science and Health, unmasks the pseudoscientific efforts that resulted in the banning of Alar and reveals the frightening gap that exists between the rhetoric of those consumer activists who try to hold the country in a state of "toxic terror" and the scientific realities about such topics as dioxin; 2,4,5-T; and radiation from high voltage power lines. In this book you will get the facts behind the headlines about Love Canal, Times Beach, the nuclear power industry, and food safety. This book may make you angry—indeed it should outrage you—because you have been the victim of a hoax. You have been told that as a result of your country's high state of technology and economic development, your environment is making you sick, when the exact opposite would be closer to the truth.

In the United States in 1900 life expectancy at birth for the total population was 47.3 years, with the male and female life expectancy at birth 46.3 and 48.3 years, respectively. By 1940 life expectancy at birth had increased to 62.9 years for the total population with 60.8 and 65.2 years for males and females, respectively. By 1988 life expectancy for the entire population had increased to 74.9 years with the male and female life expectancy reaching 71.4 and 78.3 years, respectively. Moreover, life expectancy at birth continues to increase despite the doomsday predictions of the toxic terrorists.

Ironically, self-styled health activists foment fear about industrial chemicals that appear in trace amounts around us, causing no known hazard to health, while ignoring most of the real, major hazards to our health today. For instance, some 500,000 Americans die each year as a direct result of cigarette smoking. Yet, curiously, our nation's toxic terrorists seem unconcerned about this, the leading cause of premature death, and are eager to focus our attention on other, hypothetical risks. Nor do they mention that many of our foods— vegetables, fruits, fibers, and grains—which have been consumed by mankind from the dawn of civilization—contain a large number of naturally occurring compounds, which when evaluated at high dosages in rodents are also found to be toxic, carcinogenic, or mutagenic. Forty years ago we were unaware of their existence in our natural foods, but vastly improved and more sensitive analytical procedures that are now available have established their presence. They are, however, present at such low levels that they apparently pose no serious health hazard.

In America in 1993, we have the luxury to worry about the "carcinogen of the week" and the "toxin of the month." We have sufficient food, housing, energy, medical supplies, and other necessities of life. But as you read Dr. Whelan's work, keep in mind the reality that a world without industrial and agricultural chemicals would be a very different world. Banning chemical fertilizers and pesticides will inevitably lead to deadly serious food shortages; it's as simple as that. Banning other industrial chemicals will likewise impoverish our nation. This is the price the toxic terrorists are asking us to pay.

Norman E. Borlaug
Distinguished Professor, International Agriculture
Texas A & M University

Special Acknowledgment

Special thanks to Kris Napier, M.P.H., R.D., for her tireless efforts in the research and preparation of the revised and updated version of this manuscript.

Acknowledgments

Many dedicated people assisted me in the original research phases of the preparation of the first version of this book during 1983 and 1984, including Kathleen Meister, M.S., Cathy Popescu, M.S., and Kris Napier, M.P.H., R.D., American Council on Science and Health (ACSH) Research Associates. Cheryl Martin typed many versions of the first manuscript.

I thank others (in addition to Kris Napier, whom I have acknowledged elsewhere) for their special assistance in the preparation of the newly revised edition of *Toxic Terror,* including Dr. Thomas Orme, ACSH's Washington representative; my special assistant, Patricia A. Keenan; and ACSH legal counsel, Charles H. Googe, Jr., of Paul, Weiss, Rifkind, Wharton & Garrison.

Thanks also to Ken Smith, from the editorial page of the *Washington Times,* for his ACSH commentaries "Alar: One Year Later" and "Alar: Three Years Later," substantial portions of which are used in the discussion here of food safety.

Introduction:

Bad News, Raw Deal

Like most Americans, I get a good deal of my information about health and the environment from books, magazines, newspapers, and the electronic media. And what I have seen, heard, and read in the past ten years has led me to believe that when it comes to discussions of health and the environment, the word *news* is synonymous with *bad news.*

Daily we are subjected to anxiety-producing reports about the "poisons" in our environment, the threat of premature death, human misery, defective children, or no children at all, caused by our careless use of technology. We are warned that calamity is on our doorstep, fresh out of a sinister test tube, and that we face an impending epidemic of disease and death. Human existence itself seems to be jeopardized, our ecology ruined, with nothing left for us to leave to future generations to come. And why is all this happening? The message is clear: our disrespect for nature and the environment and our thoughtless, unharnessed use of modern-day chemicals have spelled doomsday and ecological catastrophe for our country, and perhaps the world.

I am aware of the fact that the bad-news/end-of-the-world scenario is not unique to our times. In 1962, Bertrand Russell[1] told us that nuclear war was inevitable in the next few months. Dr. Paul Ehrlich's 1968 book, *The Population Bomb,* predicted that "the battle to feed all of humanity is over. . . . In the 1970s the world will undergo famines, hundreds of millions of people are going to starve to death in spite of any crash program embarked upon now." Early in the 1970s Jacques Cousteau[2] opined that the oceans would be dead by the end of the century. *Life*[3] reported in 1970 that by 1980 people would have to wear gas masks because of pollution, and that in the early 1980s people by the thousands would be killed in U.S. cities because of smog inversions. We were warned by many sources that rivers would reach the

17

poisoning point in the early 1980s because of nuclear power plants.[4] But the fact that pessimism has reigned in the past does not make the bad news any easier to accept today.

The spring of 1989 will long be remembered for "Alarmania": the fear that gripped the nation after the TV program "60 Minutes" promoted an environmental group's report claiming that children risk developing cancer because the U.S. apple crop was sprayed with a "carcinogen." Apple products were destroyed, and schools temporarily banned the fruit in all its various preparations. A wire service carried a story about a mother in upstate New York who, having heard the news that apples cause cancer, called the state police and had her child's school bus intercepted so that an apple could be removed from the child's lunch box. Apple growers lost an estimated $250 million as a result of this masterminded media campaign.

Dioxin, we read (in stories with subtitles like "Dioxin: In Search of a Killer"), is the "most toxic chemical known to man," capable of causing instant death in minute amounts, responsible for cancer and birth defects in laboratory animals, and threatening the life and health of residents of Love Canal in upstate New York; of Times Beach, Missouri; Newark, New Jersey; Midland, Michigan, and who knows where else.

Limits for acceptable residues of ethylene dibromide (EDB), a pesticide used on a number of agricultural commodities for some forty years, were set by the Environmental Protection Agency (EPA) in the early 1980s. Although the guidelines ensured that the risk of cancer from EDB to consumers was at worst negligible, activists continued their hysterical proclamations about EDB. The result: EDB, an agricultural chemical proven useful and safe, was banned. The EDB situation exemplifies how self-serving individuals and organizations can twist public health issues for political motives.

Women on the West Coast of the United States have repeatedly charged that the widespread use of herbicides—particularly, 2,4,5-T—has caused repro-ductive failures, including low sperm count, miscarriage, and birth defects. Vietnam War veterans assert that all their symptoms and diseases were initiated by their exposure to the defoliating chemicals of Agent Orange in Southeast Asia. Unrelenting public pressure eventually forced first a partial and then a total ban of 2,4,5-T.

Citizen groups have organized to interrupt the development of nuclear energy in this country, pointing always to their concern about the potential cancer-causing effects of low-level radiation, and solemnly noting the "tragedy" at Three Mile Island. We are told that we should not drink the water or breathe the air because it is poisoned with the "fallout of affluence," and we are advised against living in a heavily industrialized state like New Jersey (if we must visit it, we are admonished to hold our breath). Low-level environmental radiation is now blamed for AIDS, Lyme disease, herpes, and other immune-deficiency ailments.

Throughout the United States, individuals are applying for benefits and filing lawsuits claiming that their immune system has been damaged by chemical exposure.[5] Their efforts are supported by physicians who specialize in "multiple chemical sensitivity" (MCS), also called "chemical AIDS" and formerly called "clinical ecology," or who use questionable laboratory data to diagnose "immunotoxicity." Proponents proposed this diagnostic category to include people who had an "adverse reaction to ambient doses of toxic chemicals in the air, food and water at levels generally accepted as subtoxic." Sometimes multiple sensitivity is the diagnosis for those suffering from depression, irritability, muscle or joint pain, or a myriad of other symptoms; but more recently this diagnosis is made even in asymptomatic individuals who claim that exposure to trace levels of environmental chemicals has impaired their immune system and, while they are well now, leaves them open to future disease (the so-called "chemical AIDS" designation, which refers not just to the possibility of AIDS but any disease linked to immune suppression, including cancers). Clinical ecology has long been rejected by groups such as the American Academy of Allergy and American College of Physicians—but some practitioners proceeded with the diagnosis and patients, particularly those who had not found satisfaction with traditional approaches to their ailments, felt better off trying what they thought was the avant-garde remedy. In the case of psychiatric patients "diagnosed" with MCS, a sense of "you don't call me bonkers; I won't call you a quack" prevailed. Clinical ecologists and their patients seemed meant for each other.

But now MCS is becoming a societal problem because MCS patients are demanding medical insurance to cover their diagnostic and treatment costs— and they are suing their employers and neighbors for subjecting them to these alleged chemical exposures. MCS "patients" demand payment and have their own support groups and doctors willing to serve as expert witnesses.

In the most elementary quotes for a payoff, the patient does not even have to claim to be ill, setting up the so-called "unsick plaintiff" charge. Since there is no one to sue when the chemical is a natural product like pollen, the environmental chemical is always a pollutant that can be traced to a particular industry. The plaintiff then professes exposure and claims damage due to this fear of disease—"chemical AIDS" in the future.

Whole industries are being affected by the specter of this type of class action suit—and, of course, each one of them will pass the costs involved on to consumers in the form of higher prices on products. The pulp-paper industry, for instance, has made a significant effort over the last ten years to reduce the dioxin content of waste waters. Dioxin is generated during the bleaching process, thus making the claim that these trace levels of chemicals cause cancer highly unsupportable in court. Disappointed, environmentalists needed a new toxic endpoint—and they came up with MCS, and will continue to be successful in court unless mainstream scientists and physicians speak out to target what Nobel chemist Irvin Langumuir described as "pathological science" and author Peter Huber in *Galileo's Revenge* calls "junk science."

The popular theories here can be summarized as follows:

1. America is being poisoned by chemicals and radioactivity.

2. Our country's health has never been worse and is threatening to deteriorate even further.

3. Big business is responsible for the environmental nightmare and cares not at all about what it is doing, concerned only with its short-term profit margin.

4. Little people (like you and me) are the victims of this corporate greed and toxic crime.

5. This current and future wave of disease and death is the ultimate price we pay for technology and the "good life."

6. New and complex chemicals are poisons and must be either eliminated or highly regulated. The death-dealing technology must be stopped *at any cost.*

Where does all this bad news come from? It appears to emerge from diverse sources ranging from journalistic efforts of individuals with no apparent expertise in science, to a few seemingly prominent academics and opinion leaders who, one would imagine, had scientific data to back up their charges.

First, there has been a mini-epidemic of popular books on the subject of health (or rather ill health) and the environment. Although you may have been warned not to judge a book by its cover, the titles of the recent volumes (all of which were published after 1979) speak for themselves:

- *America the Poisoned: How Deadly Chemicals are Destroying Our Environment, Our Wildlife, Ourselves* by Lewis Regenstein.[6]

- *Who's Poisoning America: Corporate Polluters and Their Victims in the Chemical Age* edited by Ralph Nader, Ronald Brownstein, and John Richard.[7]

- *Malignant Neglect: The First Complete Up to Date Authoritative Report on Known or Suspected Cancer Causing Agents in Our Environment* by Robert H. Boyle and the Environmental Defense Fund.[8]

- *The Poison Conspiracy* by Karl Grossman.[9]

- *The Politics of Cancer* by Samuel Epstein.[10]

- *Hazardous Wastes in America* by Samuel Epstein, Lester Brown, and Carl Pope.[11]

- *A Bitter Fog: Herbicides and Human Rights* by Carol Van Strum.[12]

- *At Highest Risk: Environmental Hazards to Young and Unborn Children* by Christopher Norwood.[13]

- *Pills, Pesticides and Profits: The International Trade in Toxic Substances* edited by Ruth Norris.[14]

- *Love Canal: Science, Politics and People* by Adeline Gordon Levine.[15]

- *Laying Waste: The Poisoning of America by Toxic Chemicals* by Michael Brown.[16]

- *Agent Orange: The Bitter Harvest* by John Dux and P. S. Young.[17]

- *Deadly Deceit: Low Level Radiation, High Level Cover-up* by Jay M. Gould and Benjamin A. Goldman.[18]

- *Design for a Livable Planet* by Jon Naar.[19]

- *Saving the Earth* by Will Steger and Jon Bowermaster.[20]

- *The Greenpeace Book of the Nuclear Age* by John May.[21]

- *The Toxic Cloud* by Michael H. Brown.[22]

- *When Technology Wounds* by Chellis Glendinning.[23]

- *Diet for a Poisoned Planet* by David Steinman.[24]

We learn in these books that:

It is now apparent that a major potential threat to the life and health of every single American exists in the pervasive presence of poisonous chemicals in the environment. These toxic substances, many of which cause cancer, birth defects, nerve and brain damage and gene mutations, are so prevalent in our daily lives, that they are simply impossible to avoid. . . .

America the Poisoned[25]

The wave of chemical violence now sweeping the country is approaching epidemic proportions.

Who's Poisoning America (jacket copy)[26]

The merchandising of poison has become a huge global growth industry . . . the world is being poisoned . . . life is being lost on a wide scale. . . . We are people in Poisonland.

The Poison Conspiracy[27]

The time has come to consider the effect of an increasingly toxic environment on the health of the young and unborn. . . . The potential peril: fetal rats are some fifty times more likely than their mother to succumb to the same dose of certain cancer causing chemicals.

At Highest Risk[28]

In the United States there are some 75,000 chemicals in everyday use, many of which endanger the lives of millions of people who live near where they are produced, handled, transported, or dumped. Contained in pesticides, herbicides, food additives, drinking water, building materials, household goods, and many other carriers, toxic chemicals threaten every woman, man, child, and animal. We are literally poisoning ourselves to death.

Design for a Livable Planet[29]

Almost overnight, people have gotten the correct impression that the world's back is against the wall and that a multitude of environmental disasters is bearing down simultaneously. . . . While I remain hopeful about our environmental future, I believe we're facing the equivalent of World War III. It's ironic, since we always assumed the next war would be nuclear battle or a space race turned ugly. Instead we find ourselves locked in a battle between humankind and nature. And nature is losing ground fast.

Saving the Earth[30]

Exposure to benzene in gasoline products, lead in air pollution, PCBs in electrical transformers and plastics, and ozone from automobile exhaust can result in the deterioration of one's immune response, as well as cancer, leukemia, and birth defects.

When Technology Wounds[31]

Something in the air is wearing away the tombstones of Jacksonville, Arkansas. It's caused a rash of leukemia deaths in Port Neches, Texas, and dime-sized holes between the nostrils of workers in Newark, New Jersey. In rural Michigan, geese are born with their wings on backwards; in Casmalia, California, a man explodes from pulmonary swelling; in Tennessee, the Blue Ridge Mountains are turning dark brown.

The Toxic Cloud[32]

One might argue that books of this type do not have much of an impact on the general public because their circulation is probably small. But even if relatively few copies of the books are distributed (which we do not know to be true), the spin-off op-ed articles and magazine pieces are substantial and read by millions of people. Furthermore, authors of poisons-in-America books are frequent guests on radio and television talk programs, including the network shows, and thus their doomsday views are heard by millions on many different occasions.

There is another pervasive, although subtle message—not only to adults, but now to children. The message, permeating everything from cartoon-depicted environmental specials to the prime-time series "Thirtysomething," is that technology, science, and business are "bad." "Tele-environmentalism" came full force to TV in the fall of 1990, with the help of the Environmental Media Association.[33] As *Insight* magazine reported, "Critics of the Hollywood lobby say that its motives are covertly political and that it often treats scientific theory as fact."[34]

The Environmental Media Association was founded in 1989, recruiting major network entertainment division heads to its board. The president of the association acts as an environmental consultant for one of the shows, "E.A.R.T.H. Force," but has no experience in the field. The pilot episode of "E.A.R.T.H. Force" featured nuclear power as the villain, presented as a deadly "China Syndrome" threat. Environmental messages are not only the agenda of several mini-series and specials, but also issues pervading television movies and prime-time series—a part of twenty-five prime-time series in the 1990–91 season alone.[35]

The 1992-92 season was even more dramatic. Turner Broadcasting aired "One Child—One Voice," touted as an "appeal by children to begin . . . restoring and protecting our planet." Seven children present positions amounting to three points: (1) the world will end if we don't change our ways, (2) viewers must be taught this, and (3) developed nations' environmental problems threaten the Third World.[36] Even "The Simpsons" got into TV-environmentalism. As Lorne A. Reznowski wrote in March/April 1991 *Media Watch,* Homer Simpson, the father in the series, works at a nuclear power plant because, as his high school guidance counselor told him, "It's one of the few outfits around that won't require a college education." The plant is a disaster waiting to happen, thanks to employees like Homer who sleep on the job and ignore danger signs. As a result, the facility wreaks havoc on the environment, as Homer's son learns when he catches a mutated fish at a nearby lake. After hundreds of health and safety violations are found, the plant is shut down and its owner runs for governor.

Time's science editor, Charles Alexander,[37] capsulized the mood of, if not the motivation for, reporting environmental events as popular magazines do: "As the science editor of *Time*, I would freely admit that on this issue we have crossed the boundary from news reporting to advocacy."

Syndicated columnist Ben Wattenberg also summarizes the issue with[38] "Environmentalism is the nice crisis. It's the one that a civilization arrives at when there is no war, when the totalitarian threat is shriveling, when the economy is doing pretty well."

Rolling Stone magazine,[39] in the spring of 1989, went so far as to publish, in their "Saving the Earth Special Issue," their own "Hall of Shame." This was a list of people, corporations, and organizations responsible for "fouling the environment." Among the damned (including myself) were Ronald Reagan, George Bush, Bob Hope, the *Wall Street Journal* editorial page, and your own American home.

In addition to books and magazine stories, we learn about health and the environment from television documentaries, like those featured on the PBS series "Nova" and elsewhere, with such telling titles as "A Plague on Our Children,"[40] "Serpent's Fruits,"[41] "The Politics of Poison,"[42] "Poisoned by Progress: Saving Our Piece of the Planet,"[43] " 'A' is for Apple,"[44] "The Poisoning of America,"[45] and "Remote from Louisiana: The Massive Human Experiment."[46]

In the classic show of this type, "A Plague on Our Children," Harvard biologist Dr. Matthew Meselson addresses the topic of the presence of dioxin in the environment by noting that "thousands of Americans die every year from tumors which are induced because of their exposure to dioxin."

In "The Politics of Poison," another classic example, we hear that dioxin is a "fetus-deforming agent one hundred thousand times more powerful than thalidomide . . . a synthetic chemical so powerful that an ounce could wipe out a million people." In this same film, which focused heavily on the alleged link of the herbicide 2,4,5-T with birth defects and miscarriages, an Oregon woman tells of developing boils on her face after a spraying and proceeds to describe in detail her miscarriage: "When I miscarried . . . the fetus wasn't even recognizable as a baby or anything. It was just a mess. . . . It looked like hamburger, like chopped meat."[47]

Talk-show hostess Oprah Winfrey began her May 22, 1989, show with:

You are looking at the Mississippi River in Louisiana. By all appearances, it is a picturesque scene, but there are many people here who believe that the beauty is deceiving. They say they feel like human guinea pigs, and they call this area the most gruesome of names. They call it cancer alley, the massive human experiment on the bayou, and they tell us that they are afraid that this air, the very air that I'm breathing right now, is so filled with carcinogens that they have labeled the river area a national sacrifice zone, and there are many people here who believe that their lives are being forsaken.

The "bad news" views of scientists, federal officials, government documents, politicians, and consumer advocates who embrace the America-the-poisoned philosophy have been covered frequently in the press for over a decade.

In 1980 Julius Richmond, at that time the U.S. surgeon general, declared that throughout the 1980s the nation will "confront a series of environment emergencies" posed by toxic chemicals that "are adding to the disease burden in a significant, although as yet not precisely defined way."[48]* Dr. Richmond also reported to Congress that the "the public health risk associated with toxic chemicals is increasing, and will continue to do so until we are successful in identifying chemicals which are highly toxic and in controlling the introduction of these chemicals into our environment." In 1980 Gus Speth,[49] another government spokesman (head of the Council on Environmental Quality), noted grimly that "man-made toxic chemicals are a significant source of death and disease in the United States today."

A few well-credentialed scientists have also stepped forward with dire warnings about the environment adversely affecting our health. The late Dr. Irving Selikoff, director of the Environmental Science Laboratory at New York's Mt. Sinai Hospital, told *Time* that "toxic wastes will be the major environmental and public health problem facing the U.S. in the 1980s. . . . We're fouling our own nests and we can't survive if we continue."[50] A Harvard biostatistician was quoted in a 1986 *Wall Street Journal* article as saying: "More people are dying of cancer than before, and to say otherwise is to mislead the American people."[51]

And consumer advocacy groups focus heavily on the problems in the environment in their fund-raising and membership appeals. Joan Claybrook, president of Ralph Nader's Public Citizen advocacy group, went so far as to compare the environmental health disaster of today with the scourge of communicable and infectious diseases in earlier ages: "Earlier generations lived

---

*This is a particularly puzzling statement, leading one to wonder how something can be significant if it is not precisely defined. One is reminded here of an interview in 1971 with Michael Belknap, director of New York Mayor John Lindsay's Council on the Environment. In an article, "The American Way of Life: Is It Killing Us?" Belknap writes: "although proof of the cause and effect of pollutants and disease is not established, the evidence is overwhelming."

in fear of polio and smallpox. Nowadays, the most deadly epidemics we face are man-made. Chemical dump sites, radioactive wastes, acid rain, toxic shock syndrome . . . food additives and more. *These are the perils that most threaten our health today*" (emphasis added).[52]

The media propels left-wing environmental groups, not only by giving them heavy coverage, but also by failing to identify them for who they are. *Media Watch* discussed the environmental movement and the press:[53]

> Not only did newspaper reporters fail to identify their liberal tilt, but they usually failed to refer to them as partisan political activists in Washington. Reporters used the words "activist," "advocacy," "lobbying," "militant" or variations thereof, only 155 times (in 2,903 news stories) (5.3 percent). The newspaper reporters also committed bias by omission—four of the most active conservative environmental groups were mentioned only 60 times (an average of 15 mentions apiece). By contrast, the ten liberal groups merited about 290 stories each. That's almost 20 times more attention than the conservative groups received.

News stories spinning off of the 1990 Earth Day again catered to the liberal environmentalists. According to *Media Watch,* they were offered more than 30 times as many opportunities to speak as their opponents, tallying 68 talking head appearances, compared to two soundbites by one free-marketeer. Interviews were just as heavily weighted: 26 liberal environmentalists to one free-marketeer.[54]

Although the message of environmental gloom and doom comes from different sources, it does seem to have a consistent literary style. In discussing environmental issues, words are carefully chosen to convey horror and fear of the unknown. One of the most commonly used analogies is that of a time bomb, a technique that effectively introduces the concept of devastation occurring, outside our control, at an unknown time and place. A 1979 PBS-TV network report was entitled "Defusing Cancer's Time Bomb."[55] Regenstein, in a *New York Times* piece based on *America the Poisoned,*[56] speaks of "silent time bombs ticking away." Grossman in *The Poison Conspiracy*[57] writes of a "mammoth field of time bombs [which have] been planted, their full impact yet to come." Douglas Costle, a former Environmental Protection Agency administrator, used the same approach when he stated, "We don't understand that every barrel stuck into the ground was a ticking time bomb primed to go off."[58]

An analysis of the selection of words in the classic *Time* cover story, "The Poisoning of America," is revealing in that it confirms the authors' commitment to the concept of real environmental horror. In talking of chemicals, the article refers to "alchemists" whose "concoctions . . ." "ooze . . ." "seep," "brew," and "haunt" while "festering" and "fouling" in "Dantesque" horror.

The bad-news claims of the doomsdayers are not only general and far reaching in their scope, but also quite specific about the devastating impact that technology is having on the health of America.

First, those attempting to rivet our attention on environmental dangers warn us of the potential risk of cancer from the environmental exposure to toxic chemicals:

> Many sicknesses previously thought to arise spontaneously are now known to be caused by environmental pollution. This is especially true of cancer. . . .

> Toxic substances, including carcinogens, are in the air we breathe, the food we eat, the consumer products we use and the water we drink. Exposure to these chemicals has significant deleterious effects on human health, most notably the incitement of cancer. . . .

> Thus as our environment grew increasingly contaminated with synthetic pollutants, the cancer risks we bear rise.
>
> *America the Poisoned*[59]

> We have a cancer epidemic today . . . and that epidemic may become even worse in the years ahead.
>
> *Malignant Neglect*[60]

> Few people need convincing these days that we are in the midst of a cancer epidemic.
>
> *Jane Fonda's Workout Book*[61]

> Cancer, fate of one in four Americans, is now believed to be a byproduct of a way of life. . . . Prime targets are man-made chemicals . . . few have been tested for their cancer-causing potential.
>
> *Defusing Cancer's Time Bomb*[62]

> Cancer rates are rising about 1 percent every year. Childhood cancers have increased almost 32 percent since 1950. A 1978 study by the National Academy of Science estimated that pesticide residues in food alone could cause over 1 million cases of cancer by 2050. Since 1978, there have been twice as many carcinogenic pesticides found on food.
>
> *Our Earth, Our Selves*[63]

Second, those who fear for our health and the quality of the environment frequently point to our air and water as major sources of disease risk.

If I were a Russian spy and wanted to poison the American people, I couldn't plan a better way of doing it than the way the government is handling the hazardous waste issue. People's air and water is being poisoned and the government continues to lie to them about how they are being protected.

Hugh B. Kaufman, EPA "whistle blower"[64]

But now it is time to cast attention onto the less visible, more exotic threat of airborne toxic chemicals, the same kind that were found in the soil at places such as Love Canal. Unnoticed, they are wafting from our factories, our storage tanks, our incinerators and diesel engines—even from the neighborhood dry cleaner. And they are spreading through our global village like a toxic cloud.

The Toxic Cloud[65]

. . . this old planet is, in my opinion, in far greater danger of dying by air unfit to breathe, water unsuitable to drink or food contaminated by some man-made chemicals.

"Poisoned by Progress: Saving our Piece of the Planet"[66]

Third, self-appointed environmentalists consistently point to Love Canal, a community near Niagara Falls in upstate New York, as their classic example of technology gone amok, with resulting disaster to residents, and the inevitable accompanying denial of the offending industry:

Even with a situation such as the Love Canal, where damage to human health has been so thoroughly studied and well documented, the attitude of the chemical industry remains one of soft pedaling the harm, denying guilt and even shifting the blame to the victims.

America the Poisoned[67]

[In reference to hazardous wastes like Love Canal] Perhaps tens of thousands of Americans living in the northeastern part of the United States are either getting sick or dying early as a result of hazardous waste management practices.[68]

There are at least 1,000 Love Canals around the country. We know of 4,000 to 5,000 potential ones. . . . The only thing unusual about Love Canal is that it was discovered.

Hugh B. Kaufman, EPA "whistle blower"[69]

Fourth, we regularly read in environmental books and articles of the deleterious effects of chemicals on young and unborn children, and the manner in which environmental chemicals have apparently interfered with many phases of the human reproductive process.

Mother's milk has become so contaminated with banned chemicals, that it would be illegal to sell in supermarkets. . . .

[Sprayed chemicals] can attack the immunological and central nervous systems, causing cancer and other disorders, and can kill and deform unborn children. . . .

"A Plague on our Children"[70]

When 2,4,5-T or 2,4,D was sprayed from the air, a tragic and familiar and predictable pattern often emerged: pregnant women miscarried or gave birth to deformed babies.

America the Poisoned[71]

At that moment, sitting side by side with my scientist friend, I experienced pure panic. My arms and legs got limp, and my gut felt as if it were going to dissolve. I realized that PCBs and DDE and other poisons are swimming around in my body fluids just as they do in sewers and polluted streams. Worse, they are in the milk I am so conscientiously feeding to my helpless infant daughter.

Parents[72]

Or one could go to Gore, Oklahoma [where there is a nuclear fuel plant that suffered a serious leak of uranium hexafluoride in 1986] . . . and find . . . badly deformed creatures in the area, including a frog with nine legs and a litter of beagles with no ears. . . . One Indian was born with no eyes, and no sockets. . . . People tell me that's the type of deformities they found after Hiroshima.

The Toxic Cloud[73]

Fifth, we are told that industrial, domestic, and agricultural chemicals, including those defoliants used in Vietnam, are known causes of human diseases and death:

Our nations' children are being harmed by the very fruits and vegetables we tell them will make them grow up healthy and strong. These staples of children's diets routinely, and lawfully, contain dangerous amounts of pesticides, which pose an increased risk of cancer, neurobehavioral damage and other health problems.

"Intolerable Risk: Pesticides in our Children's Food"[74]

The most common American foods contain pesticide residues that constitute nearly 80 percent of the estimated dietary cancer risk for man, according to a National Academy of Sciences report released in May.

Audubon[75]

Both industry and government forfeited an opportunity to prevent our present environmental crisis with PCBs at untold costs in lives lost, people's health ruined and the environment poisoned.

The Toxic Cloud[76]

Agent Orange had devastating effects on the environment and human health. It apparently caused miscarriages, birth defects, cancer and liver damage among Vietnamese and Americans alike.

America the Poisoned[77]

[In reference to herbicides] The questions which have been raised recently concerning the hazards of 2,4,5-T and related chemicals . . . may ultimately be regarded as portending the most horrible tragedy known to mankind.

Senator Philip Hart[78]

The chemicals—chlordane, aldrin and dieldrin—have been labeled by their accusers as carcinogenic. Such claims always set off alarm bells with some of the nation's more impressionable citizens. One Long Island resident went so far as to have his house bulldozed, claiming it was contaminated by aldrin.

Wall Street Journal[79]

Sixth, having succeeded in alarming us about the effects of environmental poisons in the United States, the doomsday writers tell us of more horror to come as a result of our shipping garbage overseas.

When the chemical industry learns that one of its products is too dangerously toxic to be sold in the United States, it has found that leftover stocks can be sold and production often continued, by shipping the products overseas. This trade in unregistered chemicals, and in those that have been banned in the U.S., is resulting in death and disability of countless thousands of people in other countries.

America the Poisoned[80]

With America producing so many toxic substances and encumbered with so much toxic waste, U.S. corporations have been working to ship toxic wastes to nations in the Caribbean, South America, Africa and Asia—to dump the tons upon tons of poisons there.

The Poison Conspiracy[81]

The international trade in pesticides and pharmaceutical products, many of which are classified as toxic substances, looms for the 1980s as an international problem of potentially immense magnitude.

Pills, Pesticides and Profits: The International Trade in Toxic Substances[82]

This film is about double standards. . . . It is about certain pesticides and medications we in the United States and other industrial nations export to developing countries in the Third World, . . . products known to cause blood disorders, paralysis, blindness, sterility, even death among people.
"Pesticides and Pills: For Export Only," PBS, 5 October 1981[83]

Gloom-and-Doom Reality

It seems clear to me that a small but active group of individuals, including a few scientists, politicians, and those claiming to represent a consumer constituency, have managed to convince the American public that there is nothing but bad news about health and the environment in this country and that American industry is the culprit. Dr. Merril Eisenbud, former professor and director of the Laboratory for Environmental Studies, Institute of Environmental Medicine at New York University Medical Center, stated in 1980 that "in recent years [there has been] a sense of despair that has become widespread because of what I believe to be a misperception that technology detracts from the quality of life."[84] His words still ring true in 1992. Americans feel so threatened by technology that they are willing to pay anything to solve the problem.

What most Americans are probably *not* aware of is exactly what the costs of "stopping the technology" are, and what type of health consequences will accrue if an enormous portion of our country's resources are committed to additional attempts to remove pollutants from our air, water, and workplaces; to clean up toxic dumps; and to find replacements for chemical pesticides. Because (a) the cost of "environmentalism" is so staggering, and (b) we as a country seem to be moving toward giving environmental groups* and their representatives free rein toward achieving their goals, and (c) the desires of the environmentalists will inevitably lead to major changes in our country's economic system and standard of living, it seems worthwhile—nay, mandatory—for us to pause and evaluate the key premises, motivations, and anticipated outcomes of these so-called health and environment efforts.

It is this desire for evaluation that led me to examine closely the "America Is Poisoned" movement. I did so because I am a concerned American citizen, taxpayer, wife, and mother. I am also a scientist and committed personally and professionally to keeping public health standards high, reducing premature deaths and unnecessary disease, and extending the span of useful, productive

---

*Surely there are many sincere Americans who are understandably vigilant about preserving natural resources and America's spectacular environmental assets. There has, however, in the past twenty years emerged a vocal and militant environmental faction that demands bannings, restrictions, and other regulations with no apparent regard for the equation of health risks vs. economic benefit. It is that faction that is the focus of scrutiny in this book.

human life. I am enthusiastic about retaining both a high-quality environment *and* a first-rate health profile and our current enviable standard of living, made possible by the unprecedented advances in food, agriculture, and technology during this century.

My training and research in epidemiology and public health make me aware of the possibility that pollution and other environmental contamination can and have caused human disease and death, sometimes through accidents, sometimes through human carelessness. For example, in 1968 in Yusho, Japan, PCBs (polychlorinated biphenyls) were accidentally mixed with rice oil and a variety of symptoms, including a severe form of acne, headache, vomiting, diarrhea, fever, neurological disorders, and jaundice were noticed throughout the exposed community.[85]

In the mid-1970s industry misuse of kepone, an insecticide, led to severe kepone poisoning, and symptoms including liver damage, tremors, and blurred vision.[86] These symptoms were not seen in the public at large but were confined to the plant in which kepone was manufactured. Excess kepone reached the Chesapeake Bay after being dumped into sewers. No one has shown kepone poisoning symptoms resulting from ingesting fish or water from the bay area. Industrial dumping of mercury in Japan's Minamata Bay and the Agano River during the 1950s and early 1960s led to the contamination of fish, the main source of protein for the residents. An outbreak of "Minamata disease" occurred, the symptoms of which included loss of motor control, loss of hearing, and in some cases, blindness, coma, and death.[87] Episodes of air pollution and, specifically, the effects of an air inversion in Donora, Pennsylvania, in 1948 and in London, England, in 1952 caused an elevated death rate, particularly among the elderly.

There are additional exposures to man-made chemicals and circumstances that have not necessarily caused human disease and death, but because they have the *potential* for harm they need our ongoing attention and vigilance. The United States generates some 344 million metric tons of industrial waste each year, about thirty to forty million tons of which might be hazardous. These need to be handled in an environmentally sound fashion, with constant awareness of the fact that there have been examples of inadequate management.

The key point here is that there have *always* been environmental threats, reason for caution. As Dr. Rene Dubos wrote in his book *Reason Awake:*

> Man has always lived in a precarious state, worried about his place in the order of things. In the past he was threatened chiefly by natural forces that he could not con rol, and he experienced fear because of ignorance of the cosmos and his own nature. Now threats and fears are derived in large measure from science and its technologies, paradoxically the most characteristic products of human reason. . . . Most would agree that science and technology are

responsible for some of our worst nightmares and have made our societies so complex as to be almost unmanageable.[88]

Thus my purpose in evaluating the frightening claims about health and the environment in America begins with the acknowledgment that misused chemicals—from natural and man-made sources—can potentially do severe damage to human health as well as our natural resources. But the yet-to-be-answered questions here are:

- Is America being poisoned to the extent that the journalists, politicians, and others cited above claim?

- Are we experiencing an epidemic of disease, including cancer, that can be linked causally with the growth in American technology?

- Is air pollution in the United States making people sick, and perhaps even killing them?

- Would we be better off without pesticides and herbicides? If we ban a substantial number of them could we reduce the number of miscarriages, birth defects, cancer, and other ailments in this country?

- Is nuclear energy hazardous to our health, perhaps so potentially harmful that we would be better off turning to other sources of energy?

- Is the state of America's health as bad as the doomsday writers say?

- Is technology making us sick?

If the answer to these questions is *yes,* we do indeed have an environmental nightmare with which to contend. If our very lives, health, and future of our children are at risk, the elimination of environmental contamination must be our number-one goal. We would have to adjust to the fact that the twenty to thirty hours of leisure time we enjoy each week would be a thing of the past. We might have to return to the traditional seventy-hour work week, working at least six days, weaning ourselves from the labor-saving devices that made life easier on one hand, but might be threatening us on the other. We would have to do with less food, fuel, clothing, and other goods. After all, we are talking in this case about the survival of the American populace (and perhaps other portions of the world). When you perceive that your life and health are clearly and imminently threatened by man-made pollution, the concept of cost becomes largely irrelevant.

But what if the answer to those questions above were uniformly *no*? What if there is evidence that Americans have never been healthier, that with two major exceptions (lung cancer and melanoma), the age-adjusted cancer death rate has been *declining* over the past fifty years; that air and water pollution account for not one known death in the United States today; that pesticides, to our best knowledge, are not contributing to ill health, but rather promoting good health; and that nuclear energy is safer than any other kind currently available?

What if—while the doomsdayers are breeding hysteria about air pollution, water pollution, Love Canal, and dioxin—some five hundred thousand Americans are dying each year from a perfectly avoidable environmental cause that is of little or no interest to the environmentalists?

What if, instead of technology *threatening* us, it is offering us an opportunity for even *more* improvements in the quality of life? Suppose these "ifs" lead to the conclusions that America is being poisoned not by chemicals, but by the poisoned pens of alarmist writers and advocates. Then we would find ourselves spending unknown billions of dollars, terminating an unknown number of jobs, facing the reality of food shortages, becoming even further dependent on foreign sources for our energy needs, paying higher taxes, and witnessing a decline in our standard of living—all in the "interest of promoting health"— *but with no perceived or measurable health benefit whatever.*

If you went to a department store and spent a hundred thousand dollars for a large, beautifully wrapped box that the salesperson told you contained many highly valuable jewels and got home only to find the box was empty, what would your reaction be? Probably you would recognize you were the victim of a swindle. If you negotiated by phone with a real estate agent for a five-bedroom Florida condominium on a beach, mailed in your down payment, and then found out that the piece of property you just "bought" did not exist, how would you react? It would be quite clear to you that you had been robbed.

Similarly, if you pay an increasing proportion of your paycheck to the government to contribute to the expansion of the Environmental Protection Agency, learn that the monthly maintenance on your apartment is doubled to cover the increased taxes for stricter air- and water-pollution standards (requiring air and water to be a thousand times purer than they are now), pay higher electricity bills each month, spend substantially more at the supermarket each week, and watch your neighbor lose his job because the material his company was using to produce goods was considered "too risky" by the environmentalists, you may assume that these costs you and others take on translate into better health. But how would you feel if you learned that most of the tax revenues you pay for "environmentalism," the extra price margin on food that results when pesticides are banned, *resulted in nothing in terms of improved health* because there is no evidence that these environmental factors are adversely affecting health in the first place? You would feel robbed. You would feel swindled. And you would be right.

The title of this book makes clear the conclusions of my research into these critical environmental questions. I have reviewed literally thousands of popular and scientific articles on the topic of environmental factors and human health. Necessarily, I had to limit the scope of the review to what are classically thought of as "environmental factors," that is, pesticides, nuclear energy, PCBs, and others.

What I found in my literature review was an astounding gap between the consensus in the scientific and medical community on environmental issues versus what was being presented in popular publications, on television and radio, and in books (like the ones cited above) for the layman. Thus this work is an attempt to explode the myth created by the extreme environmentalist movement. It is an urgent call for Americans to recognize the severity of the gap between science and popular public thought, and the dramatically unpleasant side effects that a continued embracing of environmental alarmism will have for our country.

I hope the book will demonstrate clearly the stark differences between the claims in books like *The Toxic Cloud* and the views of mainstream scientists. And it will raise some specific questions:

First, why are the media so gullible when it comes to swallowing whole the utterances of the doomsdayers and then reporting those items that scientists see as "myth" or "fantasy" as if they were full-fledged news stories? Isn't good news ever news? When Sweden banned DDT in 1969, it was a major media event in this country, complete with large headlines. When the Swedish parliament rescinded its total ban one month later and reintroduced the qualified use of the insecticide to protect its vast forests, "the silence in the American press was deafening."[89] Why in the period from 1967 to 1969 did one single environmental organization (Environmental Defense Fund) receive over nineteen thousand column inches of press coverage reflecting its views on why DDT should be banned, and there was only scant coverage of those who thought DDT was a useful and lifesaving chemical? Where is that classic American investigative reporting style, and why has it not turned its inquiring teeth and skeptical glance to the environmental movement?

Second, where are the scientists in this debate? The most unsettling characteristic of the "bad-news syndrome" in the media is the fact that there do appear to be legitimate U.S. scientists who feel that the end of America is near. A handful of them repeatedly appear in interviews and are cited *ad nauseam* in articles. Why do we not hear more scientists who represent the mainstream of thought? Why haven't the vast majority of American scientists and physicians come forward publicly in defense of the truth? I am not the first person to raise this question. Indeed, in one of the very few sane and balanced books on health and the environment, *Ecological Sanity*,* Drs. George Claus and Karen Bolander note,

> One of the most obvious questions that may come to the reader is: "if the authors allege that a considerable number of the scientific claims of the environmentalists are false and some of the papers which support these claims are worthless or filled with errors, how does it happen that out of the more than 200,000 scientists in the United States, so few have spoken up in a similar vein of protest?"

Frankly this same question occurred to me some time ago, and it must be admitted that it is a tricky one.[90]

It seems to me that scientists shun the spotlight for several reasons. First, they don't speak the language of consumers and have no interest in presenting their ideas to the mass media. Further, they are often so highly specialized that they hesitate to venture outside their fields to give the media a glimpse of the "big picture" on the public health scene. A substantial number of physicians and scientific academicians are literally fearful of getting into debates on subjects such as the safety of Alar, BST, or dioxin because they fear they will be humiliated by being called a "paid liar" by their opposition. This is a real problem. Because nearly all colleges receive funding from corporations, scientists who defend the products of industry remain vulnerable to the charge that they are "hired guns," even though they are expressing their own professional views. Indeed in the 1990s, any scientist who defends technology in debate with those who target "chemicals" as the cause of all ills will be charged with funding bias. It's safer to keep silent.

Third, who are these extreme environmentalists, what do they really want, who is their constituency, and what interest group is backing them? What motivates them to bring us such bad news, willfully overlooking the obvious statistical signs of the health and vitality of America and Americans today? Are they really as selfless and interested only in the good of mankind as they pretend to be? Or are there some hidden motivations?

Perhaps, ideally, a book evaluating the environmental movement should be researched and written by a thoroughly unbiased source, whoever that is. But this one was not. I am biased—in favor of both health and technology. I think the United States is the most desirable and enviable country in the world. We have the most beautiful land, oceans, rivers, and streams; the most plentiful, varied and inexpensive food supply; the highest standard of health and living; the most leisure time; a stable political system that has ensured

---

*Others include *The Doomsday Syndrome* by John Maddox and *Environment, Technology and Health* by Dr. Merril Eisenbud.

its citizens the highest degree of personal liberty in the world; and the best potential for continued economic and humanitarian growth. I am incensed by the possibility that lies, exaggeration, and innuendo about the relationship of our health and environment might change the whole fabric of the lives of Americans. As a consumer who appreciates the current bounty and great potential this country has, as a taxpayer who is no longer willing to tolerate expenditures for problems that don't exist, and as a scientist who recognizes that the truth is the only antidote for the poisoned pens, I feel an obligation to set the record straight. I am well aware that defending technology is considered "politically incorrect," and that there are members of the media, lay public, and scientific community who will be outraged by the contents of the pages that follow, eager to shoot down the messenger who bears good news. But I also know that there are millions of Americans who are willing to consider "another view." I hope this book will stir the resentment of those who read it and that they, as I, realize that we are the victims of *Toxic Terror.*

> Elizabeth M. Whelan
> December 1992
> New York, N.Y.

NOTES

1. J. J. McKetta, "Is the Sky Really Falling?" *National Environmental Balance* (1983).

2. P. Erlich, *The Population Bomb* (Rivercity: Rivercity Press, 1971).

3. McKetta, *National Environmental Balance.*

4. Ibid.

5. S. Barrett, "Chemical Aids," *Priorities* (Fall 1989).

6. L. Regenstein, *America the Poisoned: How Deadly Chemicals are Destroying Our Environment, Our Wildlife, Ourselves* (Washington: Acropolis Books, 1982).

7. R. Nader, R. Brownstein, and J. Richard, eds., *Who's Poisoning America: Corporate Polluters and Their Victims in the Chemical Age* (San Francisco: Sierra Club Books, 1981).

8. Environmental Defense Fund and R. H. Boyle, *Malignant Neglect: The First Up to Date Authoritative Report on Known or Suspected Cancer Causing Agents in Our Environment* (New York: Alfred A. Knopf, 1979).

9. K. Grossman, *The Poison Conspiracy* (Sag Harbor: The Permanent Press, 1983).

10. S. Epstein, *The Politics of Cancer* (San Francisco: Sierra Club Books, 1978).

11. S. Epstein, L. Brown, and C. Pope, *Hazardous Wastes in America* (San Francisco: Sierra Club Books, 1982).

12. C. Van Strum, *A Bitter Fog: Herbicides and Human Rights* (San Francisco: Sierra Club Books, 1983).

13. C. Norwood, *At Highest Risk: Environmental Hazards to Young and Unborn Children* (New York: McGraw Hill, 1980).

14. R. Norris, ed., *Pills, Pesticides and Profits: The International Trade in Toxic Substances* (Croton-on-Hudson: North River Press, 1982).

15. A. G. Levine, *Love Canal, Science, Politics and People* (Lexington: Lexington Books, 1982).

16. M. Brown, *Laying Waste: The Poisoning of America by Toxic Chemicals* (New York: Pantheon, 1980).

17. J. Dux and P. J. Young, *Agent Orange: The Bitter Harvest* (Sidney: Hodder and Stoughton, 1980).

18. J. M. Gould and B. A. Goldman, *Deadly Deceit: Low Level Radiation, High Level Cover-Up* (New York: Four Walls Eight Windows Press, 1990).

19. J. Naar, *Design for a Livable Planet* (New York: Harper and Row, 1990).

20. W. Steger and J. Bowermaster, *Saving the Earth* (New York: Alfred A. Knopf, 1990).

21. J. May, *The Greenpeace Book of the Nuclear Age* (New York: Pantheon Books, 1989).

22. M. H. Brown, *The Toxic Cloud* (New York: Harper and Row, 1987).

23. C. Glendinning, *When Technology Wounds* (New York: William Morrow and Company, 1990).

24. D. Steinman, *Diet for a Poisoned Planet* (New York: Harmony, 1990).

25. Regenstein, *America the Poisoned.*

26. Nader, *Who's Poisoning America?*

27. Grossman, *Poison Conspiracy,* p. 1.

28. Norwood, *At Highest Risk,* p. 3.

29. Naar, *Design for a Livable Planet,* p. 37.

30. Steger and Bowermaster, *Saving the Earth,* pp. xv, xxiii.

31. Glendinning, *When Technology Wounds,* p. 55.

32. Brown, *Toxic Cloud* (book jacket).

33. R. Marin, "Networks Turn to Greener Staple," *Insight* (September 24, 1990): p. 59.

34. Ibid.

35. Ibid.

36. M. C. Byrne, "Honey, Ted's Warped the Kids," *Media Watch* (March 1992).

37. B. Wattenberg, "Humanity Craves a Crisis, and Now It's the Environment," *Houston Post,* November 7, 1989.

38. Ibid.

39. "Hall of Shame," *Rolling Stone,* May 3, 1990, pp. 53–56.

40. "Nova: A Plague on Our Children," (Boston: WGBH Educational Foundation, 1979).

41. "Serpent's Fruits" (New York: Public Broadcasting Service, WNET-TV, July 1979).

42. "The Politics of Poison" (San Francisco: KRON-TV, April 1979).

43. "Geraldo: Poisoned by Progress: Saving our Piece of the Planet" (August 24, 1989).

44. Ed Bradley, "60 Minutes: A is for Apple" (New York: CBS-TV, February 26, 1989).

45. H. Downs, "The Poisoning of America" (New York: ABC-TV, September 8, 1988).

46. Oprah Winfrey, "Remote from Louisiana: The Massive Human Experiment" (May 22, 1989).

47. "Politics of Poison."

48. "The Poisoning of America," *Time,* September 22, 1980, p. 58.

49. "The American Way of Life: Is It Killing Us?" *New York Times,* April 18, 1971.

50. "Poisoning of America," *Time,* p. 58.

51. M. Waldolz, "War on Cancer: New Study Disputes Claims of Progress,"*Wall Street Journal*, May 6, 1986.

52. J. Claybrook, Public Citizen, undated membership and fund-raising appeal.

53. "Tags not Planted on Green Groups," *Media Watch* (April 1990): pp. 6–7.

54. "Earth Day Without Alternatives," *Media Watch* (May 1990).

55. "Defusing Cancer's Time Bomb" (San Diego: KPBS-TV, November 1978).

56. Regenstein, *New York Times,* 1983.

57. Grossman, *Poison Conspiracy,* p. 24.

58. Regenstein, *America the Poisoned,* p. 137.

59. Ibid.

60. Environmental Defense Fund and Boyle, *Malignant Neglect,* p. 3.

61. J. Fonda, *Jane Fonda's Workout Book* (New York: Simon and Schuster, 1981), p. 238.

62. *Defusing Cancer's Time Bomb.*

63. R. Caplan, *Our Earth, Our Selves* (New York: Bantam, 1990), p. 123.

64. "Poisoning of America," *Time,* p. 61.

65. Brown, *Toxic Cloud,* p. 7.

66. "Geraldo" (August 24, 1989).

67. Regenstein, *America the Poisoned,* p. 142.

68. *Crown's Book of Political Quotations* (New York: Crown, 1982).

69. Regenstein, *America the Poisoned,* p. 142.

70. "Nova."

71. Regenstein, *America the Poisoned,* p. 15.

72. C. Ricci, "The Breast Milk Test," *Parents,* August 1988.

73. Brown, *Toxic Cloud,* p. 185.

74. Natural Resources Defense Council, "Intolerable Risk: Pesticides in our Children's Food" (1989).

75. "Death on Your Dinner Table," *Audubon,* September 1987.

76. Brown, *Toxic Cloud,* p. 295.

77. Regenstein, *America the Poisoned,* p. 19.

78. Quoted in Regenstein, *America the Poisoned,* p. 21.

79. "Warning to Homeowners," *Wall Street Journal,* March 18, 1985.

80. Regenstein, *America the Poisoned,* p. 216.

81. Grossman, *Poison Conspiracy,* p. 203.

82. Norris, *Pills, Pesticides and Profits,* p. 1.

83. "Pesticides and Pills: For Export Only" (Public Broadcasting Service, October 1981).

84. M. Eisenbud, "The Environment, Technology and Health: A Century of Progress, But a Time of Despair," *American Journal of Medicine* 68 (1980): p. 476.

85. World Health Organization, "Environmental Health Criteria 2: Polychlorinated Biphenyls and Terphenyls" (Geneva: WHO, 1976).

86. S. D. Murphy, "Pesticides," *Casarett and Doul's Toxicology,* 2nd ed. (New York: Macmillan Co., 1980), p. 364.

87. World Health Organization, "Environmental Health Criteria 1: Mercury" (Geneva: WHO, 1976).

88. R. Dubos, *Reason Awake* (New York: Columbia University Press, 1970).

89. G. Claus and K. Bolander, *Ecological Sanity* (New York: David McKay, 1977), p. 33.

90. Ibid., p. 49.

1

Environmental Premises
and Scientific Realities

The "house" of environmentalism sits on a unique foundation of premises and claims. An analysis of the various doomsday books, articles, and television documentaries—and the daily reporting on environmental issues in the American media—reveals that there are ten key elements to the environmental mindset, which, if valid, would provide the basis for an open-closed case verdict in favor of their recommendations. Additionally there are several techniques—or, if you will, gimmicks—that environmentalists consistently use to present their case for urgent regulation in the interest of promoting health.

Before looking at the validity of specific charges relative to air and water pollution, Love Canal, low-level radiation, pesticides and herbicides, and other current topics, it is worthwhile to evaluate critically each of the key environmental premises and the arsenal of strategies to which the prophets of doom turn in presenting their arguments. If the foundation is sound, this "environmental house" will stand unthreatened. If it is shaky, the house will ultimately fall.

PREMISE I: The United States Is in the Grip of a Cancer Epidemic and Technology Is to Blame.

Oprah Winfrey opened her May 22, 1989 show by calling the Mississippi "cancer alley . . . the massive human experiment on the bayou, and they tell us that they are afraid that this air, the very air that I'm breathing right now, is so filled with carcinogens that they have labeled the river area a national sacrifice zone, and there are many people here who believe that their lives are being forsaken."

Industry's wastes are continually blamed for the cancer of both today and tomorrow, as did the book *Who's Poisoning America* when discussing Love Canal: "Love Canal doesn't end with this generation's cancer or even with the next generation's birth defects. For many residents, the damage is permanent in their genes and their children's. The mutated genes will affect all of their descendants, one generation after another."[1]

Cancer is also foremost in mind as you fertilize your lawn and kill the weeds: "According to the National Coalition Against the Misuse of Pesticides, an advocacy group critical of the lawn-care industry, nine of the pesticides may be carcinogenic. . . ."[2]

Even food is a potential cause of cancer, as described by a 1987 *Audubon* article: "The most common American foods contain pesticide residues that constitute nearly 80 percent of the estimated dietary cancer risk for man, according to a National Academy of Sciences report released in May."[3]

Drinking water is similarly tainted, according to many sources, such as the *The Politics of Cancer:* Drinking water in New Orleans, derived from the Mississippi River, contains over 200 synthetic organic pollutants, including a wide range of known chemical carcinogens and many yet unidentified and untested chemicals.[4]

And the press would lead most people to believe that the nuclear industry is spewing out cancer-causing radiation, as described by Dr. Gofman: "The nuclear industry has been killing people every day for years in the form of cancer leukemia deaths for the workers, and because we haven't declared the workers to be lepers, we let them procreate and thus they spread their radiation damage into the population at large.[5]

A 1986 *Wall Street Journal* article, "War on Cancer: New Study Disputes Claims of Progress,"[6] opened with "Three decades of medical research have failed to stop the rising rate of death from cancer among Americans," and went on to quote the author of the study, John C. Bailer III, a biostatistician at Harvard University's School of Public Health:

> The bottom line is that despite all the billions of dollars, the promises, and the claims of success, more people are dying of cancer than before, and to say otherwise is to mislead the American people into believing we are beating this problem.

IS THERE A CANCER EPIDEMIC?

An analysis of United States cancer incidence (number of new cases) data and cancer death rates over the past few decades indicate clearly that the answer to this question is no. To make a valid comparison of cancer rates over time in this country, one must first keep in mind that it is the *rate* of cancer, not the *number* of cases, that is critical to the evaluation of a trend. Obviously there are more cancer deaths and cases in 1991 than there were in 1900, but our population base has more than doubled as well. Second, the age distribution of the U.S. population over time has shifted, with our society aging significantly in the last few decades. Because a larger portion of the 1990 population is over age sixty-five than was the case twenty, forty, or sixty years ago, and older people are more likely to develop cancer, it is necessary to "age adjust" cancer rates to establish a meaningful trend. Third, we have to recognize that cancer is the name for many diseases, each of which could have different causes and origins. So we must, in discussing cancer rates, make note of the types of cancer that are occurring with greater or lesser frequency.

Fourth, when comparing epidemiological studies we must take care to ensure that data collection methods have been constant over time. In general, this has been true with one major exception that involves a comparison of data collected in two recent studies: (a) the National Cancer Institute's (NCI) *Third National Cancer Survey,* 1969–1971 (TNCS), and (b) Cancer Surveillance Epidemiology and End Results (SEER) program, an ongoing study of cancer incidence that began in 1971.

Combination of data from these studies was the basis for the conclusion of Dr. Epstein and the Council on Environmental Quality that cancer incidence has increased in recent years. Pooling the data from these two dissimilar studies, however, gives an erroneous impression of trends in cancer incidence. According to a 1981 review of the TNCS and SEER reports that appeared in the *Journal of Fundamental and Applied Toxicology,* the studies "cover discontinuous time periods and nonidentical geographic population. . . . They may not, as they were, be pooled for time trend analysis."

To be able legitimately to compare two sets of data collected in different surveys, three important statistical criteria must be fulfilled. The study indicated that the TNCS and SEER data *did not fulfill* these criteria. Therefore, according to accepted statistical protocol, the data from these two surveys cannot be combined.

There are several factors that could have biased the results from the two surveys, making them incomparable. The TNCS data misstate the population at risk of developing cancer by using 1950 census material to estimate the incidence of cancer from 1969 to 1971. Since the populations in the areas sampled may have changed significantly during this period, this could result in errors in calculating the incidence rates.

One of the biggest problems with the SEER report is that data collection procedures have changed over time and that updating of information has apparently been inconsistent. Another group of independent evaluators under

NCI contract concluded that "there are no uniform standards for data completeness and validity . . . ," and that procedure changes "have been far too numerous, insufficiently thought out and poorly timed." These flaws seriously undermine the usefulness of such data in determining time trends.

In addition, University of Oxford cancer researchers Sir Richard Doll and Richard Peto (generally regarded as two of the world's foremost epidemiologists) have pointed out that combining the TNCS and SEER data produces incidence figures that are incompatible with cancer mortality trends over the same time period, which are not so large as is commonly assumed.

When they looked at three major cancers for which treatment and survival have not changed appreciably since 1950, they found that the inconsistency remained. For example, while mortality caused by intestinal cancer declined gradually, comparison of TNCS and SEER data indicated a very rapid increase in incidence. Likewise, while breast cancer mortality rates remained nearly constant, when data from TNCS and SEER were compared, bizarre fluctuations were evident in incidence rates during the 1970s. For prostate cancer, the researchers found the trend suggested by comparison of the TNCS and SEER data with each other to be "absurdly incompatible with the mortality data."

Overall, Doll and Peto reported that "quite fantastic and irregular variations in incidence are suggested by such comparisons (either between the two studies or within SEER), ten times greater than could plausibly be attributed to chance, and a hundred times greater than corresponding annual changes in mortality over the past few decades."

Doll and Peto felt that a comparison between the SNCS (Second National Cancer Survey) and TNCS data might be reasonably accurate in elucidating the time trends in cancer incidence, since the studies were similarly conducted and such a comparison produced results that were fairly consistent with mortality trends. (They pointed out, however, that this argument was rather circular.)

A comparison of SNCS and TNCS data indicates that composite age-adjusted cancer incidence rates *declined* slightly from 1947 to 1987. About all that can be said with any degree of certainty about the TNCS and SEER data is that neither of these studies separately shows any increase in cancer incidence. Readers are urged to interpret apparent time trends with caution, and to realize that many of the "increases" may not, in fact, be real. Thus, recent allegations that there has been a significant increase in cancer incidence during the decades of the 1970s and 1980s are open to serious question.

Taking into account age adjustment and the type of cancer, and comparing data from similar surveys over time, the national cancer data* on incidence and mortality show the following about the U.S. cancer picture:

---

*Cancer mortality statistics are available yearly through the National Center for Health Statistics. Incidence data are available through occasional national surveys (see appendix).

1. There is no general epidemic of cancer, that is, no sudden dramatic rise in cancer incidence or mortality, as a whole, over the past forty years.
2. The most important absolute increases in cancer incidence and mortality during this time period have been cancer of the lung, known to be caused largely by cigarette smoking. In 1992, the Centers for Disease Control said that 30 percent of all cancer deaths and 87 percent of lung cancer deaths are attributable to tobacco use.[7]
3. The most important absolute decreases have occurred in cancer of the stomach and cervix. Cancer of the liver has also shown a steady decline.
4. Other than the above, there seem to be no significant changes in the incidence of other forms of cancer over the past fifty years.

The appendix at the back of this book carries a full description of cancer trends by site. The *"cancer epidemic" is limited to lung cancer* and is particularly marked for males, but now is rising steeply for females *because the rate of smoking has increased among females.*

IS NEW JERSEY CANCER ALLEY?

It may be tempting to link elevated cancer death rates with the presence of the petrochemical industry in that state, but a closer look at this subject reveals that the primary characteristic of New Jersey that explains its relatively high cancer death rate is the fact that it is so urban in character. If one compares the cancer death rates, by site, of New Jersey with those of cities and metropolitan areas, instead of other states, one finds that the cancer mortality rate for New Jersey* is about the same as that in Chicago, San Francisco, New York, and Philadelphia. Why is the "urban characteristic" a risk factor for cancer? It in itself is not a risk factor, but lifestyle differences—particularly the increased frequency of cigarette smoking among city dwellers—largely explain the rural/urban differences in cancer pattern.[8]

In 1987, newspaper reports speculated that there was a connection between environmental factors at the Meadowlands sports complex in East Rutherford, New Jersey, and four cases of cancer that developed in players on the Giants football team over an eight-year period. An expert panel found no link between the four cases, which did not meet the usual definition of a cluster. An environmental survey of the area around the sports complex revealed low levels of possibly carcinogenic chemicals, typical of those found in urban areas throughout the country.[9]

---

*New Jersey's Salem County does have an elevated rate of bladder cancer, which is believed to be linked to the use of carcinogenic chemicals in the manufacture of dyes during the 1950s and earlier. The problem was confined to those who were occupationally exposed.

There is no evidence whatever that air or water pollution, or any other "environmental factor," contributes to cancer in the general population in New Jersey.[10]

PREMISE 2: 80–90 Percent of Cancer Is Caused by Environment.

Since 1970, professional and popular articles have frequently cited an estimate that "80 to 90 percent of all cancers are environmentally induced" and "thus preventable." The implication, of course, is that the "environment" refers to a virtual army of cancer-causing chemicals in our air, food, water, and workplace. Talk show host Geraldo, in point of fact, reworded this to "Ten years ago, the head of the Environmental Protection Agency said that almost 90 percent of our cancers are due to chemicals in the environment."[11] The message is particularly self-serving in government reports because it lends support to the idea that we need more regulations and regulators to deal with all those hazardous chemicals.

Unfortunately, it is a misunderstanding of the definition of "environmental cancer" that is causing the general public to believe that there are easy solutions. The 80–90 percent figure, and its variations, has its origins in the work of John Higginson, founding director of the World Health Organization's International Agency of Research on Cancer. During the 1950s Dr. Higginson compared the incidence of certain types of tumors among blacks in Africa and America and concluded that about two-thirds of all cancer had an environmental cause and were, therefore, theoretically preventable.

Dr. Higginson, regretful of the misinterpretation of his statistics, notes: ". . . when I used the term environment in those days, I was considering the total environment, cultural as well as chemical. By cultural, I meant mode of life . . . environment is what surrounds people and impinges on them." He complains that his statistics have "been misinterpreted, funnily enough, not among the majority of scientists with whom I have contact, but by the chemical carcinogen people and especially by the occupational people."[12]

Our environment is not limited solely to our physical surroundings and man-made chemicals. Many scientists now believe that cultural and personal habits contribute more to cancer causation than environmental pollutants or toxic chemicals. In its broadest sense, then, our environment encompasses such factors as smoking, diet, sexual and reproductive patterns, alcohol consumption, sunbathing, and other aspects of lifestyle, as well as our purely physical surroundings.[13] Specifically, cigarette smoking accounts for one-third of all cancers, including cancer of the lung, esophagus, bladder, pancreas, and cervix. Unhealthy diet, according to the Centers for Disease Control, is responsible for approximately 35 percent of all cancers, but not in the manner that the popular press would lead you to believe. They are referring to diets high in fat and low in fruits, vegetables, and grains, which increase the risk of several types of cancer, including cancer of the colon, breast, and uterus.[14] Overexposure to sunlight and/or ionizing radiation can result in superficial skin tumors, and more dangerous melanomas and leukemia. Alcohol abuse, particularly if coupled with cigarette smoking, can lead to esophageal and mouth cancers. Specific sexual behavior by young women who are exposed to multiple sexual partners increases the risk of cervical cancer, and delaying child-bearing to near the menopause is associated with a somewhat higher risk of breast cancer.[15]

The English medical journal *Lancet* in 1977 once referred to the 90 percent figure as "rumor" and concluded that the figure was unsubstantiated.[16] But whether it is rumor or not, the estimate does exist and has become absorbed into the popular wisdom. What needs to be clarified at this point is that the word *environment*, when used by epidemiologists and others seeking the causes of cancer, means everything except heredity. Personal habits are therefore considered an environmental factor, foremost among those being cigarette smoking. Other environmental causes of cancer include sunlight (responsible for most cases of superficial skin cancer), alcohol abuse (in synergism with cigarettes, responsible for most cases of esophageal and mouth cancers); exposure to drugs like diethylstilbestrol (DES) (which caused a rare type of vaginal cancer in a small number of daughters of mothers who used it during pregnancy); exposure to certain occupational factors (asbestos and vinyl chloride, among others); high-dose exposure to radiation; sexual and reproductive patterns (cervical cancer is frequent among prostitutes and extremely rare among virgins; women who have their first child late in life or have no children at all have a somewhat higher risk of breast cancer than do other women); and the broad components of our diet (we are still uncertain as to the exact relationship between dietary components and cancer risk).[17]

Sir Richard Doll and Richard Peto, in their classic work *The Causes of Cancer*, neatly dismiss the notion that the estimates of environmental cancer focus on pollution, toxic wastes, and "chemicals" listed in table 1. Whereas the percentage of cancer traceable to tobacco is 25–40 percent, the estimated percentage traceable to pollution is 1–5 percent.[18] Thus the environmental-cancer theory to justify more stringent control of chemicals in the environment constitutes the misuse of a legitimate estimate. By playing on the public's misunderstanding of the full implications of the word *environmental* to describe cancer etiology, and omitting the reality that some one-third of the "90 percent" figure refers to cigarette smoking, the scaremongers have successfully duped their victims into believing that the scientific community has identified a major problem, caused by man-made chemicals, when indeed chemically induced cancers account for a very small proportion of all environmentally induced cancer deaths. Higginson, Doll, Peto, and other epidemiologists who

Table 1. Proportions of Cancer Deaths Attributed to Various Factors

Factor or class of factors	Percent of all cancer deaths	
	Best estimate	Range of acceptable estimates
Tobacco	30	25–40
Alcohol	3	2–4
Diet	35	10–70
Food additives	<1	-5^a–2
Reproductive and sexual behavior	7	1–13
Occupation	4	2–8
Pollution	2	<1–5
Industrial products	<1	<1–2
Medicines and medical procedures	1	0.5–3
Geophysical factors[b]	3	2–4
Infection	10?	1–?
Unknown	?	?

[a] Allowing for a possibly protective effect of antioxidants and other preservatives.

[b] Only about 1%, not 3%, could reasonably be described as "avoidable" (*see* text). Geophysical factors also cause a much greater proportion of nonfatal cancers (up to 30% of all cancers, depending on ethnic mix and latitude) because of the importance of UV light in causing the relatively nonfatal basal cell and squamous cell carcinomas of sunlight-exposed skin.

have looked at environmental causes of cancer have *always* emphasized just the opposite—that man-made chemicals contribute relatively little to the total cancer burden.

The consumer is terrorized in a number of ways by the constant misuse of the phrase "environmentally caused" cancer. First, the carcinogens-around-us philosophy leads to a sense of fatalism, expressed in that bumper sticker that reads "Life Causes Cancer." If 90 percent of cancers are caused by the environment, why should we bother to modify habits such as cigarette smoking? Second, continued focusing of attention on unproven or minor causes of human cancer serves only to divert justified concern about the known causes and squanders our limited research and regulatory dollars on efforts that yield no measurable benefit in preventing cancer.

PREMISE 3: Occupational Cancer Is Now Rampant in the United States and, Once Again, Industry Is to Blame.

During the early eighties, there was a tremendous surge of interest in the topic of occupationally induced cancer. This is good because a poor understanding of the dangers of high-dose, long-term exposure to some chemicals in the workplace led to the tragedies involved with asbestos, vinyl chloride, beta-naphthylamine, and a number of other substances. Unfortunately, though, the issue was carried too far, leading one to conclude that occupationally related cancers are common. Indeed, statements about an "epidemic" of occupationally induced cancer are common in alarmist environmental rhetoric and almost always are based on what is commonly referred to as the Califano "estimates paper." Although this paper dates to 1978, let's take a look at it in considerable detail, as it explains the roots of current sentiment about occupationally induced cancer.

THE ESTIMATES PAPER

In September 1978, Joseph A. Califano, Jr., then secretary of Health, Education, and Welfare, told an AFL-CIO conference on occupational safety and health, "At least 20 percent of all cancer in the United States—and perhaps more—may be work-related. . . . It is estimated that 10 to 15 percent of all cancer deaths in the United States each year will be associated with previous exposure to asbestos."

Califano's numbers came from a draft report, "Estimates of the Fraction of Cancer in the United States Related to Occupational Factors," dated September 15, 1978. According to its title page, the report was "Prepared by the National Cancer Institute (NCI), the National Institute of Environmental Health Sciences (NIEHS), the National Institute of Occupational Safety and Health (NIOSH)." The "contributors" are listed in "alphabetical order" and each person's institutional affiliation follows his name: Dr. Kenneth Bridbord, NIOSH; Dr. Joseph F. Fraumeni, Jr., NCI; Dr. David G. Hoel, NIEHS; Dr. Robert N. Hoover, NCI; Dr. David P. Rall, director, NIEHS; Dr. Umberto Saffioti, NCI; Dr. Marvin A. Schneiderman, NCI; Dr. Arthur C. Upton, director, NCI. Dr. Nicholas Day, NCI, is listed as a contributor to the appendix.

These cancer figures continue to be quoted and no rebuttal has yet caught up with them. Instead, they are appearing with disturbing regularity in federal policy documents. For example, the Toxic Substances Strategy Committee report to the president of May 1980 based its chapter on cancer prevention policy on them. The Office of Technology Assessment's publication entitled "Assignment of Technologies for Determining Cancer Risk from the Environment"

(1981) also utilized these figures.

The estimates paper has been the focus of unrivaled professional criticism and scorn among all recent government health documents. Although some activists were repeating Mr. Califano's remarks as a means of bolstering their positions, the scientific community, for starters, was unsure of exactly who the authors were. A number of well-known researchers have been listed as contributors, but no one has ever been publicly identified as an author.

A review of some of the comments on the estimates paper emanating from the scientific community confirms the fact that Califano and the alleged authors dramatically overstated the proportion of cancer traceable to occupational sources:

> The American Council on Science and Health found in an investigation that 7 of the 10 scientists apparently responsible for these statistics believe they may be incorrect. Only one of the scientists, Dr. Bridbord, whose name was on the draft, defends them as reasonable [two could not be reached].
>
> ACSH News and Views[19]

> This report immediately received wide publicity; it was quoted by the Secretary for Health, Education and Welfare and obtained coverage in the world news. Yet its frame is insubstantial . . . it is sad to see such a fragile report under such distinguished names.
>
> Lancet[20]

> I regard it [the estimates paper] as scientific nonsense.
>
> Richard Doll[21]

> It shows how a group of reasonable men can collectively generate an unreasonable report.
>
> Richard Peto, Nature[22]

> It seems likely that whoever wrote [the estimates paper] . . . did so for political rather than scientific purposes, and it will undoubtedly continue in the future as in the past to be used for political purposes by those who wish to emphasize the importance of occupational factors.
>
> Doll and Peto, The Causes of Cancer[23]

During the period 1978 to 1984, the National Institute for Occupational Safety and Health conducted sixty-one investigations of such cancer "outbreaks," most involving five or fewer cases. A higher number of cancer cases than expected, based on national or local cancer rates, was documented in only sixteen (26 percent) of these investigations. In eleven of these instances, there was no identifiable occupational factor that could account for the excess. In five of the clusters, there was a plausible occupational etiology. Thus, the largest majority of occupational cancer cluster investigations did not result in identification of environmental causes of cancer.[24]

PREMISE 4: If It Causes Cancer in Animals, Then It Causes Cancer in Humans.

Throughout the last two decades there has been an increasing use of the word *carcinogen* in the popular press. Generally no reference is made, for example, when noting that "PCB is a carcinogen," as to whether that designation refers to the cancer-causing potential for laboratory animals or man. Many journalists and a few scientists today do not make this distinction because of their commitment to the premise that if a chemical causes cancer in animals, it must be also assumed to be a human carcinogen. Dr. Samuel Epstein, for instance, writes that "there is overwhelming agreement by most qualified scientists that if a chemical caused cancer in well-designed animal tests, then there is a strong likelihood* that it will also cause cancer in exposed humans."[25]

What is fascinating here is that so much credibility is placed in a methodology, namely, animal testing, that is relatively new and still fraught with many uncertainties. Dr. David Rall, director of the National Toxicology Program, told the *Wall Street Journal,* "We're dealing with a science that's only two decades old. It's a baby compared to other biomedical sciences. I think we'll be in much better shape with the experience of another ten years."[26] But the accuracy of animal testing, despite its relative novelty, provides the pillars of support for an elaborate governmental regulatory apparatus affecting every worker, every consumer, every employer, and every product made in America. Decisions directing the flow of countless billions of dollars are determined by this "baby."

There are a number of reasons for the enthusiastic development of animal testing in the past twenty years. First, the World Health Organization estimates of 70–90 percent of cancer being environmentally caused stimulated many researchers to focus their attention on the etiology of human cancer and practical measures to reduce its incidence. If extrinsic cancer-causing agents can be identified and if exposure to these agents can be reduced, it should be possible to prevent many cases of human cancer.[27]

Second, the alternative to animal testing, which is epidemiology—the study

---

*This is an amazing statement, which is quite different from saying: "It is prudent to *assume* that chemicals causing cancer in animals can cause cancer in man too." This later formulation is what most scientists would concur with. No scientist who understands statistics would agree with Epstein's phrasing.

of the distribution and cause of disease in human population—has its own limitations. Epidemiologists have excelled in identifying cancer-causing substances like tobacco, asbestos, vinyl chloride, diethylstilbestrol, and others, but only *after the fact*. Epidemiology does not allow us to predict in advance the cancer risk of a new substance to humans. The reality is that cancer can first appear decades after exposure to a carcinogenic substance begins; that is, cancer has a relatively long latency period. Smokers, for instance, don't usually develop lung cancer until some twenty or more years after they begin smoking, and asbestos workers develop cancer only several decades after their occupational exposure. This long latency period makes epidemiological investigations difficult and cumbersome, because the search for causes of current cancer has to focus on exposures that took place two or three or even four decades ago, and thus has to rely on faded memories and lost records. More important, however, one must necessarily wait for decades to know whether a current exposure may result in cancer in the future. Clearly, valuable as epidemiology has been, it is useless in assessing the effects of the many new chemicals that a modern industrial economy constantly generates (a thousand a year in the United States alone). No one wants to wait until dead bodies start dropping before acting seriously to curb carcinogenic exposures.

These circumstances necessitated the search for alternative means of assessing potential carcinogenic hazards. Small laboratory animals—typically, rats and mice—thus were selected as proxies for humans. Indeed, animals have long stood in for man, whether it was sending canaries into coal mines or having the cat try the new harvest of mushrooms.

Until relatively recently, there was no standard approach to animal testing, and individual experimentation involved many routes of exposure, including oral, inhalation, through the urethra, intravaginally and intrarectally, and by various sorts of injections, skin painting, and implantation. Only in the 1960s was a standard experimental design set forth by the National Cancer Institute for its large program of cancer bioassays on suspect chemicals. It has been continued by the National Toxicology Program, the federal agency that is the successor to the NCI in carrying out this program.

A typical test for a suspected carcinogen is performed on both sexes of two species (rats and mice). The animals are exposed to the chemical for their entire lifetime (typically, two years), usually through their diet, although sometimes in their drinking water, by inhalation, or by stomach tube. The exposure route is selected to mimic as closely as possible the route of human exposure.[28] Normally two doses are used (low and high) in addition to the undosed controls, and there are fifty animals in each sex/species dose group, for a total of six hundred. Such tests take three or more years to run and cost about $1,000 per animal; that is, about $600,000 to test a single chemical.

LIMITATIONS OF ANIMALS TO HUMAN EXTRAPOLATION*

Numerous factors suggest the need for caution in extrapolating laboratory results to humans.

A substance is considered carcinogenic in animals, and hence a potential human carcinogen, even if the animals die of old age rather than cancer, as long as a statistically significant increase occurs in tumors visible under the microscope. A single finding of increased incidence of tumors in only one species is sufficient for a substance to be judged a carcinogen for regulatory purposes; negative results in other animal species (even with lifetime administration at maximal doses) are discounted, on the "prudent" ground that humans might be as sensitive as the most sensitive animals. Indeed because of the limited sensitivity of epidemiological studies, even negative human evidence cannot reverse the regulatory judgment that a substance found to cause tumors in a single animal test is a carcinogen and hence a potential human hazard. Actually, there are three reasons to reject the assumption that rodents are miniature humans.

First, given the relatively short lifespan of the test animals, and the desire to maximize the chances of detecting even a weak carcinogen, the standard approach is to use very high doses of chemicals. The logical limit to this reasoning, of course, is to use the largest dose that the animal can tolerate without dying prematurely from ordinary poisoning. Called the maximum tolerated dose (MTD), it is now the standard practice in these tests.[29]

Maximum dosing in animal testing is the most controversial aspect of this issue, both among laymen (who frequently make jokes about animals drinking a thousand bottles of diet soda a day) and among scientists. The central question is whether the use of doses that are nearly toxic can by itself predispose the animals to develop cancer. It is very possible that physiological events occur in such metabolically stressed animals that do not happen at all at the much lower doses typical of human use.

Second, in designing animal carcinogen studies, scientists often maximize the chances of "positive" results by choosing the types or strains of animals most likely to respond to the chemicals being studied. Moreover, negative findings—no increased risk of cancer found—are rarely reported.

Thus, there is increasing reason to believe that a good number of "false positives" probably exist in animal studies; that is, chemicals causing cancer in laboratory animals, but not humans. Actually, we do not know how often false positives occur, because a vital piece of information is missing; a list

---

*Perhaps the most complete analysis of the limitations of animal to human extrapolation is found in Edith Efron's book, *The Apocalyptics: Cancer and the Big Lie* (New York: Simon and Schuster, 1984).

of chemicals that have been thoroughly examined in epidemiological studies in man and shown to yield negative results. For the great majority of chemicals that have been tested in animals, no human data whatever are at hand. The International Agency for Research on Cancer estimates that it has at least some human data on only 14 percent of the chemicals it has evaluated.[30] There is, then, no way to discover the fraction of chemicals testing positive in animals that are falsely positive vis-a-vis humans. Those who want to ignore the reality of the likelihood of false positives frequently point to the opposite finding— that most (but not all) chemicals known to cause cancer in humans also cause cancer in animals. They then reason that the reverse is also probably true— that all chemicals shown to cause cancer in animals also cause cancer in man. But that inference is logically incorrect, a type of backward thinking. That most human carcinogens are animal carcinogens offers no credibility to the argument that all animal carcinogens are human carcinogens. It would be like arguing that because all lima beans are vegetables, all vegetables are lima beans.

Third, we now know that animal carcinogens (as defined above) are numerous rather than few. We also know that many naturally occurring substances that can cause cancers in laboratory animals are normally present in our food and that human exposure to most of these substances cannot be eliminated. The more that natural products have been tested, the more it has become apparent that Mother Nature's own foods (and natural environment) abound in animal carcinogens. For example, beets, celery, lettuce, spinach, radishes, and rhubarb all contain toxicologically substantial amounts of nitrate that, in the intestine, is converted to nitrite and then to nitrosamines, which are known animal carcinogens. And chemicals in edible mushrooms (hydrazines), spices (safrole), parsley (psoralens), bread (ethyl carbamate), soybeans and alfalfa (estrogenic substances such as genestein) have also produced cancers in laboratory animals. Dr. Bruce Ames, a leading United States biochemist, asserts that there are so many plant toxins that are carcinogenic that synthetic chemical carcinogens can be ignored.[31]

A similar argument could be presented to those who claim that animal teratogens (see premise 7) are therefore capable of causing birth defects in humans. Ironically, the investigation of teratogens that began in the mid-1940s first implicated in excessive quantities in teratogenic activity essential vitamins such as A, D, and E. Additionally, it has been determined that a number of external factors when applied at critical times of gestation will increase the rate of birth defects. For example, air transport of mice on the twelfth and thirteenth days of pregnancy will increase the number of malformed fetuses.[32] Fasting for twenty-four hours during critical periods results in defects, as do even transient deficiencies of vitamins. Restriction of movement, an environment that is too warm or too cold, subcutaneous injections of sodium chloride and a few grains of sand in an incubating egg cause animal birth defects.

All in all, there are a number of reasons to be skeptical about extrapolating from animal experiments done under extreme conditions to man. This is not to say that animal testing is not useful; it is and is necessary. But we must reject the doomsdayer's simplification that "man is a little mouse" and critically assess the results of animal experiments, asking questions like, "Is there a dose-response relationship?" (see premise 5 below). That is, did the number of tumors increase as the dose was increased? Has the chemical been shown to cause cancer in more than one animal study? In more than one species? For example, if a dozen or more well-controlled animal studies showed that a substance could cause cancer not only in rats, but also in mice, guinea pigs, and perhaps rhesus monkeys, there would indeed be reason for concern about that chemical's use for man. Unfortunately, an analysis of newspaper reporting on environmental issues such as dioxin and PCBs does not reveal any interest in finding consistency of results. Many reporters seem willing to rely on a cancer finding in a single experiment as proof.

An important contribution of Edith Efron's book *The Apocalyptics: Cancer and the Big Lie* (New York: Simon and Schuster, 1984) is her demolition of the validity of animal testing as a means of extrapolation to man. According to Efron, the "apocalyptic scientists," as she refers to them, in their effort to eliminate every last trace of industrially produced carcinogens, do not make allowances for the varying potency of chemicals tested in the lab, operating on the premise that if it causes cancer under any circumstances in animals, it must cause cancer under normal circumstances of human use. And in gathering and interpreting data on which they make regulatory decisions, the apocalyptics stack the deck, apparently operating on the assumption that a chemical is guilty until proven innocent. For example, in testing chemicals in the laboratory, the apocalyptics:

1. Choose the sex and species of animals that are particularly sensitive to specific chemicals, maximizing the chances of "positive" results being produced.

For example, mice are often used in such experiments, although scientists disagree over the reliability of this species because laboratory mice have a high spontaneous incidence of tumors; that is, they develop tumors whether or not they are exposed to chemicals. Frequently a chemical will cause cancer in mice, but not in rats.

2. Use the highest dose of a chemical they can without killing the animal, thus creating a situation that bears little resemblance to human exposure. Certainly, toxicologists agree that high-level exposures in laboratory tests are necessary, given the relatively short lifespan of test animals and the need to find tumors quickly if they are to occur. But use of the "maximum tolerated dose" as the basis of judging the carcinogenicity of a substance in humans remains highly controversial.

For example, Herman Kraybill of the National Cancer Institute has explained (his own terms are far more technical than these) that all mammals have "thresholds" for chemicals, that there are doses that the metabolic process can generally handle, but that the process of high-dose testing, by drenching the metabolic process with poison, violates this basic threshold principle of toxicology. According to Kraybill, high-dose testing may falsify the testing in one of two ways: it can poison the cells and tissues so severely as to prevent a cancer-causing response, or it can so overload and change the metabolic processes as to cause a carcinogenic response.

A recent paper by researchers at the University of Southern California verified this model of an increase in cell division (as caused by toxic levels of a substance), increasing the risk of cancer development.[33]

Dr. Bruce Ames, a leading authority on cancer causation, summarizes the issue:[34]

> Given the high proportion of carcinogens among those natural chemicals tested, human exposure to rodent carcinogens is far more common than generally thought; however, at the low doses of most human exposures (where cell-killing and mitogenesis did not occur), the hazards may be much lower than is commonly assumed and often will be zero. Thus, without studies of the mechanism of carcinogenesis, the fact that a chemical is a carcinogen at the MTD in rodents provides no information about low-dose risk to humans.

3. Declare a study showing an increased rate of cancer in animals more important than a dozen tests showing no such effect.

For example, a National Cancer Institute committee chaired by Dr. Umberto Saffiotti (the same NCI scientist who in 1976 declared cancer a "social disease . . . derived from our technology") declared in 1970 that "evidence of negative results . . . should be considered superseded by positive findings in other tests." And the National Cancer Advisory Board said in 1977, "Negative results obtained in the one species do not . . . detract from the significance of clear positive results obtained in other species." The Office of Science and Technology Policy said in 1979, "Assuming that appropriate testing procedures are followed it is generally sound to let positive results supersede negative results in tests involving different species." Arthur Upton, director of the NCI, noted in 1980: "I believe that a reproducible carcinogenic response in any species of test animal must be considered sufficient to describe the test compound as a carcinogen. . . . Negative results in a second or even third species of test animal do not in my mind establish that the test agent is not a potential threat for human beings."

4. Give greater credence to positive *animal* studies than they would to negative data emerging from the study of *human* populations.

For example, in the case of saccharin, whereas male rats exposed to high doses of saccharin while in their mother's womb and throughout their own lifetime, did develop an increased rate of bladder tumors, detailed studies of diabetics who consumed large amounts of saccharin for many decades revealed no unique cancer pattern that could be attributable to saccharin use. Yet, in the views of the apocalyptics, the animal data prevailed, and in 1977 a ban on saccharin was proposed. This ban has been postponed many times, with the latest until 1997, through intervention of Congress, motivated by the outrage of American consumers.

5. Accept the results of laboratory cancer-producing studies even if the consensus is that the experiment is botched.

As Efron notes, the FDA set out to do the master safety evaluation study of Red Dye No. 2 "with a huge number of rats, 500 in all. It was an ambitious enterprise. Unfortunately the scientist in charge of the 500 rats left the agency and the rats were left unsupervised for a long time. When, finally, some scientist picked up the experiment in midstream, their work was performed slovenly. An unknown number of control rats got mixed up with the test rats, and dead rats, instead of being dissected immediately, were left to rot in cages." But botched or not, the FDA maintained that this study had not proven the safety of the food color, and thus Red Dye No. 2 was banned.

6. Ignore a number of realities of basic science.

For example, different animal species respond differently to chemical exposures. Species variation could account for a chemical causing cancer in one animal experiment, but not in another. One such chemical, penicillin, is lethal to guinea pigs and hamsters, but not to other mammals. The anesthetic fluoroxene, used safely in humans for years, is lethal to dogs, cats, and rabbits. "Hence animals are not always reliable substitutes for each other, let alone humans," notes Efron. Further, the apocalyptics ignore those aspects of basic science that have shown us, as far back as 1929, that whereas certain chemicals can cause cancer in animals, still others *prevent* cancer, or *reverse* the process once it has begun. The apocalyptics, screening the results of animal experiments, however, seemed interested only in the bad news.

7. Contradict themselves in reporting on carcinogens and noncarcinogens.

Government regulators, Efron reports, when announcing that yet another chemical has been shown to cause cancer in animals, attempt to soothe the nerves of worried consumers by saying that only a small percentage of chemicals tested are shown to cause cancer in animals. This would lead most logical minds to conclude that if there is only a small percentage of tested chemicals that are carcinogenic, then there must be a large percentage of chemicals that are noncarcinogenic. But this is not the case. Efron shows that in "regulatory science" (a term she uses to distinguish the apocalyptics' activity from academic science) there is no such thing as a noncarcinogen. Once something is shown to be negative—that is, one that does not cause cancer in animals—it is treated as if it were never tested and put back into the "potential carcinogen" file.

For example, a document from Occupational Safety and Health Administration states, "If the available evidence indicates that the chemical is not positive for carcinogenicity OSHA's position on that particular chemical is the same as if the chemical had never been tested for carcinogenicity." Comments Efron wryly, "OSHA is thus asking the public to believe in a phenomenon, the existence of which the agency refuses to acknowledge. This is not just crying wolf—it is assuring people that most creatures are not wolves, while declaring only wolves exist."

8. Accept uncritically the notion of "zero tolerance"; that is, the belief that since no one knows what amount of a carcinogen is required to trigger the growth of a malignancy, it must be assumed that there is no threshold level. But this view is coming more and more into dispute from evidence that all human carcinogens have a dosage level below which there is no evidence of increased cancer risk. For example, we are all surrounded by low-level, naturally occurring radiation, yet we do not believe this poses a general cancer risk. Even cigarette smoking apparently has a level where no increase in cancer risk can be measured (under about five cigarettes per day). Recent studies of animals exposed to potential and known carcinogens have consistently challenged the no-threshold levels only.

Again, in defending this deck stacking of animal experiments, the apocalyptics were acting not on knowledge but on "prudence," declaring that if there was any doubt that a synthetic chemical in any dose caused cancer, they thought it was prudent to label it a carcinogen and regulate it accordingly. Such prudence toward synthetic chemicals assumes two things. First, no risk is associated with the regulation and/or banning. This is clearly naive.

For example, when a series of pesticides is banned, not only is there chaos in the agricultural community as produce or other commodities with traces of the now outlawed chemical are destroyed (and obviously these costs are passed on to consumers), but both consumers and workers also face whatever new, and perhaps greater, risks are associated with those pesticides that are used in its place. Beyond that, it is obvious that a continued banning of pesticides based on prudence would ultimately threaten our plentiful food supply, leaving it vulnerable to destruction and contamination by pests. The apocalyptics' prudent approach to regulation appears to overlook the reality that chemicals used in industry are there for some specific purpose, and banning or restricting them on the basis of a mere thread of evidence is going to have a cumulative negative effect on this country's standard of living, manifesting itself in the form of less food, fewer lifesaving drugs, fewer jobs, a diminished selection of consumer products, and, inevitably, a depressed rate of economic growth.

Perhaps, it might be argued, such social changes would be worth it if they were the price to pay for reducing this country's cancer toll. But the ultimate irony—the tragedy—is that there is no evidence whatsoever that the practice of prudence has reduced America's cancer rates. Indeed, it might well be argued that the constant cancer alarm sounded over food additives, pesticides, and environmental chemicals has raised the cancer rate by diverting our attention from known causes of cancer, like cigarettes, to purely hypothetical ones, like EDB.

Animals are essential in biomedical research, but so is common sense. The major problem with animal cancer tests does not lie with the numerous scientific limitations in animal cancer bioassays, but rather with the legal and regulatory use that the tests serve. The disregard of sound toxicological concepts and the inappropriate protocols for some studies tend to discredit animal cancer testing.

When properly understood and applied, animal cancer studies can be valuable in evaluating human cancer risk. But the present nondiscriminating policy that fails to distinguish real risks from trivial ones leads to lumping major human health hazards with minute, hypothetical ones. This results in the inability of regulatory agencies to set sensible priorities and formulate wise policies to protect the nation's health.

But the results of animal testing are taken so seriously that mouse terrorism* has resulted. Mouse terrorism is defined as

> the engendering in the public mind, through scientific studies involving laboratory mice as subjects of experimentation, of an unwarranted fear of potential health hazards.

The mouse-vs.-man analogy is essential to those who seek to terrify us about food additives, pesticides, and other trace-element chemicals. The time has come for us to recognize that mouse terrorism poses a serious problem in terms of maintaining both our high standard of living and our good health. The continuation of policies that require chemicals to be banned "at the drop of the rat" threaten both our quality of life and our health. If we continue to ban everything that causes cancer in rodents, we will reduce our food supply (by banning pesticides), raise taxes (to pay for chasing down trace chemicals), and otherwise burden our economy and diminish our standard of living without preventing any cancer cases—while diverting attention from real causes of human cancer.

The solution to "mouse terrorism" and the "carcinogen of the week" phenomenon is not to abandon animal tests. Instead, we must:

---

*According to the October 1990 *Atlantic Monthly,* the term mouse terrorism is being tracked by the editor of the *American Heritage Dictionary* as a term that exhibits sustained use.

- Acknowledge that exposing animals to near-fatal doses of chemicals itself causes tissue changes that predispose to cancer. If the alleged effect occurs only in the highest dose, the results should be considered suspect.

- Before automatically issuing the label "carcinogen," ask relevant questions: Does this cause cancer in more than one species or sex? In multiple experiments? The Alar scare, for example, was triggered on the basis of one study on mice alone.

- Avoid an exorcist approach to purging our environment of every trace of the chemical in question. Instead, prudent and safe tolerance levels of exposure should be set as we do with known human carcinogens (radiation, sunlight exposure) and with known natural carcinogens.

Animal studies are critical in biomedical research—but so is common sense in interpreting the implications and applications for humans.

PREMISE 5: If High Doses of Something Cause Cancer, Then Low Doses Do Also. There Is No Safe Level of a Carcinogen.

The so-called no-threshold theory is a cornerstone of the environmentalist-alarmist dogma. And it is completely adrift from the realities of science.

All human carcinogens have a dosage level below which there is no evidence of increased risk of cancer. This lower-limiting dosage is termed the threshold level. However, we must be careful not to confuse a threshold level with the limits of sensitivity of a particular test. For the relatively small number of tests that have produced good dose-response data, the curves of dose versus response show strong evidence of upward bending (nonlinearity) in dose ranges well removed from the range in which the test loses sensitivity. Hence, the apparent thresholds are biologically real, not accidents of the sensitivity limits of the test. For example, we are all surrounded by low-level, naturally occurring radiation, yet we do not believe that this poses a general cancer risk. Cigarette smoking apparently has a level where no increase in cancer risk can be measured. A graph of risk versus number of cigarettes smoked per day predicts "zero risk" at about five cigarettes per day: five cigarettes then become the threshold level for smoking. Recent studies of animals exposed to potential and known carcinogens have consistently challenged the no-threshold philosophy, pointing to dramatic increases in tumors at higher exposure levels (that is, strongly nonlinear responses that, within the sensitivity of the tests, were compatible with threshold models).

How do scientists account for nonlinear dose-response curves? To understand this, it is necessary to know a little about how chemicals can act as cancer-causing agents in the body.

Most of the chemicals that induce cancer appear to act by damaging the genetic material (DNA) of cells. In theory, this might be accomplished by a single molecule of a DNA-damaging chemical, but of course it first has to get inside cells to the DNA, which is sequestered in the nuclei. To do this, a chemical has to be absorbed by the body through the lungs, the digestive tract, or other means, just as oxygen, water, and nutrients must be. And like them, DNA-damaging chemicals are subject to the body's uptake, transport, biotransformation (biological change, causing either activation or detoxification), distribution, and excretion mechanisms. Indeed, many chemicals are not carcinogenic in themselves but must be changed by the body into "activated" forms before they are able to damage DNA. These various pharmacological processes can be nonlinear with respect to administered dose.

In particular, the body's normal means of handling a specific substance can be overloaded at high doses, and the overflow may be handled in other, quite different ways. Thus, the array of metabolites of an administered chemical seen at high dose may well be different in nature and/or relative amounts from that which predominates at normal physiological levels. If this array of high-dose metabolites happens to include activated, DNA-damaging forms of the chemical, or if the body is unable to excrete the activated carcinogens as efficiently at maximal doses as at normal levels, then the common experimental finding that high doses of carcinogens are disproportionately more powerful than low doses, can be explained.

There are other sorts of carcinogens, however, that do not seem to act by damaging DNA. These are called nongenotoxic or epigenetic carcinogens. One class of these is called promoters, because they seem not to be fully potent carcinogens in themselves but do have the ability to enhance—or to promote—the carcinogenic activity of others. Some promoters may act by easing the entry of DNA-damaging chemicals into the cell. Others appear to act at later stages in the development of cancer after the initial DNA damage has occurred, for example, by irritating tissues and causing their component cells to multiply faster. Such extra multiplication seems to increase the chances for cancer to appear in already damaged DNA. Some nongenotoxic carcinogens, such as DES, act hormonally. For all of these nongenotoxic carcinogens, there is no reason even in theory for believing that single molecules might be able to cause cancer indirectly. These effects seem more akin to ordinary toxicity, and hence it is probably wrong to estimate the low-dose risk by linear extrapolation of the cancer risk visible only at high dose.

Other chemicals that induce cancer at high doses are normal components of the body's biochemistry (such as formaldehyde) and for this reason seem unlikely to be a cancer hazard at doses comparable to that which the body itself generates every day. And others, like vitamins A and D, are normal, indeed, necessary, parts of our diet; again it seems likely that our bodies can handle physiologically normal amounts of these substances without hazard.

Many scientists also believe that certain substances are carcinogenic only at doses that are toxic to that species. In the words of the late Dr. William R. Havender:

> Moreover, recognition is growing that the use of high doses in animal tests may artifactually promote a carcinogenic outcome. Recent work suggests that many chemicals "causing" cancer in rodents at high doses work through toxicity-induced cell proliferation and consequent promotion, a threshold process. In other words, absent incipient toxicity, there is no apparent carcinogenicity. Thus, some "positive" animal findings may merely be high dose artifacts having zero relevance to the low doses of normal consumer exposure.

The bottom line, according to Dr. Havender, is that toxicity-caused promotion of tumors implies that the relation between cancer risk and dose cannot be linear.[35]

Interestingly, there is a double standard operative when it comes to discussions and decisions relating to the zero-tolerance philosophy on carcinogens versus other chemicals. For example, the general procedure for assessing non–cancer-causing chemicals calls for doing a dose-response study in animals, establishing a "no observed effect level," and applying a large safety factor (typically, a hundredfold) to allow for possible metabolic differences between test animals and humans, and also for variations among human populations. This is how "acceptable" levels have been set for decades for ordinary chemicals such as food additives, and the method has had admirable success. One wonders why some environmentalists and some government scientists set different, often much lower, standards and will not admit that there can be minimal or nonexistent risk when exposed to low levels of carcinogens.

Dr. Samuel Epstein writes, "There is . . . no evidence at all of the existence of thresholds for the irreversible process* involved in carcinogenesis."[36] Thus, he and others would demand that our air, water, and workplace be free of even traces of carcinogens. This is an unrealistic, unattainable goal. About eighty or one hundred elements (and many more compounds made from these elements) occur in every bite of food, in every drop of water, and are present in every cell of the living organism. There is nothing that is "pure" in the sense of having no trace of potentially toxic or carcinogenic chemicals.[37]

---

*Here Epstein is presumably referring to mutation or the altering of a cell's genetic material. But mutation is highly reversible since cells have elaborate mechanisms through which many mutations can be repaired.

PREMISE 6: Natural Is Better Than Synthetic.
A Chemical-free Environment Is Safer Than a Chemical-ridden One.

An underlying theme, almost on a philosophical or religious level in environmental literature, is that technology is inherently life-threatening, chemicals are by definition dangerous, and the health of Americans would be far better if we lived more naturally, free from the deleterious spewing from irresponsible "alchemists."

The fascination with "natural," "nonsynthetic" materials goes way beyond environmentalism. Indeed, we have witnessed an explosion of natural, organic foodstores, and an increase in natural childbirth. As Dr. Helen B. Hiscoe, from Michigan State University, observes in the *New England Journal of Medicine,* "The underlying assumption of those who value things because they are natural is their belief that nature is a benign force whereas human power tends to be evil. They equate naturalness with goodness."[38] Obviously the natural versus synthetic dichotomy of good and evil, or health-promoting and health-threatening, is misleading and absurd. Epidemics of disease are natural, as are earthquakes, volcanic eruptions, floods, and droughts. So are the airborne pollens from a wide variety of allergenic plants. Beyond that, many natural substances, including food, contain toxins, otherwise known as poison. Carrots contain carotatoxin, a fairly potent nerve poison. Radishes contain goitrogens— chemicals that promote goiter by interfering with our body's use of iodine. Shrimp are a rich source of several minerals, among them arsenic. (The ocean contains natural traces of arsenic. If extracted, there is enough in a bay to kill every person on earth.) Pepper and nutmeg contain myristicin, a powerful hallucinogen.[39]

A number of different natural substances have been shown to cause cancer in animals—and, in some cases, in humans. For starters, tobacco is natural. It is particularly highly carcinogenic when it is burned and inhaled, but is also hazardous when it is chewed, and when the condensate of cigarette smoke is rubbed on the skin of animals. Ergot is a natural fungus that grows on rye and other grasses.[40] Ergot contains many alkaloids and other physiologically active substances and has been shown to cause cancer in laboratory animals.[41] Safrole, a component of the natural sassafras plant and oil of sassafras, has been shown to be a cancer-causing agent causing liver damage in some animals. Aflatoxin molds, which can grow on a variety of natural substances, including peanuts, rice, corn, soybeans, whole oats, and wheat, particularly shredded wheat, have been shown to increase the risk of cancer in rabbits, guinea pigs, cattle, ducks, mice, and rhesus monkeys, and there is much circumstantial evidence that exposure to aflatoxins may play a role in human liver cancer. Braken fern, a tender, tasty sprout with an appearance much like asparagus (eaten widely in Japan), is a powerful cancer-causing agent, even after it is cooked. Cows feeding on this natural delight suffer damaged bone marrow and polyps (swollen membranes) of the bladder.[42]

In *The Apocalyptics,* Edith Efron leaves the unprepared reader breathless with her stunning rejoinder to those who deny the existence of natural carcinogens. In a forty-page list of Mother Nature's own cancer-causing agents, she documents her case that the world is chock-full of natural carcinogenics. Even oxygen has been implicated as the cause of many types of malignancies. Natural foods contain chemicals that are carcinogenic or mutagenic, many of which have been reported to be radioactive, and many of which contain reportedly carcinogenic metals. As Efron writes:

> Man cannot digest . . . nutrients without saliva and digestive bacteria, both of which, according to the data, have been implicated as carcinogens, or as producers of carcinogens. Man cannot function as a sexual being or reproduce his own kind without sexual hormones, and they too have been reported to be carcinogenic. Finally, man cannot seek shelter from the elements or from predatory beasts, or cook many natural foods in order to detoxify them, without fire, but combustion is said to produce . . . carcinogens. . . . If the "prudence," no-threshold theory were to be invoked, crucial physiological functions might have to be medically prohibited. A theory which, according to the scientific literature, would kill off the human species cannot be accepted as prudent.

Efron stresses that the designation *carcinogen* for a naturally occurring chemical is based on *exactly* the same criteria—animal experiments using high doses, sensitive animals, assuming one positive test carries greater credence than many negative ones—as is the designation for synthetic chemicals. And she asks the obvious question: Why, if the regulator scientists are truly interested in protecting us from any chemical that causes cancer in animals, have they focused only on synthetic carcinogens? Why, if they assume that any level of a carcinogen can be dangerous, have they operated under a double standard, allowing naturally occurring carcinogens to remain unfettered? One might want to offer the immediate rejoinder here that environmental regulations have control over man-made carcinogens, and none over natural ones. But indeed, if we really believed a natural chemical caused cancer, we would presumably make an effort to control it. Efron's point is that apocalyptics are willing to overlook incriminating animal data if they apply to natural substances, apparently only interested in focusing on potential harm done by the synthetic products.

It is this double standard in regulatory science that suggests to Efron that the apocalyptics' agenda is not entirely scientific. In listing the natural carcinogens, Efron writes, "The reported carcinogens in question are marvelously invulnerable to ideological prejudices; all are attributes of the planet and the universe in which we live. No sinful Faust or economic system can be blamed for creating these carcinogens. The moral stature of their inventor can't be threatened." And the apocalyptics are thus not interested.

The irony of the natural-is-good/synthetic-is-bad argument is that because of our "unnatural" technology we are living longer than ever before, with an unprecedented control over infectious and communicable diseases. And it is that unnatural technology to which we must turn for the hope of further advances, particularly in the area of both preventing and treating cancer.

PREMISE 7: **Reproductive Failure—Infertility, Miscarriages, and Birth Defects—Is Caused by Environmental Factors.**

In the past few years, we have read a good deal about alleged epidemics of reproductive failure purportedly caused by factors in the environment. Vietnam War veterans blame the birth defects in their children on their exposure to Agent Orange. Women in Alsea, Oregon, and Love Canal are pointing to a high rate of miscarriage, relating it to exposure to the herbicide 2,4,5-T, or its contaminant, dioxin. The most interesting factors about these charges are that (a) they assume that there is a scientific precedent, supported by a large body of literature, for the claimed link between environment and re-productive failure, and (b) they maintain that the environmental damage can emanate from either gamete (sperm or egg) of the prospective mother or father. What are the facts here?

First, it is well known that human reproduction is affected by environmental factors, including climate, altitude, social class, number of previous births, infections, smoking, and some chemicals, particularly in the form of drugs. Researchers at the Centers for Disease Control report that in recent years use of infertility services has increased among American couples. The reason for this rise is attributed to numerous factors: the baby-boom generation has aged, more women are entering the work force and are therefore exposed to potential occupational hazards affecting reproduction, the avoidance of early childbearing has enhanced the age-related biologic risks of infertility, use of oral contraception has lengthened the time to conception after discontinuing its use, and desired reproduction has been condensed into a shorter interval.[43]

Second, male and female infertility characterized by low sperm count, poor sperm mobility, failure to ovulate, or diseases such as endometriosis are hardly rare in this country, and never have been. Some 10 to 20 percent of U.S. married couples over the course of this century have been childless, and the overwhelming majority of cases are suspected to be involuntary. While lifestyle factors (overuse of alcohol, marijuana smoking) have been suspected of causing some cases of infertility, examples of chemical-induced infertility are rare. One major exception here is the chemical DBCP (1,2, dibromo-3-chloropropane), a widely used nematocide between 1955 and 1977. It was banned in September 1977 from both production and field application in the United States when male factory workers extensively exposed to it were found to be infertile.[44] Further studies revealed that only the factory workers and the applicators involved in irrigation setup work and in the calibration of equipment were affected. It is likely that high-dose, long-term exposure to other occupational chemicals could also have a depressing effect on male fertility, and perhaps female infertility as well, but there is no evidence that chemicals dispersed in air or water in the general community have ever caused or increased risk for human infertility. The birth rate did decline after the dioxin accident in Seveso, Italy, although this finding may or may not have been caused by the dioxin (see chapter 8).

Third, miscarriage, technically known as spontaneous abortion, is very common in all human populations. It is estimated that 60 percent of all conceptions end in this manner.[45] There is no easy way to measure the rate of miscarriage because we do not have access to the denominator of the rate, that is, the number of pregnancies. Thus if you hear of an "increased" miscarriage rate at Love Canal or elsewhere, you should be suspicious immediately, because reliable data simply do not exist for that locality or the nation as a whole. Beyond that, there is no evidence in the scientific literature to indicate that exposure to general environmental factors has ever caused miscarriage. Anyone who makes a claim of a cause-effect relationship between, for example, herbicide spraying and elevated miscarriage risk is basing it on personal opinion and pure conjecture.

Fourth, although there are six hundred to eight hundred agents known to be teratogenic—causing birth defects in laboratory animals—only twenty-five to thirty are known to be responsible for human malformations.[46] Thalidomide, used as a means of controlling nausea of pregnancy (and offering a sedative effect), even though shown not to cause birth defects in mice and rats, did increase the risk of a deformity characterized by extremely short legs and arms in the offspring of some human mothers who used it.[47] Dilantin, a drug used for control of seizures, is associated with a wide spectrum of fetal effects.[48] In its most severe form the disorder consists of prenatal growth deficiency, mental retardation,[49] and craniofacial abnormalities. Trimethadione, another anticonvulsant used in the control of epilepsy; warfarin, an anticoagulant; diethylstilbestrol (DES), a synthetic estrogen given to pregnant women during the 1950–70 period in an attempt to prevent miscarriage;[50] certain anticancer drugs (antineoplastics); the antibiotic tetracycline; exposure to radiation; ingestion of mercury (as in the case of the contaminated Minamata

Bay in Japan)—all have been shown to cause human birth defects. Beyond that, certain aspects of lifestyle—for example, cigarette smoking and alcohol abuse—have also been linked to human birth defects, low birth weights, and spontaneous abortion.[51] And indeed, these lifestyle factors account for the majority of preventable birth defects occurring today.

There is currently no evidence that exposure of the general population to environmental contaminants—except in the cases mentioned above, of high-dose, generally long-term exposure during a critical phase of gestation—has caused reproductive failure. Again, if a Vietnam War veteran, or a resident of Alsea, Oregon, claims that his birth-defected child, or his wife's second trimester miscarriage was caused by dioxin or any environmental chemical, it is pure speculation on his part and is not consistent with what we know about environmental teratogens. All allegations should never be taken to be true until responsible scientific studies provide proof. As British scientist Peter Medawar states in his work, *Advice to a Young Scientist,* "I cannot give any scientist of any age better advice than this: the intensity of a conviction that a hypothesis is true has no bearing over whether it is true or not."[52]

As is very often the case in allegations of environmentally induced disease, one cannot prove that a link *doesn't* exist, as it is impossible to prove a negative. All that can be said in these cases is that there is no evidence that such a link is based on fact.

PREMISE 8: Chemicals Are Being Found in Human Fat Tissues and in Mother's Milk—A Clear Indication of a Health Hazard.

Claudia Ricci wrote in *Parents* magazine: "At that moment, sitting side by side with my scientist friend, I experienced pure panic. My arms and legs got limp, and my gut felt as if it were going to dissolve. I realized that PCBs and DDE and other poisons are swimming around in my body fluids just as they do in sewers and polluted streams. Worse, they are in the milk I am so conscientiously feeding to my helpless infant daughter."[53]

As Regenstein tells us in *America the Poisoned,* "deadly synthetic chemicals are now present in our food, air, and water, and even our own bodies—including mother's milk—where they remain and accumulate." He continues, "Dieldrin has been found in the flesh of 99.5 percent of all human tissue samples tested . . . now we know that almost every American carries detectable traces of several generally banned carcinogens. We must await the inevitable effects. How long can our bodies continue to accumulate such lethal poisons before succumbing to cancer?"[54]

Obviously it is emotionally unsettling to think of our bodies being contaminated with toxins, and our children being nourished with tainted milk. But the reality is that you can literally find traces of any fat-soluble material in any source of fat, like flesh tissue and breast milk. There is no known relationship between these traces and risk of disease.

When dealing with trace levels of contaminants in the body, we are unfortunately entering an area filled with many more questions than answers. Medical and toxicological researchers are currently attempting to understand better what, if any, health risks are posed by the body burden of unwanted chemicals. What the scaremongers don't tell us is that toxins occur naturally in the human body.

In some cases, a substance that is lethal in high doses is in fact an essential trace element, that is, a substance that is needed in tiny amounts to prevent a serious health problem. Selenium, a liver carcinogen, is one such element. Sex hormones, substances present in all people, can cause cancer when not present in the proper balance.

In the absence of extensive scientific data, when we attempt to determine health risk we must put the parameters in proper perspective. For those compounds that are environmentally stable and have the capacity to accumulate in our bodies faster than we can excrete them, we must carefully investigate the possibility of a hazard. But to assume that the presence of such chemicals in minuscule amounts indicates a massive health threat is foolish and irresponsible.

PREMISE 9: The Environment Is the Cause of Most Human Diseases. Our Own Behavior and Lifestyles Have Very Little to Do with Disease Risk. Don't Blame the Victim; Blame the Society.

If there was ever any "classic" reaction to human disease and death, it was one like "it was God's will" or "it was my fate; it was meant to be"—a passive reaction to maladies affecting ourselves or our loved ones.

But as John Leonard wrote in the *New York Times* in 1978, "Scientists have reduced the number of calamities we can blame on God."[55] We are learning more and more that science can provide rational explanations to once unexplained and now extremely emotional questions. Indeed, today there is almost a militancy about disease and death, a prevailing feeling that we have come so far in modern medical research that we know the cause of—and how to prevent—most all human ailments. A woman who suffers a miscarriage, a man who develops bladder cancer, parents who lose their child to leukemia demand to know *why? What caused it?* With increasing frequency, the victims vent their rage about "the environment," pesticides, food additives, air pollution, or simply living in New Jersey.

The environmentalist literature cultivates this feeling that we are in a sense helpless victims of the toxic chemicals around us. This has led to the enactment of unnecessary and scientifically unfounded legislation, such as Super-Fund. "SuperFund" is the shorthand name for a sprawling government project that purports to protect the public's health by cleaning up old, allegedly hazardous waste sites at an extraordinary cost to taxpayers.

The budget of SuperFund is approximately $1.7 billion annually, about what the National Cancer Institute has for research and development on the causes and treatment of human cancer. In addition, SuperFund authorizes the Environmental Protection Agency to order "cleanups" that cost American industry another two to three billion annually. This expense, justified by self-appointed consumer advocates, as a "polluters must pay" tax, is passed onto consumers in the form of higher prices in the marketplace. Since 1980, about $16 billion has been spent on cleanups. If the program is allowed to continue, about 2,000 sites will be cleaned up at a cost of $40 million per site, or $80 billion (conservatively) in total.

What are we getting in terms of better health for this expenditure? The best estimate is "nothing." While $80 billion is being spent under the guise of "public health" to "prevent" alleged premature death and illness from trace environmental exposure to chemicals from these sites, one million Americans are dying prematurely from known and preventable causes of diseases, including those caused by smoking cigarettes, other illicit drug use, sexually permissive behavior, failure to use life-preserving technologies like seat belts and disease-detection tests, and more. SuperFund is a perfect example of a cumbersome bureaucracy in place, being nurtured by its authorization to extract money from industry to sustain a program of overzealous abatement of hypothetical risks.

SuperFund is a direct result of the panic at a dumpsite in Love Canal in the Niagara Falls section of New York state in 1980. Yet despite this reality, the government pursues this project, with the EPA estimating that sites are the cause of 1,000 cancers per year—a purely speculative number.

Complicating the main problem of SuperFund—the diversion of enormous amounts of our limited resources toward a nonexistent problem—is the fact that most of the allocated monies have ended up in the pockets of lawyers and others involved in a staggering array of litigation about who should clean up what. One might argue that these sites are potentially dangerous or simply that they are unpleasant from an aesthetic point of view. But both of these arguments could be satisfied by (a) prioritizing, giving attention to the most offensive sites, and (b) unlinking the efforts with "public health" and downgrading the expenditure appropriately.

The SuperFund program will be debated and probably reauthorized in 1993–94. But I hope this time the selling of SuperFund will be difficult. Just as the collapse of communism will make it more difficult for the Air Force to get all the B1 bombers it wants, the failure to find a credible health threat associated with living near a dumpsite should curtail enthusiasm for totally unjustified SuperFund spending.

Consistently, the doomsdayers place the emphasis for disease prevention *outside* the individual's control; for example, amazingly excluding cigarette smoking as a cause of disease. *Malignant Neglect,* in proceeding to lay blame for cancer on the petrochemical industry's production, "which increased by more than 2,000 percent since 1945,"[56] downplays smoking by saying "cigarette smoking is hardly the sole menace." Samuel Epstein notes in a comforting fashion that "smoking is not a significant cause of the increased incidence of cancer in the past decade."*[57] Regenstein, in discussing the causation of lung cancer, says that "people living in urban areas . . . die of lung cancer at nearly double the rate of those in rural areas. In fact, there are strong statistical correlations between cities with high industrial pollution levels and death rates from lung cancer."[58] He makes no mention of the role of cigarette smoking (in particular, the fact that urban people smoke more) or the fact that air pollution has never been shown to cause human cancer. Grossman, in *The Poison Conspiracy,* uses essentially the same tactic, talking of rapidly increasing cancer death rates, but never mentioning cigarette smoking, presumably because it would weaken his case against the "environmental poisons" around us.[59]

The technique of blaming the society rather than the victim is perfectly compatible with human psychology; it is always easier to blame someone else for misfortune than to be introspective and assess one's own role in determining fact. But it is also completely out of line with scientific knowledge to recommend that a consumer focus his or her cancer prevention measures on stopping the spraying of agricultural chemicals, instead of noting the dramatic effect cigarette smoking has on the risks of many different diseases; or on another level, the dramatic effect of exposure to ultraviolet radiation from the sun and its impact on skin cancer risk.

PREMISE 10: If You Disagree with Us, You Are Dishonest and Paid Off by the Very Industries Poisoning All of Us.

For the past decade, those of us in the scientific community who, after a thorough scientific evaluation, designate a consumer product "safe," or dismiss charges

---

*Here Dr. Epstein is obviously overlooking the lagged nature of cancer induction. The cancer increase we see today reflects the increase in smoking that took place thirty years ago. So this statement of his, in the words of Richard Doll and Richard Peto, is a "simple error to be corrected, not a new scientific hypothesis to be considered."

that an environmental chemical poses a human health hazard, stand accused of the charge that we are "hired guns" for industry.

It has reached the point that groups such as the Natural Resources Defense Council, the Ralph Nader–inspired Center for Science in the Public Interest, and their allies in the media routinely dismiss those with whom they disagree, not on the basis of scientific criticism, but through innuendo, the clear implication that corporate funding dictates an organization's conclusions. Even other neutral journalists frequently feel compelled to include a statement about corporate funding—but only, of course, if the group or spokesperson in question is defending the safety of a product.

As Regenstein observes in *America the Poisoned* in his section entitled "Science for Sale?" in rejecting the conclusions of an Oregon State University study that cleared 2,4,5-T as a cause of reproductive failure, "[the university] receives large sums of money from the users and producers of these chemicals"; he averred that the university has been carrying on a "love affair with industry for many years." Grossman laments the fact that the first appointees under President Reagan in the area of environmental protection were all from "industry," which immediately in his mind made them suspect and untrustworthy.

A classic example of the "if you don't agree with me, you're a hired gun" approach involved Dr. Thomas Jukes, a professor of medical physics at the University of California at Berkeley, who was and still is an avid defender of DDT. Replying to an article in the *New York Times* in which Dr. Jukes had said that withdrawal of DDT from the WHO malaria eradication programs would be "tantamount to genocide," R. A. Cameron of the Environmental Defense Fund attempted to dismiss Jukes as a credible source by referring to his "having worked for over twenty years for the pesticide industry."[60] Actually, Dr. Jukes directed the Department of Nutrition and Physiology Research at Lederle Laboratories, a subsidiary of American Cyanamid, working on vitamins, antibiotics, and anticancer drugs—not pesticides. And American Cyanamid never produced DDT in the first place.[61] But one needs no evidence to support charges of conflict of interest when the object is to dismiss the opposition. An even more extreme example of the environmentalists' attempt to discredit those opposing their views by questioning their motives was the case of Robert Arbib, editor of *American Birds*, who wrote to the *New York Times* to protest the "misuse" by the "pesticide industry's spokesman" of the data resulting from the Audubon Society's annual Christmas bird counts. He said that such spokesmen were "being paid to lie" when they stated that bird life in North America is thriving despite the use of DDT. As authors George Claus and Karen Bolander note, this illustrates "the desperate reaction to which some environmentalists are driven when their claims are refuted by their own data. . . . We wonder whether Arbib really expects people to believe that these gentlemen, a Nobel laureate included, can be bought off for a few pieces of silver."[62]

During the Great Apple Scare of 1989 and the debate about palm oil as a "poison," the American Council on Science and Health (ACSH) felt the full brunt of the funding question as a weapon used in lieu of debate.

- The Center for Science in the Public Interest (CSPI), apparently outraged over the council's full-page newspaper advertisements that proclaimed "Our Food Supply Is Safe!" complained to the *Washington Post* (April 21, 1989) that ACSH was not a "consumer education agency." Why? Because "ACSH is funded largely by companies . . . [that] are the very producers of the pesticides and other agricultural chemicals ACSH was defending" and "many of ACSH's scientific advisors have consulted for or received research grants from the food and chemical industries." CSPI felt that the *Post* should never have published ACSH's ad "without disclosing . . . [ACSH's] conflict of interest."

- An article about ACSH in the *Los Angeles Times* (April 6, 1989) ("Scientific Group Wages Crusade to Ease Food Safety Concerns") noted that "ACSH receives up to 35 percent of its funding from corporations. . . . Critics contend that many of the Council's scientific advisers have worked for or received grants from drug, chemical or other manufacturers whose products the Council defends."

- The *Des Moines Register* (March 6, 1989), in writing of ACSH, notes "it regularly comes down on the side of business. . . . Whelan points to ACSH's opposition to cigarettes as proof that her organization is not in the pocket of corporate America. That argument is like contending that opposition to earthquakes establishes one's credentials as an environmentalist."

- A letter to the editor of a Tacoma, Washington, newspaper (April 5, 1989) urged readers to use "caution" in reading articles from ACSH because "it is supported by millions from the food and chemical industry. . . ."

- In an otherwise neutral article, a staff reporter for the *Wall Street Journal* (April 5, 1989) notes that "ACSH gets some funds from chemical and other companies."

- Similarly, an editorial in *Medical World News* recently referred to "the industry-sponsored American Council on Science and Health."

- In early April 1989, ACSH scientists were tentatively booked to appear on a national television morning program to discuss food safety. The afternoon before the interview, the producer in charge of the segment expressed concerns about ACSH receiving funding from the chemical industry and canceled the segment.

- During a ninety-minute interview with me on the subject of the safety of pesticides for "60 Minutes," CBS host Ed Bradley's first question to me was "Let's go right to the issue of funding. . . . You get a lot of money from the chemical industry. A lot of people who've looked at your contributors' list accuse you of being little more than a hired hand for the companies that make chemicals and pesticides."

ACSH AND FUNDING

Before exploring some specific implications of the "funding issue as a weapon," a few points about ACSH seem pertinent:

1. ACSH is a not-for-profit consumer organization exempt from income tax under section 501(c)(3) of the Internal Revenue Code. ACSH's budget for FY 1990 was approximately one million dollars. Roughly 40 percent of its funding is derived from private foundations, 40 percent from corporations and corporate foundations, and the balance from sales of literature and individual memberships.

2. ACSH addresses a full variety of public health issues, including AIDS, cigarette smoking, the safety of video display terminals, microwave ovens, the risk factors of cancer, heart disease, hypertension and more—hardly fitting the image of "industry's hired gun." Further, ACSH reports are reviewed by at least a dozen scientific advisors (who are not compensated for this service), and even if ACSH staff wished to transmogrify data to please funders, this would never survive the scientific review process.

3. ACSH seeks to keep its funding list diversified and has funding from corporations representing a full spectrum of interests. ACSH funders include the American Medical Association, Liberty Mutual Insurance, Alliance of American Insurers, many private individuals, and a spectrum of food, chemical, energy-producing, and pharmaceutical companies. Some of ACSH's supporters are in clear competition with each other—for example, ACSH funders include the manufacturers of aspartame (NutraSweet), saccharin (Cumberland Packing), and the Sugar Association. ACSH accepts only unrestricted grants from corporations.

4. Indeed ACSH has lost significant funding for not complying with the interests of some of its funders, making clear the organization's commitment to remain independent, and acknowledging that corporations do try to influence policy on occasion.

For example, a metal conduit manufacturer withdrew funds from ACSH when the organization defended the safety of PVC piping; some of the larger pharmaceutical and distribution firms, displeased about ACSH's refusal to endorse megadosing of vitamins, have withdrawn or withheld funding. A major pesticide manufacturer canceled its funding because ACSH's scientifically reviewed position statement failed to support its marketing claims for the alleged superiority of its type of pesticides; a large diversified corporation, which owns an insurance company, discontinued funding after ACSH refused to endorse airbags in automobiles enthusiastically; and of course, ACSH has consistently and immediately lost funding from food companies upon takeover by cigarette firms.

While ACSH believes that the funding of nonprofit organizations should be a matter of public record (ACSH has for ten years regularly published its funding list), I suggest that the knee jerk reaction of "if you take industry money, you are a paid liar" is the means by which some of our critics try to choke the open and free debate of scientific issues.

Even our harshest critic, CSPI, noted in an article they prepared on ACSH: "It is important to note that there is no indication of any direct quid pro quo between the money the Council receives and the results of its studies. There is also no indication that the contributors have any say as to what studies are carried out."

What Are the Implications?

First, the funding question is only raised for those of us who defend the products of technology.

It seems clear that if ACSH were to have the same funding list, but deplored the use of pesticides and anguished over parts per trillion of PCB or dioxin in drinking water, then the funding issue would not be raised. Funding information is almost never presented for groups such as the Natural Resources Defense Council (NRDC) (the group that brought us Meryl Streep and the apple-Alar panic in the spring 1989). If funding and finances as topics of possible conflict were universally of interest, one would think a member of the media would raise an editorial eyebrow about the fact that the NRDC, which claims to be promoting public health by pointing the finger of cancer causation at pesticides, holds one thousand shares of R. J. Reynolds common stock in its endowment fund as of 1985, the last time we checked.

Second, the reference to ACSH funding (or industrial consulting on the part of ACSH scientists) is always raised in veiled innuendo.

Third, in using the "funding weapon," groups have created a self-serving dichotomy: either you agree with them that, for example, pesticide residues pose an "imminent hazard" and that all the evils of the human race can be laid at the door of industry, or you are a paid liar. Nice and neat.

What is a reporter really trying to say when he or she adds that ACSH "is supported in part by chemical companies"? That itself means nothing. What we would appreciate, if this is the belief of the journalist or ACSH critic, is a direct statement of what is clearly implied, namely, that "ACSH is a paid liar for industry." And after they say what the industry-funded tag lines imply, they better stand prepared to prove it with specific examples of how and where funding has caused ACSH to distort scientific realities. Forget the innuendo. Innuendo is the weapon of a wimp.

Fourth, why the hypocrisy? When a publication gratuitously introduces us as the "industry supported" American Council, do they consider their own funding (advertisements from the same companies that fund ACSH)? When commercial television programs cast a skeptical eye on an organization or individual who might have an "industry connection," do the producers ever consider where their funding (salary) comes from? Perhaps, again, what we have here is a double standard, as expressed best by Ed Bradley on "60 Minutes." When I raised the question about CBS's advertising dollars, he was outraged, claiming "we are neutral here." And I stand by my response to him, "So then you are saying that it is OK to take money from industry as long as you don't defend their product?"

Fifth, and finally, the reality of this whole funding question is that what ultimately matters is not funding, but scientific accuracy and legitimacy.

Consider this example:

The Tobacco Institute claims that cigarette smoking has never been "proven" to cause human disease and death. The Tobacco Institute is exclusively funded by cigarette companies. Is the Tobacco Institute credible? No, of course not! But why is it not credible? Is it because of its funding base? No, if the institute were funded by the Easter Bunny, its pronouncements would still be scientifically outrageous because the "controversy" about cigarettes as the number-one cause of premature, preventable death has long disappeared, and there is a medical consensus that cigarettes are a threat to human health. Only the Tobacco Institute feels otherwise.

We invite our critics, the ones who claim that our food supply is contaminated, that there is a "cancer epidemic," a scourge of industrially caused disease, to step forward for real dialogue and debate, to lay aside the weapons of wimps and stand up to the scientific issues. Perpetuation of the myth that scientists who are corporate advisors, or groups that take unrestricted industry funding, are by definition mouthpieces for commercial interest groups will only continue to have a chilling effect on the free exchange of ideas because only one side of the issue—the anti-industry side—would be permitted the status of "credible." He who pays the piper does not always call the tune.

Techniques, Strategies, and Gimmicks

One might wonder how the doomsdayers have managed to be so successful in conveying their message about the environmental horrors to come when what they say is so far removed from the mainstream of scientific thinking.

They do so by regularly employing a series of tactics that allow them to evoke sympathy through descriptions of specific personal tragedies; following the questionable journalistic motto "All the News That We Think Is Fit to Print"; citing each other and the same handful of "expert" witnesses; referring to studies that have long been rejected by the scientific community; avoiding at each juncture any mention of the possible benefits of, say, an agricultural chemical; never alluding to the costs involved in regulation and to what we *might* use to replace a banned chemical, and casting their recommendations in a setting of urgency, ridden by the anxiety about what might happen. Let's take a close look at each of these techniques.

TECHNIQUE 1: USE ANECDOTAL EVIDENCE.

Henry David Thoreau (1850) is on record as saying "some circumstantial evidence is very strong, as when you find a trout in the milk."

And indeed circumstantial evidence does play a role in the early stages of scientific research. For example, when the first case of a rare form of vaginal cancer was discovered in the Boston area in the early 1970s, the diagnosing physician had "circumstantial evidence" that the cancer was the result of the young woman's *in utero* exposure to DES during her mother's pregnancy. It was only after other such cases were identified, and statistical analysis involving established scientific criteria yielded consistent results, that it became apparent that *in utero* exposure to this drug did cause this rare form of malignancy in a small number of the offspring daughters.

Anecdotal evidence is of rather limited value in itself, but one would never know that from reading the environmentalist literature. In the "environmental nightmare" scripts we are presented with a full range of human horror stories. Karl Grossman tells us of a Vietnam War veteran named Michael Ryan, whose daughter was born with eighteen separate genetic defects.[60] Grossman writes of a woman who lived near Love Canal and developed cervical cancer, then leaves the reader to conclude that there must be some connection, an allusion that would leave any epidemiologist bewildered.

The "60 Minutes" special on Alar and apples declared that Alar was causing childhood cancer and, to underscore the horror of the situation, showed scenes from pediatric cancer wards. A very effective means of connecting cancer to Alar.

"The Plague on Our Children" documentary gives time to Lois Gibbs, a former resident of Love Canal who, like Bonnie Hill, did her own survey of the health effects of the chemical residues in her area. She told in detail of her son's ailments: "Since he attended the school, he developed many, many illnesses; respiratory problems, liver problems, urinary problems. . . . I believe there is definitely a cause and effect. Our problem is trying to prove this."

Regenstein presents what was probably the most incredible use of anecdotal material when he tells the story of a husband-wife antiherbicide team whose home was burned to the ground, killing all four of their children. He observes grimly that "it was commonly believed that the house was deliberately set on fire because of the activists'* leading role in the fight against aerial spraying."[64] The technique of using anecdotal evidence is aptly summed up by British businessman J. M. Martin, who was quoted in *Industry Week* as saying that "no matter what occurs, there is always someone who believes it happened according to his pet theory."[65] And obviously, we tend to feel great sympathy for those who have undergone such suffering. But that is emotion, not science. Individual personal experiences, good or bad, in themselves make no contribution to the effort to establish cause and effect.

TECHNIQUE 2: ALWAYS QUOTE THE SAME HANDFUL OF SCIENTISTS AND FEEL FREE TO CITE DATA REJECTED BY A CONSENSUS OF THE SCIENTIFIC COMMUNITY.

The extremists among the environmentalist movement always look to the same coterie of scientists when a quote or witness is needed to back up a specific claim. These scientists include:

1. *Dr. Samuel S. Epstein* is a professor of occupational and environmental medicine at the University of Illinois Medical Center in Chicago. He has written two major popular books, *The Politics of Cancer*[66] and *Hazardous Waste in America*,[67] both published by Sierra Club Books. Epstein is one of the foremost of those who assert that the role of occupational exposure in cancer causation

---

*Steve and Carol Van Strum; Mrs. Van Strum later wrote *Bitter Fog: Herbicides and Human Rights* (Sierra Club, 1983).

is underestimated (see premise 3). His books and papers make wide-ranging claims on this topic. The premise of most of Epstein's work is that cancer is essentially a preventable disease and that the route toward cancer prevention is through the pressure of public-interest groups and organized labor—an interesting point of view for a scientist. Accordingly, the ultimate goal should be stricter government regulations and victory in court battles that set precedents for industry regulation or worker protection. Epstein recommends: Don't buy bacon, avoid all processed foods, and don't buy any food containing additives labeled "FD&C."

Writing in the scientific magazine *Nature,* Richard Peto, an authority on cancer epidemiology, pointed out a list of erroneous claims that Epstein made in *The Politics of Cancer,* but that are typical of Epstein's work in general:

- The discussion of alcoholism and cancer is entirely erroneous because of failure to standardize properly for age.

- There is idealization of the value of long-term animal tests with concomitant denigration of the value of the Ames test and other short-term tests. This is one of Epstein's most inexplicable errors of scientific judgment, unless he wants cancer tests to be difficult and expensive for industry.

- He is irritatingly puritanical, sneering at "the plastic age that symbolizes how the value of our lifestyle has been degraded."

- He seeks by stylistic tricks to attribute to oral contraceptives some of the established hazards of hormone replacement therapy and of diethylstilbestrol.

- He claims that cancer costs the U.S. economy over $25 billion per year. (In fact cancer must be prevented for humane, not for economic reasons; without cancer there would be three or four million more retired North Americans to support, costing us $25 billion per year.)

- He seems so certain about everything—how can anybody be justified in being so certain about so many details? Sometimes I know he's wrong, but more often (especially in the many places when inconclusive scientific results are presented as established fact), I know that nobody knows for sure.

- In support of his claim that saccharin causes cancer in rats even in very low doses, he presents in tabular form the control and 0.01 percent [low saccharin dosage] data for selected cancers from certain multi-group feeding experiments, leaving out the observations from those same experiments that would have refuted it. This appears to be a deliberate attempt to deceive the reader. It is not a casual slip in a 600-page book, as Epstein devotes twenty pages and two full-page tables to saccharin.[68]

Additionally, at the EPA hearings on the banning of the insecticide DDT (see chapter 2), Dr. Epstein was the only scientist to contend that DDT presents a high cancer-causing risk in human beings. Apparently, Epstein submitted into the record "an incomplete summary of an unpublished mouse study which he contended was significant in determining whether DDT, in fact, causes liver tumors in mice." Attorneys discovered that Dr. Epstein submitted only a portion of the study; that the results were erratic; that in some instances the control animals developed more liver tumors than those fed with DDT; and then, most remarkably, that the investigators lost control of the study and instead of feeding 110 ppm of DDT to the animals, as the summary suggested, the animals were fed 300 ppm for a substantial portion of the study.[69]

2. *Dr. Melvin D. Reuber* is a pathologist who, several years ago at the National Cancer Institute, reviewed the safety data on twenty-three pesticides that had already been licensed and designated safe. Reuber said that the data actually showed those pesticides were unsafe and carcinogenic in virtually every case, in contradiction of the conclusions of the scientists who actually carried out the studies.

Reuber received a sharp censure from his supervisor for failing to adhere to the strict rules of scientific and peer review before making his findings public. The letter of reprimand from Dr. M. G. Hanna, director of the Frederick Cancer Research Center, stated:

These actions are unfortunate; your carelessness and lack of professional expertise in dealing with these issues have seriously prevented any real technological issues from being addressed in a sound scientific manner.

The allegations which have been brought against you (which I have investigated and have found to be true) are that you have reinterpreted slides that were part of several bioassay carcinogenicity tests including those associated with malathion, malaoxon, and picloram. With regard to malathion and malaoxon, your statement in a letter to Mr. Rominger, the director of the Department of Food and Agriculture in Sacramento, California, was that your reinterpretation was based on "examination of every histological slide" (up to 24,000 slides) of the three studies. Based on this statement, and assuming that a competent pathologist would spend a minimum of five minutes per slide in order to adequately reinterpret a previous diagnosis, you spent a total of 333 days in the repository reading these slides. I have checked the repository records and you have not spent that amount of time in the repository. Therefore, I can only assume that your statement regarding your thorough evaluation of these slides was incorrect and misleading. On the other hand, you may have spent considerably less time per slide, thus raising a question of whether your interpretation is scientifically valid.

You exploited the privilege of scientific communication in an unrestrained manner. You have pontificated and criticized other scientists in a manner that excited the public in areas of immediate national concern. Rather than using the forum accepted by scientists, you have used an unreviewed forum to gain easy and immediate voice to the media where public health issues are most easily sensationalized. You may be correct in your interpretations, but the rest of the scientific community, and the public, has not had the advantage or privilege of learning and evaluating your view since you declined to pass it through the standard review procedure established for this purpose. Therefore, neither the scientific community nor the public has adequately benefited from your important information and viewpoint. This is counter-productive at all levels.[70]

Soon after this letter of reprimand, Dr. Reuber quietly resigned his government position.

3. The late *Dr. Wilhelm Hueper* was one of the first and foremost investigators of the role of occupational hazards in cancer causation. He first went to work for DuPont in 1934 in order to attempt to establish a link between beta-napthylamine exposure and bladder cancer in workers. In 1942 he published *Occupational Tumors and Allied Diseases*. As Larry Agran writes in his book *The Cancer Connection,* "Dr. Hueper's book became the scholarly weapon that he used, time and again, in a lifelong battle to encourage effective control measures to match the dangers of what he termed 'the new artificial environment.' "[71] In 1948 Hueper became chief of the Environmental Cancer Section of the National Cancer Institute, and with his ongoing emphasis of environmental chemicals as the cause of human disease—and, most important, his lifelong denial of the role of cigarettes in human disease—he became a great ally of the fledgling environmentalists and is widely quoted and praised in Rachael Carson's *Silent Spring.*

4. *Dr. Matthew Meselson* is a biochemist at Harvard and a longtime skeptic of pesticides in the environment. Studies done by Meselson were instrumental in the banning of phenoxy herbicides.[72] Recently Meselson has stated in the press that dioxin is probably the most toxic small molecule known to man.

In the television documentary, "A Plague on Our Children," Dr. Meselson stated that "thousands of Americans die every year from tumors caused by dioxin exposure." In chronic doses to humans, dioxin (TCDD) causes, at worst, chloracne (see chapter 9). Even though Meselson is justified in his concern over the health effects of dioxin exposure, no studies have ever shown that anyone has died from dioxin-caused cancers.

5. *Dr. Theodore Sterling* is currently professor of computing science at Simon Fraser University, Victoria, British Columbia, Canada. Sterling is a vigorous proponent of occupational factors in cancer causation. In a paper given before the American Association for the Advancement of Science, Sterling attacked the surgeon general's reports on smoking, saying that "clearly inadequate information is provided." According to a June 1983 issue of the *Tobacco Observer,* the tobacco industry's newsletter, Sterling notes the "growing adversary issue" over the extent to which workers' smoking histories have been used "to divert attention away from hazardous occupational exposures."[73] Sterling charged that the surgeon general's reports emphasized studies linking smoking to cancer and omitted important findings about occupational exposure. "It was apparent to investigators familiar with occupational factors related to cancer that the surgeon general's reports did not include a considerable body of important data. . . . These reports did not always appear to correctly discuss the occupational studies which were studied."[74] A computer sciences expert and statistician for thirty years, Sterling has served as consultant to the U.S. Public Health Service, the Environmental Protection Agency, the Federal Trade Commission, and the American Lung Association.[75]

In citing potential hazards related specifically to the use of nuclear energy, another small handful of alarmist scientists and physicians are consistently cited, a fact that implies that they represent the consensus of scientific views on the subject. Of course, they do not.

6. *Dr. John W. Gofman,* a physician with a doctorate in nuclear/physical chemistry, is on record as stating "there is no known amount of radioactivity that can be proclaimed safe."[76]

He has often expressed sentiments such as, "The decision to build and operate a nuke [nuclear power plant] is nothing less than premeditated random murder upon this and future generations."[77] In describing the risks from release of low-level radiation from nuclear power plants and from plutonium releases, Gofman has calculated that thousands of Americans are being sacrificed annually by the nuclear power industry. According to Dr. Bernard Cohen of the University of Pittsburgh's Department of Physics and Astronomy, "At least five devastating critiques of Gofman's work have been published, and I have never encountered a radiation health professional who takes Gofman's risk estimate seriously."[78]

7. *Dr. George Wald,* a Harvard professor of biology and winner of a Nobel Prize in the field of color vision and physiology of the retina, tells us that "every little bit of radioactivity hurts." (Wald made that statement on television in front of the Three Mile Island plant in the days when the antinuclear hysteria was at a high point because a nuclear plant had done what it was supposed to do: shut itself down without hurting anyone when its vast power went out of control.)[79]

8. *Dr. Helen Caldicott* avers that "the scientists who work for nuclear power and nuclear energy have sold their soul to the devil. They're either dumb, stupid or highly compromised."[80]

Dr. Caldicott approaches nuclear power as a problem best left to the medical community to solve. Since radiation causes disease and nuclear power releases radiation, she believes that nuclear power is quite dangerous. Physicians, therefore, are obliged to oppose it as a means of practicing preventive medicine.

Although an articulate speaker, Dr. Caldicott rarely gets her facts straight when speaking about nuclear power. In fact, her impassioned speeches frequently have little to do with reality.[81] In *The War Against the Atom,* Samuel McCracken explains the effects of Caldicott's blunders:

> Her speeches serve little purpose but to spread serious misinformation to the American public. And since the object of her speeches, which they must often attain, is to terrify, she terrifies for no good reason. And, finally, because her misinformation is used by herself and by others to encourage the adoption of suicidal energy policies, she is effectively working to hasten a time when this country will suffer, and suffer terribly, from energy shortages and from escalating public health problems growing out of increased reliance on coal.[82]

9. *Dr. Ernest Sternglass* of the University of Pittsburgh has during the past few decades conducted a crusade to convince the world that the scientific and health communities are hiding from the public the dangers of nuclear radiation. In his books, which include *Secret Fallout; Low Level Radiation from Hiroshima to Three Mile Island,* he charges that "several hundred" infant deaths occurred as a result of TMI (contrary to the epidemiological studies by the state health agency showing that the accident caused no human fatalities, or hazard at all to humans or animals). He further states that nuclear-weapons testing conducted in the atmosphere by the United States Atomic Energy Commission in Utah in 1957 damaged the brains of babies born that year and subsequently caused Scholastic Aptitude Test (SAT) scores to decline.[83]

The scientific community continues to reject his statements. For example, British epidemiologist Alice Stewart, whose research led to tighter standards for prenatal X-rays, once told a hearing board that was examining plans for a nuclear plant on Long Island that she had reviewed Sternglass's work and found "his approach null and void. . . . He has done what many people have done before. They have assumed that it is quite easy to be an epidemiologist."[84] The American Academy of Pediatrics, after reviewing his charges that low-level radiation from nuclear power plants caused infant deaths, said that "his conclusions are completely unfounded and unsubstantiated."[85]

Science magazine commented, "Few reputable scientists believe Sternglass has the evidence to support his contention. But that hasn't stopped Sternglass from making an unusual public impact. Indeed for a man who is so widely regarded as wrong, Sternglass has achieved surprising exposure on the nation's airwaves and in the mass media."[86]

The following passage from *The War Against the Atom* is particularly illuminating. It points out how hypocritical an "expert" such as Dr. Sternglass is when he takes the microphone and rallies an antinuclear crowd with "facts" that he knows are misleading:

> After he was through (speaking at a debate), a pregnant woman came up. She was, she said, planning several trips to California before delivery. She had heard from Peter Beckmann that airline travel increased one's exposure to radiation. Ought she to postpone her travel? Dr. Sternglass might have been a reassuring family physician. Yes, he said, there was a slight increase in radiation. But it was trivial—only a millirem or so, between Chicago and Los Angeles. There was no reason to change her plans and no reason to worry. That is, he was confessing to her that what he and the anti-nuclear movement repeatedly tell us is not so, that there is in fact a safe level of radiation.
>
> And since he called "trivial" the 3 or 4 millirem she would have gotten from making the three trips, he was also calling "trivial" the no more than 3 or 4 millirem she might have gotten from a nuclear reactor by living next door to it and standing naked before the fence twenty-four hours a day for a year.
>
> It appeared to me, standing there watching, that although Dr. Sternglass the media figure did not hesitate to terrorize people in crowds with fabrication, Dr. Sternglass the man was incapable of terrorizing an expectant mother face to face and therefore told her the simple truth.[87]

Not only are the same scientists cited over and over again, but the scaremonger authors are also fond of quoting each other. Some day literary historians will sit down and lump all of the scare books together, finding stylistic facsimiles produced by the same word processor's apprentice.

Another common and related alarmist technique is the use of rejected data to back environmentalist claims. For example, Regenstein, in his 1982 book, cites as authoritative proof of the "disaster" at Love Canal Dr. Beverly

Paigen's study, which supposedly showed more birth defects, miscarriages, and other disorders in the Niagara Falls region.[88] In October 1980 a blue-ribbon panel of physicians, appointed by Governor Hugh Carey of New York, had rejected the Paigen statistics as "literally impossible to interpret." Yet another often-quoted "rejected study" that pops up frequently in the environmentalist literature is the so-called Califano estimates paper, which was discussed previously. Like the child's song "The Cat Came Back," rejected flawed data do not fade very easily when they serve the interest of an environmental activist.

TECHNIQUE 3: DON'T EVER MENTION THE ADVANTAGES
OF A CHEMICAL; ONLY STRESS ITS POTENTIAL DISADVANTAGES.
WHEN IN DOUBT EXAGGERATE THE DISADVANTAGES,
STEER CLEAR OF DISCUSSION OF THE COST OF AN
ENVIRONMENTAL REGULATION, AND ONLY CRITICIZE,
DON'T OFFER SOLUTIONS—UNLESS THEY IN SOME WAY
TARGET "INDUSTRY" AS THE CULPRIT.

Dr. Merril Eisenbud writes in the *American Journal of Medicine,* "It is certainly true that the detrimental effect of many forms of technological advances are to be seen everywhere, but on balance we are a fortunate generation that enjoys a variety of advantages that would not have been possible in former times. We must not lose sight of the ways in which we have benefited because of science and technology."[89]

But that is exactly what the environmentalists have lost sight of: the way technology, including agricultural technology, has improved our standard of living and our health. Any doubt in one's mind about the polemical nature of environmentalist writers is erased when one studies their discussions of pesticides, like DDT. Nowhere in the rantings against DDT, that it caused cancer in animals and damaged ecology, do we ever find the environmentalists pointing to the fact that DDT has saved millions of lives. Where is the acknowledgment that until 1940, when DDT was introduced on a worldwide basis, two hundred million people a year were stricken with malaria, with an average of two million deaths annually?

Environmentalists are remarkably naive, or cunning, when it comes to the cost of the regulations they propose. They seem eager to promote bans and restrictions but rarely talk about the potential downside risk of such regulations, the cost to the consumer, and what alternative would remain to do the job.

When the extremists were raving about the carcinogenic threat posed by EDB in our food supply, we often heard that there were alternative safer pesticides to keep stored grain free from insect and mold infestation. What the environmentalist fanatics did not tell the public was that none of the available substitute chemicals had ever been given a "clean bill of health" after thorough toxicological testing. And now that EDB has been tried and found guilty by the media and public, we are left with (1) the recently-found-to-be-carcinogenic methyl bromide, which Dr. Epstein enthusiastically endorsed on ABC's "Nightline" program; (2) carbon disulfide, a compound that is explosive if not mixed with the flame-retardant carbon tetrachloride, which is, of course, carcinogenic; (3) phosphine, a chemical that has not been subjected to chronic toxicity testing. So much for the protection of public health through the banning of a useful pesticide.

After immersing oneself in the environmental literature, one is left with the nagging suspicion that the preservation of human health and the quality of the environment may be secondary to some other goal, one that is ultimately focused on the destruction of technology, the American economic system, and the way of life as we now know it. Dr. Eisenbud raises a number of interesting questions:[90] If environmentalists are committed to protecting human health by preventing exposure to pesticides, why are they focusing on banning agricultural chemicals that have never been shown to cause disease or death when used as intended? Why instead don't they give higher priority to the problem posed by toxic household chemicals, left within easy reach of curious children? Thousands of youngsters in the United States are injured, or killed, through such accidental poisonings. Is this not an environmental problem?*

Dr. Eisenbud asks:

> Why is it that there is so little concern with the influences from our social environment that we know to be the causes of death and disease? . . . Why is it that so much attention has been given to the need to eliminate lead from gasoline and to reduce exposure to airborne lead, which has not been identified as a health hazard, whereas peeling lead paint in ghetto buildings has received only minor attraction, despite the fact that we know infants are being poisoned?

TECHNIQUE 4: TIME IS RUNNING OUT.
WHETHER OR NOT THE DATA ARE IN, LET US TAKE ACTION.
ONE CAN NEVER TELL WHAT MIGHT HAPPEN.

The standard cry of the environmental movement of recent years seems to be, "There is no time. The ship is sinking and the appointment of research teams to study the matter will not prevent her from going down."[91]

The sense of urgency and the resulting panic are enhanced by the promotion

---

*In the nutrition area, similar questions have been raised about individuals, allegedly dedicated to reduction of tooth decay, who ask for government restrictions on sugar-containing products for children, but never mention the most effective way of preventing tooth decay: fluoridation of water.

of fear of the unknown: we might not have data now that indicate that it causes cancer, but just in case. . . . We are left paralyzed by anxiety, because the unknown is actually scarier than the real thing, given the ability of our imagination to run wild.

As Donald R. Stephenson, an executive with Dow Canada, noted in *Vital Speeches,* "A threat of disaster can create more alarm than an actual catastrophe. It lends itself to speculation of the most sensational and irresponsible kind. That makes an impending disaster potentially more disastrous to an organization than an actual disaster that happens and is soon over with."

Rachael Carson in *Silent Spring* proved to be a master of stirring up fears of the unknown, anxieties about what might characterize our future. Her book begins with what she calls a "Fable for Tomorrow":

> All life seemed to live in harmony with its surroundings. . . . But then a strange blight crept over the area and everything seemed to change. Some evil spell had settled on the community, mysterious maladies swept the flocks of chickens. . . . There had been several sudden and unexplained deaths, not only among adults but even among children, who would be stricken suddenly while at play and die within a few hours.

Of course, in the context of Carson's book, all this bad news is caused by pesticides. Oh, and also, all of this horror hasn't yet happened. Still she pseudo-innocently informs us as we shiver in fright, "But it might happen in the future." In using this "it might happen" approach, Carson set an example that alarmists are today following. Interestingly, in books like *America the Poisoned* and *Who's Poisoning America,* the qualifiers "could," "apparently," "seemingly," "possibly" appear frequently, as if the authors *knew* that the problems they were addressing were only hypothetical.

Indeed, in the long run, instilling fear of unknown disaster is by far the most effective route environmentalists have taken in capturing the interest of journalists and consumers alike. Veteran Canadian broadcaster Gordon Sinclair once said that four elements make news: love, money, conquest, and disaster. One might add to that list—the fear or threat of disaster. Or, as a *Time* cover story put it, "The most sinister side of the chemical waste threat may be the very uncertainty of its ultimate impact."[92]

Modern-day environmentalism is thus suffering from what might be called the Chicken Little phenomenon. Chicken Little was hit by a falling acorn and interpreted this to mean the sky was falling. She panicked her little neighborhood for a good time, but fortunately a cooler head prevailed and the community lived happily ever after. Right now, the United States needs some cooler heads to enter the dialogue, until now dominated by Chicken Little environmentalists and their spurious premises and questionable techniques.

NOTES

1. R. Nader, R. Brownstein, and J. Richard, *Who's Poisoning America* (San Francisco: Sierra Club Books, 1981), p. 305.

2. J. Skow, "Can Lawns be Justified?" *Time,* June 3, 1991, p. 63.

3. "Death on Your Dinner Table," *Audubon,* September 1987.

4. B. Epstein, *The Politics of Cancer* (San Francisco: Sierra Club Books, 1987), p. 34.

5. J. W. Gofman, testimony before California Assembly, April 1979, as quoted by Bernard L. Cohen in "Radiation Fantasies," *Reason* (March 1980): p. 24.

6. M. Waldholz, "War on Cancer: New Study Disputes Claims of Progress," *Wall Street Journal,* May 6, 1986.

7. *Morbidity and Mortality Weekly Report* (June 19, 1992): p. 417.

8. American Council on Science and Health, *ACSH News and Views* (November–December 1979), p. 6.

9. American Council on Science and Health, *Cancer Clusters* (New York: American Council on Science and Health, 1989).

10. American Council on Science and Health, *New Jersey: Garden State or Cancer Alley?* (April 1981).

11. American Council on Science and Health, *Cancer in the United States: Is There an Epidemic?* (New York: American Council on Science and Health, 1988).

12. "Interview with John Higginson," *Science* (September 28, 1979): p. 1363.

13. American Council on Science and Health, *Cancer in the United States.*

14. *Morbidity and Mortality Weekly Report* (June 19, 1992): p. 417.

15. E. M. Whelan, "How to Reduce Your Risk of . . . Cancer," *Priorities* (Summer 1990): p. 36.

16. David Halberstam (column), *Washington Post,* January 16, 1979.

17. E. M. Whelan, *Preventing Cancer* (New York: W. W. Norton, 1978).

18. R. Doll and R. Peto, *The Causes of Cancer* (New York: Oxford University Press, 1981).

19. American Council on Science and Health, *ACSH News and Views* (November–December 1979): p. 6.

20. Ibid.

21. Ibid.

22. *Nature* (March 1980): p. 284.

23. Doll and Peto, *Causes of Cancer.*

24. P. A. Schulte, et al., "Investigation of Occupation Cancer Clusters: Theory and Practice," *American Journal of Public Health* 77 (1987): p. 52.

25. Epstein, *Politics of Cancer,* p. 21.

26. "Toxic Waste Fights Start in the Laboratory, But How Good Are the Testing Methods?" *Wall Street Journal,* June 21, 1983.

27. American Council on Science and Health, *Of Mice and Men: Benefits and Limitations of Animal Cancer Tests* (March 1984).

28. American Council on Science and Health, *Of Mice and Men.*

29. J. Rocericks and M. Taylor, "Application of Risk Assessment to Food Safety

Decision Making," *Regulatory Tox. Pharm.* 3 (1983): p. 14.

30. International Agency for Research on Cancer, "An Evaluation of Chemicals and Industrial Processes Associated with Cancer in Humans Based on Human and Animal Data; IARC Monograph Vol. 1-20," *Cancer Research* 40 (1980): p. 6.

31. W. Lijinsky, "Environmental Cancer Risks—Real and Unreal," *Environmental Research* 50 (1989): pp. 207–09.

32. G. Claus and K. Bolander, *Ecological Sanity* (New York: David McKay, 1977), p. 233.

33. S. Preston-Martin, M. C. Pike, R. K. Ross, et al., "Increased Cell Division as a Cause of Human Cancer," *Cancer Research* 50 (1990): pp. 7415–21.

34. B. N. Ames and L. S. Gold, "Too Many Rodent Carcinogens: Mitogenesis Increases Mutagenesis," *Science* 249 (1990): pp. 970–71.

35. W. R. Havender, "A Foolish Way to Predict Human Risk" (letter to the editor), *Wall Street Journal,* February 20, 1986.

36. Epstein, *Politics of Cancer,* p. 67.

37. Claus and Bolander, *Ecological Sanity,* p. 212.

38. H. B. Hiscoe, "Does Being Natural Make It Good?" *Journal of American Medical Association* (June 16, 1983): p. 1474.

39. E. W. Whelan and F. J. Stare, *Panic in the Pantry* (New York: Athenum 1975), p. 100; R. Hall, "Safe at the Plate," *Nutrition Today* 12 (no. 6): pp. 1–4.

40. National Academy of Sciences, "Toxicants Occurring Naturally in Foods" (1973): p. 515.

41. Ibid., p. 528.

42. Whelan and Stare, *Panic in the Pantry,* p. 97.

43. S. O. Aral and W. Cates, Jr., "The Increasing Concern with Infertility: Why Now?" *Journal of the American Medical Association* (November 4, 1983): p. 2329.

44. D. Whorton, et al., "Infertility in Male Pesticide Workers," *Lancet* (December 17, 1977): pp. 1259–61.

45. G. P. Oakley, "Birth Defects in the Search for the Evaluation of Possible Human Teratogens," *Journal of Environmental Path. Tox.* 2 (1979): pp. 211–16.

46. T. H. Shepard, "Detection of Human Teratogenic Agents," *Journal of Pediatrics* 101 (1982): pp. 810–15.

47. C. M. Rennert, "Drug-induced Somatic Alterations," *Clinical Obstetrics and Gynecology* 18 (1975): p. 245.

48. J. W. Hanson and D. W. Smith, "The Fetal Hydantoin Syndrome," *Journal of Pediatrics* 87 (1975): p. 285.

49. E. H. Jackai, "Fetal Trimethadione Syndrome," *Journal of Pediatrics* 87 (1975): pp. 280–84.

50. A. L. Herbst, et al., "Adenocarcinoma of the Vagina," *New England Journal of Medicine* 284 (1974): p. 878.

51. R. W. Smithells, "Environmental Teratogens of Man," *British Medical Bulletin* 32 (1976): pp. 27–33; J. G. Wilson, "Present Strategy of Drugs as Teratogens in Man," *Teratology* 7 (1972): pp. 3–16.

52. Quoted in J. Greene, *Morrow's International Dictionary of Contemporary Quotations* (1982): p. 221.

53. C. Ricci, "The Breast Milk Test," *Parents,* August 1988.

54. L. Regenstein, *America the Poisoned* (Washington: Acropolis Books, 1982), p. 246.

55. Greene, *International Dictionary of Quotations,* p. 216.

56. Environmental Defense Fund and R. H. Boyle, *Malignant Neglect* (New York: Alfred A. Knopf, 1979), p. 19.

57. Epstein, *Politics of Cancer,* p. 22.

58. Regenstein, *America the Poisoned,* p. 191.

59. Grossman, *Poison Conspiracy,* p. 191.

60. *New York Times,* August 18, 1971.

61. Claus and Bolander, *Ecological Sanity,* p. 299.

62. Ibid., pp. 299–300.

63. Grossman, *Poison Conspiracy,* p. 57.

64. Regenstein, *America the Poisoned,* p. 28.

65. Greene, *International Dictionary of Quotations,* p. 221.

66. Epstein, *Politics of Cancer.*

67. S. Epstein, et al., *Hazardous Waste in America* (San Francisco: Sierra Club Books, 1982).

68. R. Peto, "Distorting the Epidemiology of Cancer: The Need for a More Balanced Overview," *Nature* (March 27, 1980): pp. 297–300.

69. R. L. Ackerly, "DDT: A Re-evaluation, Part II," *Chemical Times and Trends* (January 1982).

70. "Dr. Mel Reuber, Pathologist, Gets Sharp Censure, Warning from his Supervisor," *Pesticide and Toxic Chemical News* (April 15, 1981): pp. 22–23.

71. L. Agran, *The Cancer Connection* (Boston: Houghton Mifflin, 1977), p. 177.

72. "The Politics of Poison" (San Francisco: KRON-TV, 1979).

73. "Sterling Asks Accountability for 'Inadequate' Reporting," *Tobacco Observer* (June 1983): p. 3.

74. Ibid.

75. Ibid.

76. P. Beckmann, *Doctors Against Health* (Colorado: Golem Press, 1982).

77. B. Cohen, "Radiation," *Reason* (March 1980): p. 24.

78. Ibid., p. 29.

79. Ibid.

80. Ibid.

81. S. McCracken, *The War Against the Atom* (New York: Basic Books, 1982), p. 115.

82. Ibid., p. 116.

83. Book review in *Chemical Engineering News,* August 24, 1981.

84. Ibid.

85. Zivic, letter to *Ms.,* July 1979.

86. R. E. Lapp, *The Nuclear Controversy* (Greenwich: Fact Systems, 1975), p. 15.

87. McCracken, *War Against the Atom,* pp. 132–33.

88. Regenstein, *America the Poisoned,* pp. 138–140.

89. M. Eisenbud, "The Environment, Technology and Health: A Century of Progress

but a Time of Despair," *American Journal of Medicine* 68 (1980): p. 476.
    90. Ibid., p. 477.
    91. Claus and Bolander, *Ecological Sanity,* p. 151.
    92. "The Poisoning of America," *Time,* September 22, 1980, p. 61.

2

The DDT Debate and the
Birth of Environmentalism

False facts are highly injurious to the progress of science, for they often endure
long; but false views, if supported by some evidence, do little harm, for everyone
takes salutary pleasure in proving their falseness.
—Charles Robert Darwin, *The Descent of Man*

It is no easy task to define exactly what is meant by the term *environmental
movement*. It has occasioned various connotations and perceptions, and varying
degrees of both respect and contempt, often dictated by the time period and
individuals the term refers to. The environmental movement is not the same
as the conservation movement or the preservation movement.

What we call environmentalism was born in the early sixties, but in some
respects it has roots going back well over a hundred years. The birth of
environmentalism in the United States, and what it has come to represent,
presage a stormy day ahead for the movement. The reasons for this require
a look into environmentalism's history, politics, and future.

One might well argue that if it is defined broadly, environmentalism has
always been an inherent part of all human societies. Until relatively recently,
much of the world's population had not enough to eat, was in constant search
of drinkable, non–disease-producing water, and was perpetually seeking ways
to protect itself from the elements. In these cases, the "environmental" forces
that threatened life and health were from natural sources. Dr. John Snow
in 1849 noticed that there was a sudden increase in the number of cases of
cholera in London. He was alarmed and agitated enough to investigate and
eventually concluded that the victims were not evenly distributed around the

city; rather, they all lived in one geographic area. Once he made that observation it did not take him long to implicate the sewage-contaminated water flowing from the infamous Broad Street pump. In identifying and acting to prevent an environmentally caused disease, Dr. Snow was in a sense an early environmentalist.

There are other examples of early environmental gains that helped to rectify much of the damage that was inflicted upon human health during the Industrial Revolution and the years thereafter. Referring to the Industrial Revolution in Britain, John Maddox writes in *The Doomsday Syndrome:*

> The public water supply had been progressively improved in quality since the 1840s when health officials recognized that impure public water could quickly spread typhoid through a community. Other infectious diseases have been increasingly controlled by medical advances. Diphtheria, for example, has been virtually eliminated in the advanced societies of the world. Tuberculosis is similarly vulnerable to present medical technologies. Poliomyelitis is now eradicable.[1]

A drastic reduction of occupational hazards, both chemical and physical, has yielded remarkable gains in the past century. Indeed, as Maddox explains, it is a common failure of environmentalists to recognize the advances that have been made in this area, and this becomes damaging to even their own cause.[2]

Conservation as we know it today was formalized around the turn of the century by Gifford Pinchot, the German-trained forester who was born in Connecticut. Pinchot became the pioneer of scientific forestry in the United States. To him the object of forestry was not to preserve the forests solely for their beauty and wildlife but, more importantly, to ensure the availability of wood as an important commodity long into the future. Pinchot was a member of the "doomsday" movement in that he was convinced that the United States timber reserves would be exhausted in thirty years, and that soon thereafter our other raw materials, such as iron ore and natural gas, would be depleted. (He sounded very much like his environmental the-end-of-progress-has-come colleagues today.) But Pinchot sought a way out of this predicament. He believed in a single approach: "The use of foresight and restraint in the exploitation of the physical sources of wealth as necessary for the perpetuity of civilization, and the welfare of the present and future generations."[3]

This theory of forestry in a more generalized area was carried over by Pinchot into the administration of Theodore Roosevelt. It was President Roosevelt who spearheaded the belief that science and technology provided the best avenue for the management of the country's natural resources.

The Roots of Modern-day Environmentalism

Environmentalism, as Dr. Merril Eisenbud, professor and director of the Laboratory for Environmental Studies at the Institute of Environmental Medicine at New York University Medical Center, describes in his book *Environment, Technology, and Health,* is concerned about pollution, population control, and resource conservation. Preservation and protection play an important role as well.[4]

As early as 1874, before the days of Pinchot conservationism, G. P. Marsh wrote that human activity would eventually affect the earth's topography. Loren Eiseley, writing in a 1962 issue of *Saturday Review,* spoke of D'Arcy Thompson, the great British biologist of the late nineteenth century, who "commented astutely in 1897 that the increasing tempo of human cultural revolution produces a line of evolution of chance itself—an increasing dissonance and complexity beyond what one finds in the world before man came. . . ."[5]

Herbert Quick in 1913 asserted in *The Good Ship Earth* that life on earth depended on a closed system of living things and physical objects. Edward A. Ross in the 1920s continued with the same pen as did Thomas Malthus (1766–1834), writing about population problems.[6] Apparently, then, the ideas that began to concern the environmentalists in the 1960s were tossed about much earlier.

Dr. John Maddox, author of *The Doomsday Syndrome* (and now editor of the prestigious British science publication *Nature*), believes that the movement in its present form can be traced to the widespread and understandable fear of radioactive debris from the atmospheric nuclear-weapons tests in the 1950s and the legitimate concern about the effects of radioactivity on the environment in general and human health in particular.

In the 1950s, frequent testing of nuclear weapons and general disregard of the potential health implications for the public at large resulted in the threat of worldwide radioactive dust contamination.

The first atomic test in New Mexico in the summer of 1945 sent radioactive dust drifting eastward. Subsequently, X-ray film was damaged after being packaged in cardboard made from cornstalks that had been contaminated by the fallout in Indiana.[7] In the early 1950s, the Soviet Union, the United States, and Great Britain were testing so many weapons that fallout began to be seen as a public health hazard. The anxiety became particularly intense in the case of a test explosion by the United States in the South Pacific.

On March 1, 1954, the United States tested a fifteen-megaton hydrogen bomb on the Marshall Islands, and, as explained by the antinuclear education group Ground Zero in *Nuclear War: What's in It for You,* "Unexpected winds spread a plume of radioactive fallout from the test site . . . over a 20,000-

square-kilometer area of the South Pacific. Within this area were several inhabited islands and—at the time of the explosion—the Japanese fishing vessel *Lucky Dragon,* whose crew all suffered radiation sickness. Eventually one of them died—very much in the public eye."[8]

Subsequently, it became well known among laymen that radioactive constituents from the fallout of nuclear explosions could be "assimilated" by the food-chain organisms and passed on to humans. For example, it was discovered, and well publicized, that strontium 90 has a chemical activity similar to that of calcium and can be passed up the food chain, by way of grass, to cows, and then to humans. Maddox feels that "the discovery of radiostrontium in the skeletons of young children was a more powerful assault on the public conscience than even the discovery of DDT in the liver and fatty tissues of people as well as other mammals a decade later."[9] Maddox notes that "in retrospect, it is curious how comparatively slowly people recognized the potential destructiveness of nuclear weapons. The fact that a single explosion at Hiroshima killed close to 140,000 people was an awesome piece of information. . . ."[10]

Not surprisingly, the 1950s saw the formation of organizations to deal with the potential health hazards of high-level exposure to man-made radiation. Foremost among these organizations was the Federation of American Scientists, now known as the Federation of Atomic Scientists. The distinguished founding scientists of this group frequently urged in their publication, *Bulletin of Atomic Scientists,* that the U.S. government create laws that would control nuclear energy in such a way that the military authorities in the United States would not have sole charge of the manufacture of nuclear weapons and that the United States would do everything humanly possible to prevent the spread of nuclear weapons overseas.

The lobbying efforts of the scientific group were successful. The McMahon Act placed responsibility for construction of nuclear weapons in the hands of a nonmilitary agency, the United States Atomic Energy Commission. As Maddox explains, "This piece of legislation made it much easier for a strictly civilian nuclear industry to grow up alongside an industry for the development and manufacture of nuclear explosives."[11]

Nevertheless, the general public felt a large degree of helplessness about the whole issue of the fallout from nuclear-weapons testing. Indeed, the *British Army Journal* in 1948 observed, in a resigned fashion, that "the best defense against the atomic bomb is not to be there when it goes off."[12] Even this begs the question since it was widely known that one need not be near a nuclear explosion to be affected by it. That same sense of doomsday was simply summarized a couple of decades later by Susan Sontag, the American essayist, in her *Styles of Radical Will:* "Cogito, ergo, boom."[13]

But fallout fears were largely laid to rest when the series of atmospheric testing ended first in 1958, when the United States, the Soviet Union, and

Britain agreed to a voluntary test ban. This moratorium held until 1961, when the USSR tested over fifty devices. The United States followed with a rash of atmospheric tests of its own. There was great public concern worldwide. In 1963 the United States, the Soviet Union, and Britain signed the Atmospheric Test Ban Treaty, which has held ever since.[14] Maddox stresses that at least in some people's minds the movement against nuclear testing was the framework on which current environmentalism was built:

> Dr. [Barry] Commoner now says that the partial test ban should be regarded as the first victorious battle in the campaign to save the environment and its human inhabitants from the blind anarchy of technology. For him, at least, there is no doubt where the roots of the environmental movement are to be found.[15]

It thus appears that once the problem of uncontrolled nuclear testing was "solved," there was somewhat of a void: a structure and a precedent existed for citizens and scientists effectively to organize to protect health and the environment, but a viable cause did not. By the early 1960s, however, a new cause was identified: pesticides and other alleged environmental contaminants took the place of nuclear fallout in the discussions and controversies about health and the environment.

Reflecting on the hypothesis of modern-day environmentalism, with its strident cries against the use of pesticides and other agricultural chemicals, and its outrage over health-threatening pollution from allegedly toxic and cancer-causing chemicals, it is remarkable how the adverse reaction to the real danger of indiscriminate use of test nuclear weapons was both mild and very late in coming, at least by today's standards. The "environmentalists" of the 1950s had a *genuine* cause for alarm, with some hard data to back up their demands for more discriminate use of nuclear testing devices. Today's environmentalists, however, seem to be constantly groping for a cause, and so often those causes turn out to be combating purely hypothetical risks. They seem to be searching for environmental problems simply to justify their existence, even if that means bypassing the scientific process. If the modern-day environmental movement does have its roots in the real problems of nuclear contamination, then it has surely forgotten its origins.*[16]

---

*George Claus and Karen Bolander in *Ecological Sanity* argue that the environmental movement as we know it today did not originate in the nuclear-fallout issue but was related more to the need of America's early-1960s youth for a "good clean cause" on which to focus their energy and attention.

Silent Spring—Or Silent Springboard?

The early 1960s proved to be an ideal time for an outbreak of furor about pesticides and other potential contaminants in the environment. Not only did there exist that void mentioned above, which was created when regulatory effects lessened the possibility of disaster from nuclear pollution, but the United States was also sailing on relatively calm waters. Environmentalism, for example, could not have come into bloom twenty years before as the country prepared for full involvement in World War II. Nor could this cause have worked up much enthusiasm even ten years before, during the country's military involvement in Korea. Furthermore, the early 1960s saw the breaking of the tragic story about the devastating effects of prenatal use of thalidomide and, as Drs. Claus and Bolander write in their book *Ecological Sanity*, "the climate of receptivity for a book about dangerous chemicals was very high."[17]

The stage was set, the audience baited and enthusiastic, for the entrance of Rachael Carson, a nature lover and author of such well-received books as *The Sea Around Us, Under the Sea Wind,* and *The Edge of the Sea.* During the late 1950s, Carson received letters from friends and associates on Long Island, New York, and those communications gave her a new cause: the case against pesticide spraying.

Carson once wrote, referring to a letter from friends that originally turned her attention to pesticides: "In it you told me what had happened to you and your feelings about the prospect of a new and bigger spraying and begged me to find someone in Washington who would help. It was in the task of finding that 'someone' that I realized that I must write a book."[18] And that book was *Silent Spring,* a half-science, half-fiction work that, when published in 1962,* gave the infant environmental movement the boost it needed. It rode the wave of interest and concern generated by Carson's book, catapulting it to a prominent and powerful position in short order.

Carson vehemently protested the way pesticides were being used and abused in the United States. In reality, there was at least some truth to what she was saying. Enthusiasm over the unprecedented effectiveness of modern-day pesticides did in some cases lead to overuse. Insecticides were being used inappropriately to clear insects from inland lakes in such a careless manner that fish were being killed almost as rapidly as the insects. Even some of Carson's

---

*A number of those advocating the America-the-poisoned philosophy claim that American industry attempted to stop the publication of *Silent Spring.* For example, Regenstein in *America the Poisoned* writes, "In 1962, Velsicol Chemical Corporation even tried to prevent the publication of *Silent Spring* because the book's arguments on pesticides might be a part of a 'sinister' communist plot to destroy American farms." But indeed, my communication from the publisher of *Silent Spring,* Houghton Mifflin, dated 12 July 1983, indicates that the allegation is untrue.[20]

strongest critics give her some credit for encouraging a more carefully controlled use of pesticides.

But in the long run, *Silent Spring* was a polemic, filled with alarmist statements, fraught with innuendo of what might happen, and replete with the questionable arts of overstatement and bait-and-switch. As Claus and Bolander appropriately put it, "One reading of *Silent* Spring is enough to throw any psychologically balanced layman into a seesaw syndrome of deep depression and hypochondriacal anxiety."

Carson's motivations are immediately suspect when one reads on an early page of *Silent Spring,* "Dedicated to Dr. Albert Schweitzer," who said, "Man has lost the capacity to foresee and to forestall. He will end by destroying the earth." She presumably knew that Dr. Schweitzer, in making this grim prophecy, was referring to atomic warfare, but the clear implications, given the context of her book, was that he meant DDT or some other insecticide when speaking of the end of the world.[21]

Carson terrified with beautifully written prose:

> The contamination of our world is not a matter of mass spraying. Indeed for most of us this is of less importance than the innumerable small-scale exposures to which we are subjected day by day, year after year. Like the constant dripping of water that in turn wears away the hardest stone, this birth-to-death contact with dangerous chemicals may in the end prove disastrous. . . . Lulled by the soft sell and the hidden persuader, the average citizen is seldom aware of the deadly materials with which he is surrounding himself; indeed, he may not realize that he is using them at all.[22]

Because Rachael Carson was a literary master, her book received bountiful praise from nonscientists. But the scientific reviews and some of the reviews written by laymen, although varied in their conclusion about the ultimate validity of the book, emphasized the inaccuracies and gross distortions of scientific facts.

Carson had already developed a reputation as one of the most impressive naturalist writers of the time; thus she was no stranger to book reviewers. Her work was classic in the sense it brought to the public's attention a subject that had not really been in the limelight before—pesticides—and it charged that our public agencies were not protecting us from this hidden danger. It had everything: novelty, literary genius, and all the elements to provoke fear and anxiety.

Thus, some reviewers lapped up the contents of *Silent Spring* with enthusiasm.

For example, Loren Eiseley, the world-renowned anthropologist, reviewed *Silent Spring* for *Saturday Review* and said that the book was a "devastating, heavily documented, relentless attack about human carelessness, greed and irresponsibility—an irresponsibility that has let loose upon man and the countryside a flood of dangerous chemicals in a situation which, as Miss Carson states, is without parallel in human history."[23]

Eiseley noted that Carson "documented her case with complete accuracy," and went on to say that the "casual spraying of the landscape with chemicals capable of mutagenic effects is regarded by some authorities as representing as great a menace as high-level radiation."[24] As will be pointed out later in this chapter, many of the claims that Carson made were indeed inaccurate and have since been shown to be untrue. But presently, even the extreme environmentalists do not go as far as to compare the dangers of pesticide use with that of high-level radiation. The supportive review of *Silent Spring* in *Commonweal* (a publication with a large Roman Catholic audience) made claims with which even Carson herself would not have agreed:

> The reader will find that she has answered point for point the broadsides of the chemical industry that her book has provoked. No, she has not exaggerated. No, these poisons are not necessary. The food and fiber production of America can be maintained better by using less lethal pesticides, and especially by using presently effective biological controls and developing others.[25]

The *Commonweal* review concluded with a plea to "reject the sprayed death" that destroys the "tremendous web of life that binds man to earth."[26]

But, fortunately, four of the most widely read magazines, *Time, Newsweek, Scientific American,* and *Science,* were more critical of Carson's work. In general these reviewers saw *Silent Spring* as purposefully one-sided, yet at the same time praised Carson's literary skill and the fact that her book had brought an important issue into the public arena for the first time.

The *Time* review (and its revealing title "Pesticides: The Price for Progress") noted that most readers would no doubt be shocked at the claims made in *Silent Spring* and that "many unwary readers will be firmly convinced that most of the U.S. . . . is already laced with poison that will be soon [taking] a dreadful toll, and that the only hope is to stop using chemical pesticides and let the age-old balance of nature take care of obnoxious insects." But, continues the reviewer, "Scientists, physicians, and other technically informed people will also be shocked by *Silent Spring*. They recognize Carson's skill in building her frightening case, but they consider that case unfair, one-sided, and hysterically overemphatic."[27]

Newsweek, in its review, titled ominously "Hiss of Doom?" quoted a national Agricultural Chemicals Association spokesman as referring to Carson as "an alarmist and a sensationalist—and she's done it beautifully." According to the review, *Silent Spring* would be beneficial because Carson's "obviously one-sided presentation may startle Americans into realizing that chemical pesticides can be misused."[28]

The two most popular scientific magazines, *Scientific American* and *Science,* not only shared the feelings expressed by the reviewers in *Time* and *Newsweek,* but also defended the scientific community that Carson had indirectly attacked. I. L. Baldwin, then professor of agricultural bacteriology at the University of Wisconsin, wrote in *Science:* "I cannot condone, however, the sarcastic and unjustified attack on the ethics and integrity of many scientific workers."[29]

All the reviews that were critical of *Silent Spring* stressed the obvious fact that Carson underplayed the importance of insecticides in disease prevention; as Baldwin wrote in *Science,* "Just as it is important to be reminded of dangers inherent in the use of new pesticides, so must our people also be made aware of the tremendous values to human welfare conferred by the new pesticides."

Norman Borlaug, "Father of the Green Revolution" in agriculture, which brought innovative food production techniques to the Third World, agreed strongly with Baldwin ten years later in a speech before the World Agricultural Association in 1971. The 1970 Nobel Prize recipient stated:

> The gravest defect of *Silent Spring* was that it presented a very incomplete, inaccurate and oversimplified picture of the needs of the interrelated, world-wide, complex problems of health, food, fiber, wildlife, recreation and human population. It made no mention of the importance of chemicals such as fertilizer and pesticides for producing and protecting our food and fiber crops. Nor did it mention that by producing more food per unit of cultivated area more land would be available for other uses, including recreation and wildlife.[30]

Thus, although broadly criticized in the popular as well as the scientific press, *Silent Spring* definitely touched a nerve and set off a wildfire of protest among the public against pesticide use. The environmental movement as we know it today was off and running.

Although the Carson book raised anxieties about pesticide use in general, it was one pesticide in particular—DDT—that the infant environmentalist movement chose as its first target. In doing so, the environmentalists launched what turned out to be the first of a series of attacks on agricultural chemicals. What is indeed shocking and ironic here, some twenty years after the fact, is that in evaluating the events that led to the banning of DDT in 1970, DDT *was in every sense the most unlikely subject for the environmentalists to choose as their flagship.* Yet it was precisely this feature that made DDT so inviting, because if the environmentalists could get DDT banned, they would have little or no trouble with other pesticides. Whereas in the 1980s and 1990s the term *DDT* conjures up the image of poisons that are dispersed widely in the air, destroying fish, birds, and wildlife, and increasing our risk of cancer, the scientific record indicates exactly the opposite: *DDT, when used as intended, did not threaten wildlife or the environment and did not cause human disease.*

Indeed, DDT prevented more human death and disease than any other man-made chemical* in all of recorded history.

DDT: An Elixir of Death?

It has been incontrovertibly shown to prevent human illness on a scale hitherto achieved by no other public health measure entailing the use of a chemical.[32]
—*British Medical Journal*

Chemicals used as sprays are like devils that create chains of poison and death.[33]
—Justice William O. Douglas

Both of these allegations refer to the same substance. And they reflect well the paradox of the saga of DDT.

DDT,† the abbreviation for 1,1,1-trichloro-2,2-bis(p-chlorophenyl) ethane, was first synthesized in 1877, but its actions against insects were not discovered until some sixty-five years later, when it was found to be highly lethal to clothes moths and ectoparasites, and highly protective of field crops. Remarkably, it was harmless to human beings when dusted on their skin to

---

*The history of DDT and particularly the events leading to its banning make fascinating reading. One is left with a number of unanswered questions about why the environmentalists were so enthusiastically anti-DDT. Dr. J. Gordon Edwards makes an impressive case to the effect that some of those pushing for the DDT ban had some rather questionable motives, specifically, the banning of a lifesaving chemical as a means of human population decimation. Edwards quotes environmentalist LaMont Cole: "To feed a starving child is to exacerbate the world overpopulation problem." He writes that during a debate in San Francisco, Dr. Van den Bosch, from the University of California, chided him about his concern for "all those little brown people in poor countries." Dr. Charles Wurster, chief scientist for the Environmental Defense Fund, responded to a reporter's question by stating that there are too many people and "this is as good a way to get rid of them as any," referring to the banning of DDT. His comments caused attorney Victor Yannacone, an early opponent of DDT, to resign from the Environmental Defense Fund in disgust.[31] (Yannacone later became involved in Agent Orange litigation.)

†The literature on DDT, both pro and con, is overwhelming. My intention here is simply to summarize how the environmental activism relative to DDT, and its eventual success in having DDT banned in the United States, set the pace and created the blueprint for the environmentalists' misuse of science in the 1980s and 1990s. For a more detailed description of the history of DDT and the events leading to the ban see: Robert L. Ackerly, "DDT: A Reevaluation, Part I," *Chemical Times and Trends* (October 1981): pp. 47–53; and "DDT: A Reevaluation, Part II," *Chemical Times and Trends* (January 1982): pp. 48–55; Norman Borlaug, "In Defence of DDT and Other Pesticides," *UNESCO Courier* (February 1972): pp. 4–12; George Claus and Karen Bolander, *Ecological Sanity* (New York: David McKay, 1977); Thomas R. Dunlap, *DDT: Scientists, Citizens, and Public Policy* (Princeton, N.J.: Princeton University Press, 1981); Thomas H. Jukes, "Insecticides in Health, Agriculture, and the Environment," *Naturwissenschaften* 66 (1974): pp. 6–16.

kill lice.[34] Dr. Paul Muller, a Swiss chemist, patented it as a contact insecticide in 1939 and was awarded the Nobel Prize in medicine in 1948 for his success in replacing (with DDT) a number of extremely dangerous chemicals then being used for pest control, including arsenic, mercury, fluorine, and lead, which were not only persistent in the environment, but also extremely poisonous and cumulative in the bodies of both animals and humans.

Until the 1940s, some two hundred million people worldwide were stricken annually with malaria, with an average of two million deaths per year. Two-thirds of the world's population lived in malaria-ridden areas.[35]

By 1946 it was recognized that DDT was one of the most important disease-preventing agents known to man, claiming its initial success in the field of public health by drastically reducing the cases and deaths from malaria. The events that occurred in Ceylon (now Sri Lanka) provide a good example of the positive impact of DDT on human health, and the devastation that occurred when it was, for highly questionable reasons, withdrawn. As is evident from the statistics below, both the impact of the spraying and the impact of the withdrawal of the spraying were enormous.

As Claus and Bolander commented, "DDT has had a tremendous impact on the health of the world . . . few drugs can claim to have done so much for mankind in so short a period of time as DDT did."[36]

Malaria cases reported in Ceylon	Year	Comment
2,800,000	1948	No DDT
31	1962	Large-scale DDT program
17	1963	Large-scale DDT program
150	1964	Spraying stopped
308	1965	
499	1966	
3,466	1967	
16,493	1968	(Jan. only)
42,161	1968	(Feb. only)
1,000,000	1968	
2,500,000	1969	

Why was there an increase in malaria in Ceylon after 1964? It is clear that the effect of *Silent Spring* was not limited to the United States. Following the publication of this book, the use of DDT was discontinued in Ceylon. Epidemic conditions reappeared and it has been estimated that between 1968 and 1969 "considerably more than two million cases occurred," all related to the campaign against DDT.[37]

DDT began its life of use as a public insecticide during World War II. It was an essential part of this country's military strategy, with the chemical employed in the fight against two devastating insect-borne diseases; malaria and typhus. General worldwide use began after 1945. At first the emphasis was on the medical benefits of the insecticide, especially its unprecedented efficiency in fighting malaria, but eventually its uses were expanded to control yellow fever, sleeping sickness, plague, typhus, and encephalitis, all of which are transmitted by insects. The low cost and effectiveness of DDT led to its later use in pest control for agriculture and forestry. DDT soon became vital in increasing worldwide production of food and fiber. In many cases, the use of DDT greatly increased crop yields, as in the case of rice production in the Philippines, Thailand, and Venezuela. In this country DDT was used, among other places, in the southern states to combat the insect destroyers of cotton, peanuts, and soybeans. DDT was also found to be an effective agent against the spruce budworm, pineweevil, tussock moth, and gypsy moth, all of which can devastate woodlands.

It is no surprise that Claus and Bolander write glowingly of the disease-prevention qualities of DDT: "With the introduction of DDT to control the vectors of disease, it seemed for the first time in human history, that man could look forward to a life of dignity, free from the scourges of maiming disease and famine. It is no wonder, then, that its applications were greeted with general high enthusiasm."[38]

THE UNIQUE BENEFITS OF DDT

Since DDT was not the only insecticide available by the early 1950s, one might wonder why it continued to dominate the scene, especially for use in public health programs. There were three reasons why DDT remained the preferred insecticide for many uses. First was its extraordinarily low cost. In 1968 one pound of DDT cost 17.5 cents. Since, for many purposes, the recommended application level of DDT was one pound per acre, enormous areas of land could be treated at a minimal expense. At the height of the DDT controversy it was generally acknowledged, even by opponents of DDT, that no available alternative could be obtained as cheaply.

Second, the overwhelming success of DDT was, ironically, ascribed to the very property that was to become ammunition for those who sought to ban its use in the late 1960s, namely, the exceptional stability and persistence of DDT in areas sprayed. Because DDT remained active on trees or crops long after application, there was no need for frequent respraying.*

---

*DDT has been shown to remain active for a period on the order of one to two weeks. Even though DDT persists longer than two weeks in the soil, it loses its toxicity to pests often

Although this made DDT efficient for both forestry and agriculture, it was in the area of malaria eradication that the persistence of the insecticide was most vital. In many cases, the homes to be sprayed were in rural areas and difficult to reach, and the need for constant respraying would have crippled antimalaria programs. The long-term indoor residual effect of DDT made it possible for three to six months to elapse between spraying of dwellings. Without the advent of DDT or some other equally effective and persistent insecticide, large scale malaria eradication programs may have never been attempted.

As it stands now, DDT has been credited with saving a hundred million lives from insect-borne diseases. In addition to Ceylon, DDT has been found incredibly effective in reducing the incidence of malaria in India. Ten years of insecticide use there reduced the annual malaria death rate from 750,000 to a mere 1,500.

Third, DDT combined high toxicity for insects with low toxicity for other organisms, including man, a fact that may well seem amazing in light of the infamous reputation that this chemical was ultimately to earn. Thousands of individuals, military and civilian, had their clothing and skin dusted with 10 percent DDT powder without ill effect. More pertinent to the safety issue was the absence of any DDT-related fatality or chronic disease among individuals employed as DDT sprayers in antimalaria programs, a group estimated at one time to consist of 130,000 men annually. Nor was any toxic effect noted in the 600 million to one billion people who lived in repeatedly sprayed dwellings. Poisoning with DDT was a rarity, and the only documented instances were the result of massive accidental (and sometimes suicidal) ingestion. Actually, in these cases it was probably the kerosene solvent rather than the DDT that caused the acute toxicity.

It is clear that the *British Medical Journal* was not overstating the case when it noted that DDT was a "miracle" chemical that "has been incontrovertibly shown to prevent human illness on a scale hitherto achieved by no other public health measure entailing the use of a chemical."[39]

DDT was also essential for the protection of fiber-producing plants, such as cotton, from the boll weevil and other devastating pests. Nobel Prize winner Borlaug emphasized in a speech before the U.N. Food and Agricultural Organ-

---

after a few days and usually within two weeks. A paper by R. G. Nash and E. A. Woolson— "Persistence of Chlorinated Hydrocarbon Insecticides in Soils," *Science* 25 (August 1967): pp. 924–27—is the basis of claims that it takes DDT seventeen years to lose 39 percent of its activity in soil (Nash and Woolson reported 39 percent of original application remaining). The experiment was performed on a small plot of soil to which DDT was applied at a concentration equaling forty pounds per acre. At this level, soil microorganisms, which usually break down DDT at one to five pounds per acre, were killed. The plot was kept dry, in the dark, and was kept free of all vegetation. The authors did a good job in their experimentation but the results should not be taken as indicative of the nature of DDT in the environment.

ization in 1970, "I have seen attempts to grow cotton without the use of insecticides in the native home of the boll weevil in Mexico, where all the native predators of this insect were present. The results were disastrous. . . . It was difficult to tell from casual observation whether the cotton was being grown for the production of fiber to clothe man or for the production of feed for a native insect."[40]

The gypsy moth has been a major nuisance in Europe for centuries and in the United States for more than a hundred years. The moth's larvae devastate trees by defoliation. Because of a well-planned program of spraying, however, the moth was virtually eliminated in the United States by the late 1950s. When spraying was stopped, the insect rapidly reoccupied most of the Northeast.[41]

Although the Entomological Society of America reported in 1962 that only 0.28 percent of the 640 million acres of U.S. timberland were treated with DDT (613 million acres were never treated),[42] the spread of foliage-destroying pests specifically harmful to timber-producing trees was effectively held under control. One pest still not under control is the bark beetle, which destroys a large proportion of forest trees in the West—probably twenty times more than the amount destroyed by fire.

THE LIMITATIONS OF THE "MIRACLE INSECTICIDE"

Despite this generally clean bill of health, DDT use was not completely problem-free. For one thing, certain insect strains began to develop resistance to DDT. By 1969 insect resistance to DDT had necessitated the use of alternative insecticides in 1 percent of the areas where DDT had originally been used for disease eradication. Of course, it should be remembered that the problem of resistance was not peculiar to DDT and has been shown to occur with repeated use of most other chemical pesticides (as well as nonchemical insecticides).[43] The occurrence of resistance in some insect species, though disturbing, cannot be considered a rationale for banning a chemical, just as few would suggest discontinuing the general use of penicillin because of the emergence of several penicillin-resistant strains of bacteria.

The greatest problem associated with DDT, however, was that, in a few instances, enthusiastic use became enthusiastic overuse, primarily in the area of agriculture. Pesticide dealers sometimes encouraged the oversale of DDT because of the obvious financial benefits to themselves. However, they received much greater benefits from selling insecticides such as malathion, Sevin, chlordane, pyrethroids, etc. The actual increase in financial benefits was ten to two hundred times more than the dealers could get from DDT sales. According to a 1963 *Reader's Digest* article, "Half of the deaths were not due to improper use at all, but were accidents in which children got hold of the toxic material. The other deaths have been traceable to careless handling and application of some pesticides, failure to heed the warning on the label."[44] In addition, concentrated pesticides found their way into lakes and streams because of accidents and/or carelessness.

On one occasion, extremely high amounts of DDT were reported in the waters off Los Angeles. The source was traced to a major pesticide manufacturer who was supposedly allowing DDT to enter that city's sewer system.[45] This was later refuted, however, by the Los Angeles Sanitary District and many scientists. Later analyses demonstrated relatively small quantities of DDT (a few pounds per day). The one day on which more DDT was "found" happened to be the first day the district began using its new gas-liquid chromatograph machine. (This technique, usually termed GLC, is a sensitive method employed by analytical chemists to detect and identify trace amounts of chemicals in various mixtures.) The measurement performed via the GLC found over four hundred pounds of DDT per day in a sewer line far from any possible source. The sanitary district later admitted, however, that that day's analyses were faulty. Nonetheless, uncorrected accounts of this incident still appear in environmentalist literature.

Although DDT opponents claimed the pesticide was killing fish, the facts clearly refute this. Reports of major fish kills are compiled annually by the Federal Water Pollution Control Administration. In 1967, a peak year for fish kills, only 3 percent of these could be traced to all pesticides. And as Claus and Bolander mention in *Ecological Sanity,* "even this small percentage originated either from applications contrary to labeling instructions or from usage which has subsequently been suspended—that is, direct spraying of waters with chemicals inappropriate for this purpose."[46] Although DDT was not specifically involved in many of these mishaps, its reputation with the public suffered from guilt by association.

Proper and responsible application and disposal of DDT were the rule rather than the exception. Even the increased applications of DDT to cropland, considered damning evidence by those opposed to the pesticide, were sometimes a legitimate, and accepted, response to the development of insect resistance. However, the incidents of carelessness and misuse, real and exaggerated, but both luridly portrayed, inevitably provided ammunition for individuals opposed to DDT use.

THE REJECTION OF A MIRACLE

DDT was banned from most uses in the United States in 1972. This action, however, wasn't the first in which people showed concern about the pesticide's safety. People started wondering about the safety of DDT when it was first used extensively as a delousing agent by the Allied forces in World War II. But mostly, before the publication of *Silent Spring* in 1962, discussions about the safety and effectiveness of DDT as an insecticide had continued in quiet scientific circles, among entomologists, toxicologists and biologists. The publication of *Silent Spring,* however, sparked the public debate. Within months, the lay public was interested in a topic it had never before dared to touch. The popular press had a heyday. The Environmental Defense Fund (EDF) was born, court actions abounded, and the press assumed an enlarged role. In the 1960s, this was a volatile combination of events.

It was not real, but only perceived pesticide abuses that gave credence to *Silent Spring's* arguments. This perceived threat also set the pace for the crusade to ban DDT, led primarily by the fledgling EDF. Ironically, as mentioned earlier, DDT was not the main focus of the Carson book. *Silent Spring* is hard on DDT, generally inaccurately so, but it is even more critical of other pesticides, which, it states, make DDT "seem by comparison almost harmless." Nevertheless, although Carson never specifically advocates a ban on DDT or any other pesticide, those using her book as a means to reach their environmental goals focused specifically and intensively on DDT. (Rachael Carson herself did not take part in this anti-DDT campaign; she died in 1964 at the age of fifty-six.)

The environmentalists' attack on DDT was based on three main erroneous arguments. First, DDT was causing a huge diminution, and perhaps extinction, of bird populations. Second, DDT was so stable that it could never be eliminated from the environment; further, it was hazardous to ecologic balance. And third, DDT might cause human disease, including cancer. Again, these three arguments were not at the core of the Carson book; but those who jumped off the "silent springboard" into the waters of litigation that soon swirled around the miracle insecticide depended heavily on them. Each needs a brief response.

1. *Did DDT harm the bird population?* This anti-DDT argument actually had two elements to it: one that the insecticide threatened birds directly, and the other that DDT interfered with their reproduction by causing them to lay eggs with thin shells. According to the environmentalist literature, these shells would eventually become so fragile that the eggs would break, causing dismal failures in reproduction. Both of these related charges were either unfounded or greatly exaggerated. Carson also claimed that large earthworms could transfer lethal doses of DDT to robins.[47] This claim, however, could not be proved by a leading researcher who was unable to kill captive robins by feeding them DDT-laced worms, neither were baby robins harmed by receiving only DDT-tainted worms.

There *were* unfortunate accidents and improper uses of DDT, such as when larger than necessary amounts of DDT were used.[48] In New Brunswick, Canada, in 1954, stream insects were killed after a forest spraying above the Miramichi River. Without a food source, the resulting salmon deaths were predictable. A spraying of nine hundred thousand acres in Montana in 1956 caused numerous trout deaths, presumably because of the loss of food organisms. Rachael Carson charged that in 1961, preventable discharges of DDT into the Colorado River caused fish deaths up to two hundred miles downstream.* Most of these wildlife deaths could have been prevented by responsible, well-directed spraying programs that were sensitive to the essentials of wildlife habitat. For example, when 430,000 acres of forest in Washington, Oregon, and Idaho were sprayed with DDT in 1974, no fish kills resulted. A well-planned program paid off.

Rachel Carson widely publicized these rare, isolated events, failing to mention that these wildlife kills were the result of poorly planned spraying programs. She went so far as to say that all uses of DDT were threatening robin and eagle populations, placing them on the verge of extinction.[49]

The facts, however, clearly refute that charge. The annual Christmas bird counts of the Audubon Society indicate that between 1941 and 1961, the heaviest years of DDT usage, there was a noticeable increase in most bird populations. These counts detailed 12 times more robins, 21 times more cowbirds, 8 times more blackbirds, and 131 times more grackles. Gulls in this time period became so abundant on the East Coast that the National Audubon Society sought and obtained permission to poison thirty thousand of them on Tern Island, Massachusetts, in 1971. The bird that Carson and other environmentalists warned was doomed, the robin, became the most abundant bird in North America during the DDT years.[50]

Since 1934, data on fifteen species of raptors have been compiled at the Hawk Mountain Sanctuary in Pennsylvania. Raptor birds are high in the food chain and should therefore be expected to rank high among other birds in DDT levels. Two of the species that the environmentalists said were in the most trouble, the osprey and the peregrine falcon, showed static populations.[51]

Whereas the peregrine fluctuated in number from a low count of 14 in 1965 to a high of 32 in 1969, the osprey actually increased in number in the Hawk Mountain Survey, from a total of 191 in 1946 to 600 in the year 1970. The total number of hawks counted increased from 9,291 in 1967 to 13,616 in 1956, to 14,818 in 1961, to 20,196 in 1967.[52] Part of this increase probably traces to better counting methods and more counters, but the survey represents the best data that we have in the area of raptor counts.

Interestingly, the research of Dr. Joseph Hickey, an authority on the peregrine falcon and a key witness for the EDF and the EPA in the DDT hearings, revealed that the peregrine population had been declining since 1890, fifty years or more before the introduction of DDT into widespread use in the United States.[53]

---

*This is extremely difficult to believe based on the fact that any amount of DDT spilled into the Colorado River would undergo such extensive dilution that the effects, if any, would be minimal.

Claims that DDT prevents the eggs of various birds from hatching and reduces reproduction rates are at best controversial. According to Dr. Thomas Jukes, thinning eggshells can have many causes, including diets low in calcium or vitamin D, fright (which may cause premature extrusion of eggs), various physiological disturbances in birds, high nocturnal ambient temperatures, toxic substances or drugs such as sulfanilamide, and certain infectious diseases, especially Newcastle disease. If indeed eggshell thinning did occur as a result of DDT spraying, it was probably confined to small geographic areas. It has always been unclear if this problem really did exist, and, if it did, whether it was because of DDT, mercury, PCBs, or actually the effects of human encroachment.

Nobel laureate Dr. Norman Borlaug succinctly summarizes the issue:

> One does not need a thin eggshell hypothesis due to DDT to explain the reduction in the population of these species. The truth of the matter is that many ornithologists have reported on the reduction in populations of these large birds of prey as far back as the 1880s, long before the time of DDT. It is almost a foregone conclusion for anyone who uses some common sense, that one or more of these species is about to flunk the imperative "evolve or perish." Their habitats are being destroyed by the encroachment of man.[54]

There is general agreement that the case of DDT causing thinning bird eggshells was greatly overplayed. In a 1981 article, "Evaluation of DDT," the editors of the *Journal of the American Medical Association* stated: "Although DDT had an effect on the thickness of eggshells, it has not yet been proven whether this is the effect of pure or crude DDT alone, or DDT in combination with something else, perhaps another pesticide. The eggshells of many bird species apparently have not been affected.[55]

2. *Was the persistence of DDT in our bodies and environment a cause for alarm?* Indeed DDT *is* stored in human fat tissue, as are many naturally occurring and man-made fat-soluble chemicals, such as other pesticides and vitamin A.

The American Medical Association reported in 1970, "Extensive studies by several investigators have shown that a small concentration of DDT and its metabolites is present in the fatty tissues of many people in all walks of life. However, there has been no significant increase in storage of DDT by the general population in the United States since it was first measured in 1950." The study went on to say that even pesticide handlers, who have been found to have up to fifty times the average amount of DDT in their fat tissue, have exhibited "no interference with their health despite long continued exposure. Injuries to humans have been observed only in persons who accidentally received acute massive doses."[56]

In one study DDT was fed to human volunteers in a federal prison by a Public Health Service scientist, Wayland J. Hayes, M.D., Ph.D. At levels of intake up to 35 mg per day, there was no noticeable effect on the subjects. This is in contrast to the average daily intake of 0.065 mg among the general population in the United States in 1968. In a second study conducted by Dr. Hayes, the same doses of DDT were administered over a period of twenty-one months. Observations for an additional twenty-seven months failed to reveal any ill health effects.[57]

In humans, most scientists stress a steady-state concept with regard to bioaccumulation of DDT in the body. This means that as a person gets older, more DDT accumulates in the fat tissues and blood serum, but after a certain equilibrium is reached, excretion of DDT metabolites eventually matches DDT uptake. On the other hand, a study of a community with exceptional exposure to DDT (Triana, Alabama) reports different findings when looking at blood serum levels of DDT.

The report about residents of Triana that appeared in the *Journal of the American Medical Association* contended that blood serum levels of DDT continue to rise with age without reaching a steady-state level. However, the authors emphasize that "no acute health effects were demonstrated" by this accumulation, although the study did not specifically address long-term effects.[58]

According to Maddox, "Human fat tends to contain between ten and twelve parts per million of DDT, which is another way of saying that each pound of fat will contain one-fifth of a thousandth of an ounce of DDT." No harm whatsoever has ever been shown to be related to those traces of DDT in human fat.

Similarly, it has been known for years that DDT is present, in trace amounts, in breast milk, again because of its solubility in fat. If animal experiments and human history can be used as a guideline, the traces of DDT present in human breast milk are harmless to infants. No harm has been detected in infants exposed to DDT in countries where the insides of houses are sprayed to control malaria and the levels of DDT in those mothers were significantly higher than those in the United States.[60]

And, yes, DDT traces can be found in our environment. DDT is decomposed by ultraviolet light in the air. Because over 93 percent of DDT (and metabolites) is broken down in sea water in thirty-eight days, it is not surprising that less than one part per trillion DDT was found in coastal seawater in the heyday of DDT use.

As to the bioaccumulation of DDT in fish, J. Gordon Edwards successfully argued in *Agrichemical Age* in 1980 that it is a myth that DDT is passed up the food chain, accumulating in greater and greater amounts the higher up the food chain the animal is. Edwards cited an experiment with fish that showed that "more than 80 percent of the DDT had been acquired through the gills rather than being extracted from the food."[61]

3. *Was DDT a cause of human disease? Specifically, is it a cancer-causing agent?* The International Agency for Research on Cancer (IARC), a group commissioned by the United Nations, has concluded that DDT is an animal carcinogen, but extensive research has never shown it to be a human carcinogen.

Studies beginning in the 1940s reported liver abnormalities in laboratory rodents fed DDT. In a 1969 study, Tarjan and Kemeny[62] reported a higher incidence of leukemia and malignant tumors in experimental mice fed DDT. This experiment was later found to be flawed. For example, even though the mice were supposed to be a leukemia-free strain, the disease was found in the control group as well as in the treated group. Tumors were also reported in the breeding stock and the controls. There were other experimental problems. A study undertaken by the World Health Organization suggested that the feed used in the Tarjan and Kemeny work was contaminated with aflatoxins, one of the most potent natural carcinogens.[63]

Also in 1969, the so-called Innes or Bionetics Report purported to show that DDT caused cancer in laboratory mice. This report, much cited by anti-DDT advocates, found that liver "tumors" appeared when neonatal mice were incubated at the maximum tolerated dose rates (that is, close to lethal). The dosages correspond to intake approximately one hundred thousand times higher than the average daily intake of pesticide residues in food for humans! Even after these tremendous dosages the Innes Report never specifically stated that the mice developed "cancer"—the report mentioned only tumors. It appears that the authors did not describe these tumors in detail, that they did not distinguish between malignant and benign tumors, and that there were serious flaws in experimental design.[64]

In stark contrast, the National Cancer Institute announced on October 9, 1978, that a two-year test failed to show that DDT caused cancer in laboratory animals.[65]

There is no evidence from human studies that DDT causes cancer. Indeed, the studies of humans heavily exposed to DDT give us assurance that the pesticide does *not* cause malignancies. Deaths traceable to liver cancer (the type expected based on animal data) in the United States have decreased about 30 percent from 1944, when DDT was introduced, to 1972, when use was discontinued.

Individuals who have been occupationally exposed to DDT at high levels have reported only transient effects, including tingling of the extremities. The World Health Organization reported that 130,000 spraymen in the malaria eradication campaign were exposed to high concentrations of DDT without observed symptoms, and that "there is at present no sound reason to believe that millions of people protected against vector-borne diseases are at tangible risk from their small exposure to DDT . . . the withdrawal of DDT would indeed be a major tragedy in the chapter of human health."[66]

As mentioned earlier, millions of people have had the interior walls of their homes sprayed year after year with DDT, sometimes for twenty years or more, all without known ill effects.* Indeed, DDT has been added to drinking water for control of yellow fever, and this type of ingestion also appears innocuous. According to the World Health Organization, "The only confirmed cases of injury have been the result of massive accidental or suicidal ingestion."[67]

Dr. John Higginson, former director of the International Agency for Research on Cancer, summed it up:

> We have had [human] exposure to DDT for approximately 20 to 25 years [without an increase in liver cancer]. We have no evidence at present that during the recent part of that 25 years there has been a significant trend or modification in cancer patterns that would suggest a reasonable association with the use of DDT in our present environment.[68]

These words are still true today, when the long-term cancer effects (due to a possible extended latency period) should be showing up.

The argument that many scientists and administrators were enthusiastic about the continued use of DDT, despite the suspicious health claims of those who followed Rachael Carson, is supported by the following quotes:

Dr. Philip Handler, president, National Academy of Sciences:

> DDT is the greatest chemical that has ever been discovered. The second generation of pesticides is a darn sight more dangerous than DDT, but because of the public outcry the government has needlessly banned DDT for most uses. . . . The predicted death or blinding by parathion, of dozens of Americans last summer must rest on the consciences of every car owner whose bumper sticker urged a total ban on DDT. (*Science,* 15 January 1971)

Dr. Wayland J. Hayes, Jr., chief of toxicology, U.S. Public Health Service:

> If we restrict DDT so as to interfere directly or indirectly with its availability and use in combating malaria, we must accept responsibility for the suffering and death of thousands of people. . . . [testimony, Washington State Hearings on DDT, October 1969]. The changes produced by DDT in the livers of rodents involved primarily the endoplasmic reticulum responsible for the formation of the microsomal enzymes of the liver; the changes are peculiar to rodents. The changes are essentially identical with those produced by the drug phenobarbital . . . and a number of other materials. (Letter to Washington State Department of Agriculture hearings officer, 11 October 1969)

---

*Spraying the interior walls of homes is the primary mode of malaria eradication because the disease-carrying mosquitoes attack sleeping humans at night, and during the day they rest on the walls.

Dr. Thomas H. Jukes, University of California, Berkeley:

> The issue of banning DDT is unquestionably a genocidal one. . . . The balance is overwhelmingly in favor of DDT. . . . I refer you to the monumental bibliography of 3,404 references on DDT compiled by the Division of Biology and Agriculture. (Letter to editor, *Science*)

Clifford M. Hardin, secretary of agriculture:

> DDT is an indispensable weapon in the arsenal of substances used to protect human health and has an amazing and exemplary record of safe use. . . . The total value of DDT to mankind is inestimable and is comprised of nutritional, economic, and social benefits. . . . Not one of five distinguished committees of professional scientists that have studied pesticides has recommended or intimated that DDT use should be summarily banned. These groups include the President's Science Advisory Committee, the Committee on Persistent Pesticides, Division of Biology and Agriculture of the National Academy of Sciences, the Secretary's Commission on Pesticides and Their Relationship to Environmental Health, the Council on Occupational Health, and the Council on Environmental and Public Health of the American Medical Association. (Brief to U.S. Court of Appeals in Washington, D.C., August 31, 1970)

Special report of the United Nations Food and Agriculture Organization:

> With no cheap substitutes available, these [developing] nations will suffer crippling agricultural setbacks if they hastily follow the example of the United States in curtailing the use of DDT. . . . The case against DDT has not been proved. On the contrary, the case for it, in controlling pests ranging from malaria-carrying mosquitoes to locusts to cotton worms, is well documented. . . . The United States in 1967 manufactured 120 million pounds of DDT, of which it exported two-thirds, using 40 million pounds at home . . . DDT costs 15 cents a pound and prices of substitutes range from twice to six times that much. The latter are often more toxic. Many developing countries simply could not afford to switch. (*New York Times*, November 29, 1969)

Dr. A. J. Lehman, director of pharmacology, U.S. Food and Drug Administration:

> DDT is not a carcinogen. ("Summaries of Pesticide Toxicity," 1965)

National Academy of Sciences:

> It is estimated that in little more than two decades, DDT has prevented 500 million deaths that would otherwise have been inevitable. (*Life Sciences*, 1971)

Dr. Jesse L. Steinfeld, surgeon general, U.S. Public Health Service:

> DDT has been instrumental in literally changing the course of history for many
> nations and continues to do so today. Its use . . . has meant the difference
> between hunger, despair, and poverty, and food, hope and the promise of a
> better life to billions of people throughout the world. . . . Few drugs can claim
> to have done so much for mankind in so short a period of time as can DDT.
> (Testimony before Environmental Protection Agency, 9 September 1971)

Dr. Donald A. Spencer (retired from U.S. Fish and Wildlife Service after thirty-
four years):

> Statements are common that the half-life of DDT is fifteen years or longer.
> . . . These are very irresponsible statements. . . . DDT is metabolized to less
> toxic and finally to harmless compounds. In most cultivated croplands in
> the southern part of the U.S. the half-life of DDT is something less than
> one year. (1970 pamphlet, "An Ecologist Views the Environment")

Dr. Hardin B. Jones, professor of medical physics and physiology, University
of California, Berkeley:

> Of all the pesticides, DDT is the safest. At high levels it is destroyed rapidly
> by body tissues; at low levels it is metabolically inactive and harmless, simply
> dissolved in body fat. (*Los Angeles Herald Examiner,* 12 February 1970)

Dr. Lee A. DuBridge, President Nixon's chief scientific advisor:

> My view is that DDT is still an extremely useful agent for many kinds of
> insects and pests, crop killers, and disease bearing insects and so on. Banning
> it would have serious effects on human life, with the spread of disease and
> the destruction of crops. (*San Francisco Examiner,* January 11, 1970)

Nearing a Judgment on DDT

As is evident from the above quotes, by 1970 the overwhelming scientific evidence
was that DDT was both safe and effective, but yet the DDT ban crusade
was in full swing. The popularity of the anti-DDT movement led a 1970 *Nature*
editorial to quip, "In the last few months, resistance to insecticides has been
growing almost faster among people than among insects."[69] In 1969 Michigan
was the first state to ban the chemical, followed by Wisconsin, Arizona, and
California. In 1969 the Environmental Defense Fund, the Sierra Club, the
National Audubon Society, and a Michigan environmental group petitioned

Secretary of Agriculture Clifford Hardin to ban DDT, alleging it to be a carcinogen. The same year, a Commission on Pesticides and Their Relationship to Environmental Health, called the Mrak Commission, was appointed by the secretary of health, education, and welfare. On the basis of the recommendations of that commission, the agriculture secretary announced a plan for phasing out the use of DDT by December 31, 1970, with the exception of uses essential to protection of public health and welfare. Under this ban, the use of DDT in health-related mosquito-control programs and on certain crops such as cotton continued to be permitted.

The ban on DDT that was recommended by the Mrak Commission was based, as was stated in the commission's report, more on "suspicion of danger" than on proof. In exempting certain essential uses of DDT from the ban, the commission was careful to note that "the current evidence is not sufficient to justify unqualified banning of the insecticide."

The partial ban of DDT, extensive though it was, did not satisfy the environmental groups, which subsequently pressed the newly formed Environmental Protection Agency (EPA) to cancel the remaining registered uses of DDT. Such an action would have amounted to a total ban on the use and sale of DDT and effectively have eliminated DDT use worldwide.

It is worth noting that, though the incidents of pesticide overuse that motivated the anti-DDT crusade occurred solely in developed nations such as the United States, the real hardship of a total DDT ban would fall on the poor and underdeveloped Third World countries, where human existence is more fragile than thin pelican eggshells. The same economic considerations that made DDT so appealing and essential for use in developing nations tended to militate against the wasteful overuse of the chemical by those poorer countries, whether in agriculture or in mosquito-control campaigns. In fact, the use of DDT for malaria control entails almost no environmental contamination, as spraying is restricted to the inner surface of the dwellings. In pushing for a total DDT ban, the American environmental elitists were pursuing a course that would punish developing nations for the occasional pesticide excesses of the United States. Time and again, the World Health Organization stated that a total ban on DDT would mean the demise of programs against insect-borne disease in Third World nations, and the death of millions of people.

It was this push for a total ban that created the real controversy. In 1971 a hearing was scheduled so that each side could present its case. It is revealing that, although the EPA was meant to decide the question of the ban on the basis of the recommendations of the hearing examiner, the EPA ultimately participated in the hearings on the anti-DDT side, along with the Environmental Defense Fund and other conservation groups.

In April 1972 the hearing examiner, Edmund Sweeney, after reviewing ninety-three hundred pages of testimony and three hundred technical documents by some 150 "expert scientists over the course of seven months," recommended to the EPA that *no more extensive ban of DDT was necessary or desirable, based on the evidence presented at the hearings.* The highlights of Sweeney's findings are summarized in the following nine points, excerpted from his final decision.

1. DDT is extremely low in acute toxicity to man.
2. DDT is not a safety hazard to man when used as directed.
3. DDT can have a deleterious effect on freshwater fish and estuarine organisms when directly applied to the water.
4. DDT can have an adverse effect on beneficial animals.
5. DDT is concentrated in organisms and can be transferred through food chains.
6. DDT is not a carcinogenic hazard to man.
7. DDT is not a mutagenic or teratogenic hazard to man.
8. DDT uses under the registrations involved here do not have a deleterious effect on freshwater fish, estuarine organisms, wild birds, or other wildlife.
9. There is a present need for the continued use of DDT for the essential uses defined in this case.[70]

With that impressive clean-bill-of-health decision, one would assume that the environmentalists had lost their case and that DDT would have survived the well-organized pseudoscientific attack. But less than two months later, on June 14, 1972, the administrator of EPA, William Ruckelshaus, who had neither attended any of the hearings nor studied the transcripts generated by the hearings, *banned all of the remaining uses of DDT with the exception of uses related to essential public health purposes.* For some mystifying reasons Ruckelshaus pointed out the following conclusions in his overturn of Sweeney's findings:

1. DDT is lethal to many beneficial agricultural insects.
2. DDT can have lethal and sublethal effects on useful aquatic freshwater invertebrates.
3. DDT is toxic to fish.
4. DDT can effect the reproductive success of fish.
5. DDT can cause thinning of bird eggshells and thus impair reproductive success.
6. DDT is a potential human carcinogen.
7. Responsible scientists believe that tumor induction of mice is a valid warning of possible carcinogenic properties.
8. There are no adequate human epidemiological data on the carcinogenicity of DDT, nor is it likely that such can be obtained.
9. DDT presents a carcinogenic risk.[71]

Additionally, there was the following incredible summary in the administrator's opinion: "Viewing the evidence as a total picture, the preponderance of evidence supports the conclusion that DDT does cause eggshell thinning."[72]

It seems obvious here that in making his decision Ruckelshaus designated the wealth of scientific data as irrelevant. Ironically, in a speech before the National Academy of Sciences eleven years after he handed down the DDT decision, and after he had returned to Washington for another try at the helm of the then–well-established EPA, Ruckelshaus stressed that policy making at the EPA would be "based on scientific evidence and scientific consensus only." He said that science and the law are partners at the EPA, and that it is important to "insure that our laws reflect . . . scientific realities." EPA is an "instrument of public policy," he states, but the standards it sets, "whether technology or health-related, must have a sound scientific base."[73] Certainly, Ruckelshaus could not have justified the banning of DDT if he believed in this philosophy during his first stint as EPA administrator. After all, if he was so convinced of the benefits of sound science during the DDT debate we would still have the benefits of the use of that chemical today.

Why Ruckelshaus ignored Sweeney's recommendations is not clear, but his action may have stemmed from a desire to establish the authority of the infant EPA through some muscle flexing. Ruckelshaus's motive was especially perplexing to those who remembered his stated position on DDT two years before:

> DDT is not endangering the public health and has an amazing and exemplary record of safe use. DDT, when properly used at recommended concentrations, does not cause a toxic response in man or other mammals and is not harmful. The carcinogenic claims regarding DDT are unproved speculation.

By making an example of DDT, Ruckelshaus may have hoped to give warning to various environmental bad boys that the new agency meant business, while simultaneously garnering brownie points from environmentalists. Indeed, Ruckelshaus and his associates for years denied that the decision to ban DDT was based on something other than science, but finally in a letter to Allan Grant, president of the American Farm Bureau Federation, Ruckelshaus admitted:

> Decisions by the government involving the use of toxic substances are political with a small "p" . . . science, along with other disciplines such as economics, has a role to play. *The ultimate judgment remains political* [emphasis added]. In the case of pesticides in our country, the power to make this judgment has been delegated to the administrator of EPA.

This politicization of Ruckelshaus became even more apparent when, having left the EPA, he agreed to sign membership solicitation letters for the Environmental Defense Fund.[74]

Regardless of the intent of the move, it set a precedent for subsequent capricious actions of the EPA.

The Aftermath

In the 1990s the DDT controversy and the furor that surrounded the call for a ban have been largely forgotten: the majority of Americans are vaguely convinced that DDT was the ultimate in dangerous pesticides and unaware of the millions of lives the chemical saved. DDT may seem an irrelevant issue today, but in considering the environmental hysteria nowadays, it is critical to keep an eye on this first victory of the environmental alarmists.

In retrospect, what we had with the banning of DDT was the elimination of a lifesaving chemical through the application of politics, emotion, and pseudoscience.* Of course, other pesticides were available at the time of the ban and were even relatively affordable. But the negative fallout of the DDT ban remains. On one level we saw misconceptions about the alleged hazards of DDT that were effectively exported to the Third World countries, discouraging use of this essential chemical. But beyond that, the DDT conflict set a pattern for environmental decisions based less on science than on histrionics, mudslinging, hyperbole, and dishonest science. The rigid dichotomizing issues and the enshrinement of The Cause are now honored traditions, stemming from the format of that prototypic contest, the DDT debate. In that sense, we are still paying in the 1990s for the 1970 ban on DDT.

NOTES

1. John Maddox, *The Doomsday Syndrome* (New York: McGraw Hill, 1972), p. 120.
2. Ibid., p. 121.
3. Samuel P. Hays, *Conservation and the Gospel of Efficiency: The Progressive Conservation Movement 1890–1920* (Cambridge: Harvard University Press, 1959), p. 123.
4. Merril Eisenbud, *Environment, Technology, and Health* (New York: New York University Press, 1978), p. 3.

---

*The "cause" of defending saccharin, in 1977, for example, against the pseudoscience allegations of the environmentalists pales by comparison with DDT's significance to the economy and human need.

5. Loren Eiseley, "Using a Plague to Fight a Plague," *Saturday Review,* September 29, 1962, pp. 18–19.

6. Eisenbud, *Environment, Technology, and Health,* p. 54.

7. Ibid., p. 55.

8. Ground Zero, *Nuclear War: What's in It for You?* (New York: Pocket Books, 1982), p. 177.

9. Maddox, *Doomsday Syndrome,* p. 12.

10. Ibid., p. 13.

11. Ibid., p. 14.

12. Jonathan Greene, *Morrow's International Dictionary of Contemporary Quotations* (New York: Morrow, 1982), p. 226.

13. Susan Sontag, *Styles of Radical Will* (New York: Farrar, Straus, & Giroux, 1969).

14. Eisenbud, *Environment, Technology, and Health,* p. 56.

15. Maddox, *Doomsday Syndrome,* p. 13.

16. George Claus and Karen Bolander, *Ecological Sanity* (New York: David McKay, 1977), pp. 7, 29.

17. Ibid., p. 7.

18. Frank Graham, Jr., *Since Silent Spring* (Boston: Houghton Mifflin, 1970), p. 17.

19. Claus and Bolander, *Ecological Sanity,* p. 7.

20. Private communication, Claudia C. Regan, assistant communications director, Houghton Mifflin, July 12, 1983.

21. J. Gordon Edwards, "Pesticides and People" (undated, unpublished manuscript).

22. Rachael Carson, *Silent Spring* (New York: Fawcett Crest, 1962), p. 157.

23. Eiseley, "Using a Plague," p. 18.

24. Ibid., p. 34.

25. James Rorty, "Varieties of Poison," *Commonweal,* December 14, 1962, p. 321.

26. Ibid.

27. "Pesticides: The Price for Progress," *Time,* September 28, 1962, p. 45.

28. "Hiss of Doom," *Newsweek,* August 6, 1962, p. 55.

29. I. L. Baldwin, "Chemicals and Pests," *Science* (September 28, 1962):p. 1043.

30. Norman Borlaug, "In Defence of DDT and Other Pesticides," *UNESCO Courier* (February 1972).

31. J. Gordon Edwards, San Jose State University, Remarks before International Meeting on Pesticides, Pakistan, August 1980.

32. "DDT in the Environment" (editorial), *British Medical Journal* (November 22, 1969).

33. H. Kelly, "The DDT Debate: The Beginning of the Big Ban Era," *ACSH News & Views* (May/June 1981).

34. Thomas H. Jukes, "Insecticides in Health, Agriculture, and the Environment," *Naturwissenschaften* 66 (1974): p. 6.

35. Claus and Bolander, *Ecological Sanity,* pp. 289–91.

36. Ibid., p. 294.

37. M. J. Grayson and T. R. Shepard, Jr., *The Disaster Lobby, Prophets of*

Ecological Doom and Other Absurdities (Chicago: Follett, 1973), p. 1.

38. Clause and Bolander, *Ecological Sanity,* p. 929.

39. "DDT in the Environment."

40. Borlaug, "In Defence of DDT," p. 10.

41. J. G. Edwards, R. A. Fusco, and C. F. Nishimatsu, "Gypsy Moth Larva Host Plant Screening and Reproduction Studies" (undated, unpublished manuscript), p. 1.

42. "Pesticides: The Price for Progress," p. 46.

43. Pimentel et al., "Environmental Risks Associated with the Use of Biological and Cultural Pest Controls," mimeograph (supported by NS, Grant PRA80-00803).

44. John Strohm and Cliff Ganschow, "The Great Pesticide Controversy," *Reader's Digest,* October 1953, p. 125.

45. "A Brown Study of the Brown Pelican," *Natural History* (January 1982): p. 40.

46. Claus and Bolander, *Ecological Sanity,* p. 308.

47. Carson, *Silent Spring,* p. 100.

48. J. J. Hickey, "Initial Songbird Mortality Following Dutch Elm Disease Control Program," *Journal of Wildlife Management,* no. 3 (1960): p. 265.

49. Carson, *Silent Spring,* p. 110.

50. R. T. Peterson, *The Birds* (New York: Life Nature Library, 1963).

51. Robert L. Ackerly, "DDT: A Re-evaluation, Part I," *Chemical Times and Trends* (October 1981): p. 52.

52. *Hawk Mountain Sanctuary Newsletter* (May 1977).

53. Robert L. Ackerly, "DDT: A Re-evaluation, Part II," *Chemical Times and Trends* (January 1982): p. 49.

54. Borlaug, "In Defence of DDT," p. 8.

55. "Evaluation of DDT," *Journal of American Medical Association (JAMA)* (May 11, 1970): p. 1056.

56. Ibid., p. 1055.

57. W. Hayes, Jr., *Annals of the New York Academy of Science* 160 (1969): pp. 40–54.

58. K. Kress et al., "Cross-section Study of a Community With Exceptional Exposure to DDT," *JAMA* (May 15, 1981).

59. Maddox, *Doomsday Syndrome,* p. 128.

60. Thomas H. Jukes, "DDT," *JAMA* (July 29, 1974): p. 572.

61. J. G. Edwards, "The Myth of Food Chain Biomagnification," *Agrichemical Age* (April 1980): p. 10.

62. R. Tarjan and T. Kemeny, "Multigeneration Studies on DDT in Mice," *Food, Cosmetics, and Toxicology* 7 (1969): pp. 214–22.

63. Claus and Bolander, *Ecological Sanity,* p. 336.

64. Ibid., pp. 346–51.

65. Thomas Jukes, "DDT and Cancer," *Clinical Toxicology* 14, no. 4 (1979): p. 461.

66. "The Place of DDT in Operations Against Malaria and Other Vector-Borne Disease," *Official Records, WHO,* no. 190 (Geneva, April 1971): pp. 176–82.

67. Ibid., p. 176.

68. J. Higginson, in *Record of EPA Hearings on DDT,* Washington, D.C., 1972, p. 1457.

69. *Nature* 226 (1970): p. 585.

70. Ackerly, "DDT, Part II," p. 51.

71. Ibid., p. 55.

72. Claus and Bolander, *Ecological Sanity,* p. 537.

73. American Council on Science and Health, "EPA Administrator Speaks on Science," *ACSH News and Views* (September/October 1983): p. 12.

74. Edwards, "Pesticides and People."

3

The "Disaster" of Love Canal

The Charges

The story of Love Canal has been etched into modern history as few other events have. It has set the pace. It is the centerpiece of hazardous waste debate.
— *Hazardous Waste in America*, p. 89

What lay beneath the surface was 43.6 million pounds of 82 different chemical substances: oil, solvents and other manufacturing residues. The mixture included benzene, a chemical known to cause leukemia and anemia; chloroform, a carcinogen that effects the nervous, respiratory and gastrointestinal systems; lindane, which causes convulsions and extra production of white blood cells; trichloroethylene, a carcinogen that also attacks the nervous system, the genes and liver. . . . The list of chemicals buried in the Love Canal seems endless, and the accompanying list of their acute and chronic effects on human beings reads like an encyclopedia of medical illness and abnormality. . . .

Love Canal doesn't end with this generation's cancer or even with the next generation's birth defects. For many residents, the damage is permanent in their genes and their children's. The mutated genes will affect all of their descendants, one generation after another.
— *Who's Poisoning America*, pp. 270, 305

The best known, certainly the most infamous, of the nation's toxic dump sites is the Love Canal area of Niagara Falls, New York. There the Olin Corporation and Hooker Chemical Corporation buried over 200,000 tons of toxic chemicals, many of which are known to cause cancer, birth defects and other disorders.

After residents of the area began to experience an unusually high number of miscarriages, deformities in their newborns and incidents of blood disease, cancer, epilepsy, hyperactivity and other ailments, it became apparent that the community was unfit for human habitation.

—America the Poisoned, pp. 137–38

Chromosome damage found in Love Canal tests.

*—*Front-page headline, *New York Times,* 17 May 1980

Love Canal is a name which until recently was relegated to the back pages of history along with the unspent dreams of a visionary for whom it was named. . . . Instead, the center of attention is an ominous array of chemicals buried within the boundaries of the unfinished canal for more than twenty-five years—toxic ingredients which are infiltrating scores of nearby homes, posing a serious threat to human health and upsetting the domestic tranquility of hundreds of families. . . . Described as an environmental time bomb gone off, Love Canal stands as testimony to the ignorance, lack of vision and proper laws of decades past which allowed the indiscriminate disposal of such toxic materials.

—Love Canal: Public Health Time Bomb, p. 3

What may be needed just as much are sharp new incentives for industry not to pollute in the first place. Making corporate officials personally and legally responsible for chemical pollution could also do the job. No one from Hooker has gone to jail. . . . Beyond discussing the problem with the local school board, the company did nothing to warn local residents of the dangers.

—Progressive, May 1980, p. 31

I live in a heavily industrial area, and I wonder just how many years it will take off my life. . . .

It is not enough for industry and government to act in good faith— their mistakes are counted in human lives.

—Glamour, November 1980, p. 31

"Someday I'm going to have to sit down with my daughter and explain to her that her mother brought up two children in this area, and she may have suffered because of it," says Barbara Quimby, who apparently has chromosome damage. "My daughter will then have to explain it to the man she loves and decide whether having children is worth the risk."

—National Wildlife, August 1980, p. 35

Only wastes would continue to be handled in dubious and dangerous ways. . . . Slowly but inevitably, they would continue to work their way into the human body. . . .

Only when we acknowledge our folly and temper our greed will our society begin to conform to the needs of the nature outside and inside ourselves.

Only then will we be sure that what rises from the ground or what is in our air and rivers will be, as it ought, the source of life and good health—and not the agents of an untimely death.

—*Laying Waste*

In the neighborhood of Niagara Falls known as Love Canal, one of these time bombs recently exploded: poisonous chemicals in great concentrations began to leak into the basements of homes and to the surface of one back yard after another. The human anguish that was a consequence is worth a very close look. . . .

[It is] "an advance briefing" on America's future of "cancerous, toxic cesspools left by callous corporations."

—Ralph Nader, review of *Laying Waste*

Love Canal Recipe:
1. Mix 82 Chemicals
2. Place in Canal for 25 years.
Yield: sickness and death.

—Sign reprinted in *Niagara Gazette,* 7 August 1978

The Facts

- Although there was chemical leakage into the Love Canal community due to the disruption of the chemical-waste-deposit area, there is no conclusive case of human illness or death during the 1960s, 1970s, 1980s, or 1990s, related to exposure to the chemicals in Hooker's waste-disposal site.

- There is no evidence of increased rates of cancer, respiratory ailments, nervous disorders, liver damage, or any other human ailment among residents of the Love Canal region.

- There is no evidence that residents of the Love Canal area are experiencing or have experienced any higher rates of genetic damage, miscarriage, or birth defects than those of other populations in the United States.

- There is ample evidence that Hooker Chemical Company followed all of the state-of-the-art guidelines for chemical-waste disposal, and that the seepage of toxic chemicals which did occur was related to the failure of the city of Niagara Falls Board of Education to heed all warnings relative to the limited use of the Love Canal area.

Love Canal has become one of the key buzzwords of the alarmist environmental dialect.

The term instantly conjures up images of oozing, noxious chemicals, helpless families being terrorized by an army of toxins and carcinogens, high rates of disease, miscarriage, deformed children, and worse—all caused by the action of an uncaring, callous industry that violated all the rules of human decency and corporate responsibility by dumping its garbage with no regard whatsoever to the impact on human health and well-being.

The 1960s Tom Lehrer song about Wernher von Braun and his out-of-control missiles immediately comes to mind: "Once the rockets go up, who cares where they come down. That's not my department, said Wernher von Braun."

Love Canal is the centerpiece of the environmental cause, which argues that (a) the government should "protect" America's health and blames almost all suffering on corporations and the allegedly hazardous materials they dump "indiscriminately" on us poor, unsuspecting people, and (b) enormous numbers of federal (i.e., taxpayers') dollars should be spent to counteract the pollution through regulatory action.

Love Canal is also another type of centerpiece. It serves well as the focal point for an expose of the questionable, indeed, immoral and dishonest tactics of those individuals who term themselves "environmentalists" but who are in fact mostly a group of anticorporation, antitechnology advocates. Love Canal is a classic story of half truths, distorted historical facts, unprecedented media exaggeration, and misguided government intervention, all of which caused substantially more human upset and misery than did even the most toxic of Hooker's chemicals. In dealing with Love Canal, the environmentalists and their colleagues in the media and the government acted about as ethically as someone falsely crying fire in a crowded theater.

Love Canal is an all-too-typical story about how both local (in this case New York State) and federal taxpayers footed the bill for coping with a disaster that never existed. It is a painfully clear example of what happens when one mixes volatile solutions of half-baked scientific data, media hype, political opportunism, and an intense phobia about chemicals that disallows any form of rational evaluation and judgment, with an underlying philosophy that seems eager—nay, anxious—to find one simple solution to a complex problem by blaming a corporate giant. It is an episode that again brings us to that yet unanswered question: Who are these people who tell us of "time bombs," corporate irresponsibility, mass poisoning and deaths, when the scientific facts clearly point in the other direction? Why is the American press (with the notable exception of the editorial page of the *Wall Street Journal*) so willing to accept, uncritically, the bad news about health at Love Canal and everywhere else in America?

Background

The serenity of the origins of Love Canal stands in stark contrast to the turbulent and frenzied atmosphere there today.

In May 1892 an ambitious entrepreneur named William T. Love arrived in Niagara Falls intent on making his financial dream come true. He wanted to build a model city that would service a massive industrial complex, and he had a big advantage going for him: Thomas Edison had just mastered the use of electricity, and since the state of the art at that time allowed for transmission only by direct current, which was uneconomical at long distances, industries were under pressure to locate near sources of electrical generation. Love was committed to creating an immense source of water power by harnessing the energy from Niagara Falls. In January 1893 Love officially announced his plans for the creation of a new city that would house some six hundred thousand people. Love was clever in promoting his idea. Indeed, he extensively advertised his model city through circulars and brass bands playing his "original" ditty, sung to the tune of "Yankee Doodle":

> Everybody's come to town,
> Those left we all do pity;
> For we'll have a jolly time
> At Love's new model city.
>
> This tale I tell is no less true
> Though in a silly ditty,
> They give free sites and power too
>
> In Love's new model city.[1]

But even original ditties could not make Love's dream come true. Although work began on excavation for the canal in 1894, the country soon found itself in the grip of a major economic recession. To complicate Love's plans even further, Nikola Tesla in 1894 came up with a system of alternating power that allowed for transmission of electricity over long distances at reasonable cost. Tesla had thus eliminated from consideration the prime advantage Love was offering at his model city.

William Love eventually gave up, and although a few others attempted to pick up where he left off, the last of the property owned by his corporation was subjected to mortgage foreclosure and sold at public auction in 1910. The only souvenir he left was a partially dug section of canal in the southeast corner of the city of Niagara Falls. In the early 1900s this canal was used as a swimming hole for children.

In 1941 Hooker Electrochemical Company began to consider the possibility of using the unfinished canal as a means for legally disposing wastes from its Niagara Falls operation. After considerable study, company officials concluded that since the canal had been dug out of clay, they were certain that the chemical wastes would remain in place indefinitely. Indeed, the canal was an ideal place to put potentially hazardous industrial wastes.

In April 1942 the company completed legal transactions to begin dumping what ultimately amounted to some 21,800 tons of company waste into the canal. The dumping continued until 1953. At the same time other wastes were also being dumped into the canal. Federal agencies, especially the army, disposed of toxic chemical wastes there during and after World War II, because the clay lining of the canal provided such an ideal spot for storing chemical waste without fear of human exposure.[2]

Around 1950, the social and demographic climate of the Niagara Falls region changed in a way that dramatically modified the history of Love Canal. The postwar baby boom had precipitated a need for new housing and, particularly, more schools. As Eric Zuesse wrote in an in-depth *Reason* magazine article, "Every available open lot or suitable site was being eyed voraciously by the Board of Ed's Buildings and Grounds Committee for possible construction of new schools."[3] The canal site seemed ideal for the financially strapped school board, as land prices around the dump site were low. Although the negotiations took a number of years, what ultimately happened was that Hooker agreed to donate the property to the school board for the token price of $1, primarily because Hooker was under considerable pressure from the board to do so, knowing that if the company didn't willingly deed the land, it would be seized under eminent domain for the building of the public school.

Hooker deeded the property to the local board with the clear warning that it could be used for the school, parking, or a playground, *but that the land should not under any circumstances be excavated,* for fear of disturbing the clay lining and allowing the escape of chemical wastes. The *Wall Street Journal* noted in its May 22, 1979 history of the Love Canal that, as the "November 1957 school board minutes and the news accounts reveal, a lawyer for what was then the Hooker Electrochemical Company twice issued strong public warnings about potential health hazards at Love Canal."

Specifically, the minutes of the board's meeting on November 7, 1957 indicate that A. W. Chambers of Hooker was present, giving specific warnings about the potential dangers of chemicals escaping if disturbed. The board was considering developing parts of the canal area and Chambers was sent to discourage such activity.

> He [Chambers] reminded the board that, due to chemical waste having been dumped in that area, the land was not suitable for construction where under-

ground facilities would be necessary. He stated that his company [Hooker] could not prevent the board from selling the land or from doing anything they wanted to do with it, but, however, it was their intention that this property be used for a school and for parking. . . . He further stated that they feel the property should not be divided for the purpose of building homes and hope that no one will be injured.

How much clearer a warning could Hooker have made to the board of education?

Thus, as the *Wall Street Journal* concludes, "Contrary to the half truths and innuendos dealt in by professional corporate baiters, the story does not provide an object lesson in unbridled corporate callousness or villainy." The greed, the callous lust for profits, was entirely on the part of the school board.

The Love Canal deed itself, dated April 28, 1953, is quite revealing, in that it emphasized that it was turning over to the board of education and the city of Niagara Falls all legal responsibility:

> Prior to the delivery of this instrument of conveyance, the grantee herein has been advised by the grantor that the premises above described have been filled, in whole or in part, to the present grade level thereof with waste products resulting from the manufacturing of chemicals by the grantor at its plant in the City of Niagara Falls, New York, and the grantee assumes all risk and liability incident to the use thereof. It is therefore understood and agreed that, as a part of the consideration for this conveyance and as a condition thereof, no claim, suit, action or demand of any nature whatsoever shall ever be made by the grantee, its successors or assigns, against the grantor, its successors or assigns, for injury to a person or persons, including death resulting therefrom, or loss of or damage to property caused by, in connection with or by reason of the presence of said industrial wastes. It is further agreed as a condition hereof that each subsequent conveyance of the aforesaid lands shall be made subject to the foregoing provisions and conditions.[4]

Moreover, according to evidence uncovered by Eric Zuesse in his investigative reporting piece for *Reason,*

> Hooker had evidently been so concerned that the board knew what it was getting into taking over the canal that the company had not left to chance whether school board officials would physically inspect the property prior to acquiring it. Instead, Hooker had escorted them to the canal site and in their presence made eight test borings—into the protective clay cover that the company had laid over the canal, and into the surrounding areas. . . . So whether or not the school board was of a mind to inspect the canal, Hooker had gone out of its way to make sure that they *did* inspect it and that they did see that *chemicals* lay buried in that canal.[5]

But ignoring this advice, the board of education took no action to prevent future movements of topsoil and construction. The city of Niagara Falls began to construct sanitary and storm sewers at the site, ignoring also the reports in a 1957 issue of the *Niagara Gazette* that "there had been an unwritten understanding at the time of the gift that the board would not dispose of the land in any way that might lead to digging or construction work . . . there are dangerous chemicals buried there in drums, in loose form, in solids and liquids. It was understood that the land would be used for a park or some surface activity if it was developed."[6]

Construction of storm sewers, roads, and utilities proceeded in 1957 and 1958, disturbing the cover of the canal and causing some chemical wastes to become exposed. In June 1958, children playing in the area developed minor skin irritations after coming into contact with the exposed chemicals. Hooker Chemical again warned the board to cover the area to prevent further seepage of the chemicals. And again the warning went unheeded.

Thus, in retrospect, those who claim that Hooker Chemical negligently and irresponsibly contaminated the Niagara Falls area with its industrial wastes are simply misrepresenting the facts. It is clear that the seepage of the toxic chemicals was related to the board of education's failure to heed the multiple warnings given by Hooker concerning the limited use that should have been made of the canal area. But works of sensational journalism, including Michael Brown's *Laying Waste: The Poisoning of America by Toxic Chemicals* (which for some mystifying reason received three Pulitzer nominations and was praised in a review by Jessica Mitford: "This extraordinary and terrifying book is one of the best examples of tenacious, dedicated journalism I ever read"), ignore the role of the city of Niagara Falls and pin the blame for the "Love Canal Disaster" on "industry," in this case Hooker. In *Laying Waste* Brown writes: "At that time [1953] the company issued no detailed warnings about the chemicals; a brief paragraph in the quit-claim document disclaimed company liability for any injuries or deaths that might occur on the site."[7] Samuel Epstein writes in a similar vein: "The deed clause failed to explain that the Love Canal waste dump site contained many chemicals known at the time to be highly toxic."[8] And Lewis Regenstein in *America the Poisoned* sings the same refrain, complaining that "when Hooker . . . deeded the land to the Niagara Falls Board of Education in 1953 . . . the company made no real effort to warn the board about the toxic nature of the chemicals buried there."[9]

Apparently Brown, Regenstein, and others either did not read the deed at all, or had on alarmist-tainted, anti-industry-shaded glasses at the time of the reading. Beyond misrepresenting the warnings Hooker set forth before the $1 sale of its property, all these authors overlook the fact that after 1953 Hooker no longer had any legal control over the property.

Ironically, not only did Hooker appear to do about all it could to warn the city of potential dangers, it apparently was also not negligent in the manner in which it disposed of its chemicals in the first place. In 1980 William Sanjour, then chief of the Environmental Protection Agency's Hazardous Waste Implementation branch, told the *New York Times,* "Hooker would have had no trouble complying with these [federal hazardous waste standards] regulations. They may have had a little extra paperwork, but they wouldn't have had to change the way they disposed of the wastes."[10]

The "Health Disaster" at Love Canal: Why Politics and Science Don't Mix

The modern-day Love Canal saga might be traced back to 1976 when residents adjacent to the canal began to complain of chemical odors from the landfill and claimed that their discomfort was related to the seepage of wastes from the Love Canal property. Beginning in about 1976, Michael Brown, a reporter with the *Niagara Gazette,* started to write about suspected cases of toxic waste-induced illness among residents of the canal area. A review of the Brown *Gazette* articles and those printed by the *Courier Express Niagara News* leaves no doubt in one's mind about why the residents of the Love Canal became hysterical and in some cases militant. The headlines to Brown's stories told it all: "Toxic Exposure at Love Canal Called Chronic" (May 25, 1978), "Vapors from Love Canal Pose Serious Threat" (May 15, 1978), and under "Wider Range of Illnesses Suspected" (August 4, 1978), Brown noted that a "random survey" conducted by the *Niagara Gazette* hinted that "through the years, residents have also suffered high rates of hearing disorders, rectal bleeding, skin problems, sinus and respiratory ills, and headaches."

On June 25, 1978, Brown introduced us to one Fred Downs, who

> does a lot of wondering these days. He has the time for it. He is on social security because he can't work construction anymore. And the reason for his disability is a nasty, often terminal affliction called Hodgkin's disease— cancer. What Downs, 33, wonders so much about is yes, the Love Canal, where suspected cancer-causing agents have been marauding the environment for years. Did chemicals buried there lead to his illness? And if so, will they claim his life?

In 1978 Love Canal became a national media event when, as a result of the emerging unsettling press reports, New York State Commissioner of Health Robert Whalan, in a document with the hardly neutral title, "Love Canal: Public Health Time Bomb," declared a health emergency. Dr. Whalan's recommendations called for the temporary relocation of families with pregnant women and children under the age of two from the first two rings of homes around the canal. If just these recommendations had been followed some twenty families might have been relocated.

But on August 9 of that year, when Governor Hugh Carey visited the area, he announced that all 236 families living on both sides of Ninety-Seventh and Ninety-Ninth streets would be relocated—permanently—at taxpayers' expense. In addition, officials decided to build a system of sewers along the sides of the canal and across it, which drained into a holding tank where a treatment plant, built on the site, detoxified the wastes before they were let into the regular sewage system of the town (where, as part of the routine treatment of sewage, they underwent a second round of detoxification). This drainage setup was also intentionally designed to lower the water table so that the groundwater flow was toward the canal rather than away from it as previously designed. And a three-foot thick, impermeable clay cap was placed over the canal to deflect rainwater away from the buried chemicals.

This, however, was not the end of the affair but merely the beginning. Residents on the three or four streets outside the inner-ring homes found that their homes had lost value because of their proximity to the canal. And the residents were worried as well that, despite official assurances that they were in no danger, there might still be insidious effects upon their health. A group of local residents organized themselves into the Love Canal Homeowners Association, which, conducting its own informal health surveys, reported elevated incidences of asthma, urinary disorders, suicides, spontaneous abortions, epilepsy, cancer, and other grievous conditions. In particular, these ills seemed to cluster along the old drainage routes that had existed long before the neighborhood had been filled in and developed with residences, suggesting that there might, after all, be a migration of chemicals out of the canal.

Nervous Conditions, Miscarriages, Birth Defects . . .

In February 1979 Dr. Beverly Paigen, a biologist with Roswell Park Memorial Institute in Buffalo, urged the evacuation of even more families following the results of her study. Among other things, she found a high rate of birth defects and miscarriages among Love Canal residents. As summarized by Regenstein in *America the Poisoned,*

> She found . . . a much higher incidence of health disorders among those living in homes above moist ground or wet areas. In testimony before the House Subcommittee on Oversight and Investigations on March 21, 1979, chaired by Congressman Bob Eckhardt (D-Texas), she recounted the astonishing history of several families who have inhabited one such house located directly above

where liquid wastes were seeping out of the dump. In her testimony Dr. Paigen noted that, in houses near the canal, "in family Number One, the wife had a nervous breakdown and a hysterectomy due to uterine bleeding. In family Number Two, the husband had a breakdown. The wife had a hysterectomy due to uterine cancer. The daughter developed epilepsy and the son asthma. In family Number Three, the wife had a nervous breakdown. Both children suffered from bronchitis. In family Number Four, who lived there less than two years, the wife developed severe headaches after moving in. She also had a hysterectomy, uterine bleeding, and a pre-malignant growth."[11]

Dr. Paigen, in her well-publicized but largely irrelevant and impossible-to-interpret findings—all of course related to anecdotal or hearsay experience, and not controlled by comparisons with other human populations (which also, whether living or not at Love Canal, undergo hysterectomies, develop epilepsy, bronchitis, and headaches)—also asserted that children were being born with an unusually high number of birth defects, and miscarriages were occurring at a "rate of 25 percent." Additionally, she reported high levels of urinary diseases, convulsive disorders, suicides, and hyperactivity.[12] There was nothing random about her sample, as she obviously selected the families on whom she chose to report. Dr. Paigen also said she had evidence that the health of the Love Canal victims dramatically improved when they moved out of the area.

Following the explosive announcement of the Paigen findings (not only quoted in the Regenstein book, but also used as "givens" in all the literature proclaiming a health disaster at Love Canal) came two more years of unsettling revelations, health alarms, confrontations, and publicity stunts. By the spring of 1980 there was a charged atmosphere of fear, financial worry over falling real estate values, and frustration, coupled with an intense distrust by the residents of politicians, health agency bureaucrats, and the scientists working for these agencies. A crisis was near, needing only a spark to set it off.

EPA Enters the Love Canal Investigations: The Picciano and Barron Studies

Enter the EPA. It had filed suit the preceding December against the Hooker Chemical Company (which was the main source of the chemicals in the canal), and early in 1980, the EPA commissioned a study of possible chromosome damage among Love Canal residents as part of its effort to develop information for use in its lawsuit. The study was carried out by Dr. Dante Picciano. On May 15 he filed his report with the EPA, which purported to find evidence of an elevated occurrence of chromosome damage. The next day the report was leaked to the press. On May 17 it was on the front pages of the *New York Times* and the two local newspapers.

Coming as it did when emotions already were brittle, it caused a sensation. Media coverage was enormous; within two days the streets were full of press and TV reporters, who, as it happened, arrived just in time to cover the reaction of residents to the results of another EPA study, this one on nerve damage, which was released that day (May 19).

This one had been carried out by Dr. Steven Barron, and his provisional conclusion was that a degree of peripheral nerve damage did indeed exist among Love Canal residents. A mob gathered, and two EPA officials were involuntarily detained. Lois Gibbs, president of the Homeowners Association, then phoned the White House, telling the switchboard operator, "We are holding two EPA officials hostage," only to be put on hold![13] Persisting, she described the situation and the hostility of the crowd. The officials were released that evening.

By the next day (May 20) the EPA had, not surprisingly, reached a decision, which was announced on May 21. On that day President Carter declared a state of emergency at Love Canal, triggering the temporary relocation of some twenty-five hundred residents at a cost of $3 million to $5 million. At that point, Governor Carey, who had previously ordered a very limited evacuation, became suspicious and belligerent but resigned to the inevitable. On May 31, he told the Long Island newspaper *Newsday* that "the costly relocations of more than 700 Love Canal homeowners is medically unnecessary but has to be carried out to assuage the panic caused by the [EPA] report."[14] And some five months later, the relocation became permanent, escalating the cost of the buyout to more than $30 million.

In 1991, when asked to comment about Love Canal, Governor Carey said:

> The psychic trauma of the situation was undoubtedly real. But several factions took advantage of a frightened, hysterical population. Washington politicians pointed a finger at us, saying Love Canal was the ultimate symbol of [state] government neglect. They then used Love Canal to pass Superfund. The federal government released the results of hastily prepared and improperly conducted studies claiming that oozing chemicals were harming human health. The media added their own hype and Love Canal became the object of pity and horror, and the condition accelerated.[15]

Hank Cox, writing for the *Regulatory Action Network: Washington Watch* in September 1980, opined—in retrospect quite accurately—that the EPA officials knew full well they were involved in a gamble when they caused the public panic of evacuation without adequate data. EPA deputy administrator Barbara Blum, the Carter appointee from the Georgia environmental movement, was very cautious in her announcement of the Love Canal evacuation—"This action is being taken in recognition of the cumulative evidence of exposure to toxic wastes . . . and of mounting evidence of resulting health effects." Actually, at that time extensive studies by the New York State Department of Health had failed to produce any evidence of unusual health patterns in the community. "Why," asks Cox, "did the EPA's second in command proceed with a publicity exercise that she must have known would generate national attention and create much fright among the people of Love Canal?" The answer, he concluded,

> may lie in EPA's awareness of the growing tide of public opinion opposed to excessive regulation and the agency's desire to deflect political pressure for reform. At the same time it was creating the Love Canal panic, the EPA came out with another report showing that there were an estimated 50,666 hazardous waste sites similar to the Love Canal around the country, thereby laying the ground work for a bill now in the Senate that would create a "Superfund" to clean up this alleged danger to the American people.[16]

Were EPA's actions at Love Canal self-serving, simply to stimulate more federal laws, activities, and, most important, budgetary revenues for itself? That is hard to say, though one becomes particularly skeptical when reviewing the scientific comments that followed the release of the unscientific data that precipitated the evacuation, data that, incidentally, were released before peer review. The kindest thing to be said was that the Carter evacuation of Love Canal was based on anything but calm, studied decisionmaking. But then, let's be fair. A speedy decision like the one President Carter made would have been justified if the dangers were real—or there was good reason to believe they could be real. If those studies of nerve damage and chromosomal destruction had some relation to scientific reality, then perhaps the evacuation and expense to the American taxpayer were legitimate. But by releasing the reports before any scientific review had taken place, panic was set off without establishing cause for concern. Let us, then, take a moment to look at those three studies: those from Beverly Paigen, Dante Picciano, and Steve Barron.

The Paigen Study

Although Beverly Paigen is cited frequently in the media as "the authority" on Love Canal health statistics, very few, if any, scientists accept her findings as valid.

Immediately after she released her charges of high birth defects and miscarriages in Love Canal, the New York State Department of Health noted, "We cannot say with certainty that the high rates found in each of the categories are directly related to chemical exposure." A governor's panel (discussed in more detail below) convened by Hugh Carey reviewed Dr. Paigen's work and concluded in 1980 that her report

> falls far short of the mark as an exercise of epidemiology. She [Dr. Paigen] believes fervently that her observations prove the existence of multiple disease states directly attributable to chemical pollution, but her data cannot be taken as scientific evidence for her conclusions. The study is based largely on anecdotal information provided by questionnaires submitted to a narrowly selected group of residents. There are no adequate control groups, the illnesses cited as caused by chemical pollution were not medically validated. . . . The panel finds the Paigen report literally impossible to interpret. It cannot be taken seriously as a piece of sound epidemiological research, but it does have the impact of polemic.

The New York State review did not validate any of Dr. Paigen's findings. All results of the epidemiologic survey were negative, with the exception of an apparent blip of miscarriages in the 1960s, but that condition had returned to normal by the start of the 1970s. It was during the 1970s, of course, that the chemical seepage started and Paigen's work refers only to the 1970s.

The Picciano/EPA Chromosome Study

What about the chromosome study? It was seriously weakened by the fact that no matched comparison group was included; one had been planned and selected, but the EPA at the last minute refused funding for this portion of the study. This meant it was impossible to process the cells from exposed and unexposed populations in a parallel manner, to score them "blind" (that is, without the scorer knowing which samples were from exposed and un-exposed people), and to compare the level of aberrations among the Love Canal residents with the spontaneous level in a group of people not resident there but otherwise matched in factors known to induce chromosome aberrations (medical radiation, drugs, viral infections, occupational exposure to chemicals, etc.). In the absence of such a matched control group, Picciano used a group from a previous, published study of his for comparison (that is, it was not matched to the Love Canal population).[17]

This difficulty aside, overall chromosome abnormalities—that is, all types lumped together—were lower (you read that right) among the Love Canal residents than among the comparison group (1.1 percent and 1.4 percent, respectively). The difference was small and probably not biologically meaningful, but such as it was, Love Canal residents seemed on the whole to have healthier chromosomes than the comparison group![18]

Then why all the media ballyhoo about chromosome damage? Of the four categories of chromosomal abnormalities looked at, the frequency of one type—known as supernumerary acentrics—appeared to be elevated. Picciano claimed that eight of the thirty-six members of the sample population exhibited this type of damage whereas only one in one hundred is expected. The comparison figure of one to one hundred came from a previously conducted, unpublished Picciano study.[19]

Not only were there no adequate controls in the well-publicized Picciano study, but there also was the additional question of how the thirty-six people in the sample were selected for inclusion in the study. They were not a random sample of the Love Canal residents. Instead, they were picked by criteria that, it was hoped, would enrich for chromosome abnormalities, if any at all were present. Persons were chosen who lived in "wet" areas (that is, along the old drainage paths), who had measurable amounts of chemicals in their homes, or, most important, who had a history of adverse birth outcomes. (According to Hank Cox, this was not the first time Picciano was involved in a controversy. "Some years before, he performed a study of workers exposed to benzene for Dow Chemical, and Dow found that study useless because of the lack of controls." Picciano later worked for OSHA and that agency used his Dow study as evidence in its hearings on the OSHA benzene standard, later thrown out by the Supreme Court.)[20]

As a result of a freedom-of-information request submitted by a newspaper chain,[21] the New York State Department of Health issued the results of its earlier epidemiological study, "Adverse Pregnancy Outcomes in the Love Canal Area."[22] At the press conference releasing these data, Dr. Nicholas Vianna of the New York State Department of Health also released information regarding various other medical studies conducted by the state.[23] His comments with regard to pregnancy outcome were revealing:

> Efforts to establish a correlation between adverse pregnancy outcomes and evidence of chemical exposure have proved negative. Comprehensive studies of three households with unusually adverse reproductive histories did not produce evidence of unusual risk of chemical exposure. . . . We have not yet been able to correlate the geographic distribution of adverse pregnancy outcomes with chemical evidence of exposure. At present, there is no direct evidence of a cause-effect relationship with chemicals from the canal.[24]

Toxic Wastes Aren't the Only Things That Leak

How is it, then, that Picciano's study got leaked? Only the EPA knows for sure, but enough facts have emerged to suggest that it is a dirty story. As

Adeline Levine explains in *Love Canal: Science, Politics, and People,* it was neither an accident nor a surprise that the report was leaked. Picciano's formal account was filed with the EPA only on May 15, but he had written a letter to the EPA on May 5 indicating that he would be reporting elevated chromosome abnormalities among the Love Canal residents. And by May 12 Jane Hansen, a White House aide, had learned not only that this report was about to be submitted, but also that "someone was going to tell the newspapers about it." That is, three days *before* Picciano's report had been received, plans were afoot (and well known within certain circles) to release it to the press.

Nothing, it seems, was done by the White House or the EPA, even with this foreknowledge, to stop this leak from taking place. (Indeed, one sour soul close to these events said in a private conversation that the leak was purposely encouraged as a way of embarrassing Governor Carey of New York, whose support for President Carter's reelection campaign was felt to be less than enthusiastic. The leak also helped set the stage for President Carter to be seen as "coming to the rescue" four days after the report's results appeared in the news. This may be just gossip, but it is not implausible.)

Whatever the motivation, it is clear that the release of the report was intentional, not inadvertent. This release had to take place *before* a government committee of scientists had had a chance to examine the report (this had been scheduled for the following week). Such a review would have made it immediately clear that the report was totally inadequate to support a declaration of a health emergency at Love Canal.

The Barron Study That "Hit a Nerve"

The nerve study is easily disputed. It had been undertaken expressly as a pilot study, and the summary statement of its results that Dr. Barron had supplied to the EPA was contained in an application for funding to conduct a much larger study.

Fourteen different nerve measurements had been made on each of the persons investigated, and one or two of these did look, by visual inspection of the data, to be sufficiently depressed among Love Canal residents compared with a control population, to warrant support for the more thorough study. No statistical analyses had been done on these data at the time the application for further funding was submitted to the EPA.

Ordinarily, Dr. Barron would not have made this claim public at this early stage, but the hullabaloo over the leaked chromosome study made him fear that his preliminary results would be leaked too, and he felt an obligation to talk over the results with the affected persons before this happened. This is what forced the premature release of the study on May 19. Later, when the statistics were finally completed and proper allowance was made for the fact that multiple measurements were taken on each person (which meant that the likelihood of at least one of them looking significant purely by chance was fairly high, hence a correction must be applied), it was concluded that there were no statistically significant findings at all; the apparent effect could have easily resulted simply from chance.

The study, then, did not find the Love Canal residents to have impaired nerves. But by the time this crucial fact was known, it was too late.

All Early Health Reports Clean

Unlike the first improperly conducted and rapidly released studies, there were a number of carefully prepared and conducted studies of the health effects at Love Canal. All found that the Love Canal disaster consisted primarily of anxiety and apprehension among residents, and *not* chemically induced health problems.

The comments of Dr. Nicholas Vianna of the New York State Department of Health, cited above, included some general—and reassuring—comments about the status of health of Niagara Falls residents:

> Our initial impression was that both the numbers and types of cancer were in no way unusual from that which would be expected in the general population. . . .
>
> Blood testing, which was designed to screen for liver and kidney abnormalities, leukemia, and other blood diseases, showed no patterns of excess abnormality. . . . None had clinical evidence of liver disease. . . .
>
> Computer analysis of the twenty-two-page health questionnaire, which elicited information on some 150 different diseases or symptoms, produced no evidence of unusual patterns of illness or other disorders. Cancer incidence was within normal limits.

A second close look at cancer incidence at Love Canal (also the work of the New York State Department of Health), one of the first to win the approval of serious scientists, was published in the respected journal *Science*. It concluded, "Data from the New York Cancer Registry show no evidence for higher cancer rates associated with residence near the Love Canal toxic waste burial site in comparison with the entire state outside of New York City."[25] Because of the long latencies involved, this finding does not rule out the possibility that cancer may appear in the *future*. It is important, however, in that it belies the allegations of Paigen that elevated cancer rates are *already* evident.

As would be expected, members of the Love Canal Homeowners Association whose homes had been bought by the state immediately downgraded the importance of the study, saying it was designed to minimize the health risks of Love Canal homes that the state plans to resell. "We've lost all our faith in government," a Homeowners official said. Stated another, "It's another big coverup."[26] As so often happens in the panic-ridden discussions relating to chemicals, environment, and health, those claiming a chemical-disease link will accept *only* studies that support their cause, and reject all others as coverups.

Additional evidence, however, indicated that residents were not being exposed, that chemicals were not migrating out of the containment area. Separate surveys of chemical contamination in the soil and groundwater outside of the inner-ring homes in 1978 by the New York State Department of Health, and in 1980 by the EPA, independently confirmed there were no outmigrating chemicals. (A sophisticated system of test wells in the Love Canal site confirms through 1991 that chemicals have been effectively contained for over a decade).[27]

Moreover, measurements inside these homes found no levels higher than would be normally expected in homes containing an oil burner in the basement, or a bicycle (the lubricant evaporates), or garden pesticides. The *highest* level of in-home contaminant was a thousandfold lower than the levels permitted workers in the normal course of their jobs. These contextual facts make it difficult, to say the least, to believe that the residents in the outer homes were ever in danger.

Then, in October 1980, a panel of scientists appointed by Governor Carey concluded that "inadequate" scientific studies might have exaggerated the seriousness of the health problems caused by toxic wastes leaking at Love Canal. The panel, chaired by Lewis Thomas, M.D, chancellor of Memorial Sloan-Kettering Cancer Center, and including such dignitaries of the scientific-medical world as Arthur C. Upton, M.D., chairman of environmental medicine at New York University Medical Center, and former director of the National Cancer Institute declared:

> As a result of this review, the panel has concluded that there has been no demonstration of acute health effects linked to exposure to hazardous wastes at the Love Canal site. The panel has also concluded that chronic effects of hazardous wastes exposure at Love Canal have neither been established nor ruled out yet.[28]

The expert panel was also critical of the September 1978 booklet *Love Canal: Public Health Time Bomb,* which described the Love Canal situation as an "environmental nightmare" capable of causing "profound and devastating effects," and constituting a condition of "great and imminent peril."[29] The panel noted that there was a reason . . . [for *Love Canal: Public Health Time Bomb*] but not a good enough reason. There ought to be a better mechanism for convincing the federal government that a certifiable disaster area exists . . . [rather] than to arouse such fears of imminent peril as swept through the Love Canal area in this case.

In conclusion, the governor's panel wrote, "The scientific evidence, incomplete though it is, reveals no state of population damage justifying the terms 'imminent peril' and 'profound and devastating effects.' "[30]

As a result of this report, even the *New York Times* felt snookered. A June 20, 1981 editorial explained:

But from what is now known, Love Canal, perhaps the nation's most prominent symbol of chemical assaults on the environment, has had no detectable effect on the incidence of cancer. When all the returns are in, years from now, it may well turn out that the public suffered less from the chemicals there than from the hysteria generated by flimsy research irresponsibly handled.

And, we might add, irresponsibly picked up by major newspapers like the *New York Times*.

Continuing Health Studies Also Clean

Reports about "no health effects" at Love Canal continued. In the May 27, 1983 issue of *Morbidity and Mortality Weekly Report*, the Centers for Disease Control (CDC) notes that the frequency of chromosomal aberrations did *not* differ significantly between residents of Love Canal and control residents—yet another blow to the already mortally wounded Picciano study. It is of interest to note that the frequency of supernumerary acentrics, the allegedly elevated aberration, was not found to be high. In June 1983, the CDC noted no excess illness among persons who live close to the Love Canal.

Similar results were reported in an American Medical Association news release on March 16, 1984 and in a subsequent issue of the *Journal of the American Medical Association*. Chromosomes of residents from houses suspected of having high levels of chemical contamination and members of the Picciano/EPA study were compared with controls from other areas in Niagara Falls. Investigators at CDC found "no increase in the frequency of chromosomal abnormalities . . . of residents in the Love Canal area."[31] Not surprisingly, subjects in all groups who smoke cigarettes were found to have increased frequency of particular defects in their chromosomes.

Further analysis of pregnancy outcomes was done by Vianna and published in *Science* in 1984. This analysis looked at birth weights by more limited time periods (the original analysis was of the total period 1940–78) and revealed a significant excess of low birth weight for white infants born during 1940–53, a time when there was active dumping at the Love Canal. Encouragingly, though, the study also found that infants born in Love Canal during 1960–78 were at no greater risk of low birth weight than were those born in upstate New York (where there was no chemical dumping) during 1954–78.[32]

An unpublished study[33] of low birth weight, prematurity, and birth defects found that infants born to mothers living in Love Canal during pregnancy had a greater risk of weighing less than 2,500 grams at birth (independent of the following factors known to cause low birth weight: weeks of gestation, race, maternal smoking, alcohol consumption, illness, socioeconomic status, and maternal age). It should be noted that birth weight was provided by recall in 74.5 percent of the cases and from birth certificates in only 25.5 percent. These same authors published an abstract[34] reporting a statistically significant difference in anthropometric measures in children who were born and who had lived in the Love Canal area for 75 percent of their lives. Their decreased height and weight could not be accounted for by differences in midparent stature, socioeconomic class, nutrition, birth weight, or chronic illness.

The lack of evidence for damage to human health was confirmed by a thorough analysis of all published and unpublished studies by the Committee on Environmental Epidemiology of the National Research Council, who published their review in 1991. They found that there was no definitive evidence for harm to human health at Love Canal as a result of the leaking chemicals, with the possible exception (and only possible) of the decreased height and weight of some Love Canal children.[35]

Stress: A Real Health Effect

Without a doubt, the stress induced by the fear of disease was very real and very damaging. Consider, for example, Picciano's study about chromosome abnormalities. One resident who had had breast cancer five years prior to the 1978 activity at Love Canal had her fears reignited when the study revealed that she had abnormal chromosomes. Prior to the study, she had thought her prognosis was good; after the study she wasn't so sure.

There was the fear that the government was suppressing positive results, or, in the case of the Picciano study, declaring results invalid in an attempt to cover up problems. As Sheldon Wolff, Ph.D., of the University of California's Laboratory of Radiobiology and Environmental Health concluded upon the release of the 1984 study showing no chromosome abnormalities:

The residents of the Love Canal area should take heart since no significant differences in [chromosome abnormalities] were found in their chromosomes when compared with those in the concurrent matched controls. Furthermore, the study should allay fears resulting from the appearance of rare supernumerary acentric chromosomes, since they were also found in the controls.

The muddied scientific waters have now been cleared. The emotional climate at the Love Canal is such, however, that it is problematic whether the residents will be relieved or will reject the new evidence as part of a government coverup to deny that they indeed have genetic damage.[36]

A 1980 *Science* article compared the psychological damage of Love Canal with that of two other situations: the accident at Three Mile Island and the belief of some Vietnam veterans that their exposure to the dioxin-containing herbicide Agent Orange has led to cancer, birth defects, and a variety of other disorders. Love Canal was like the former in that

despite the fact that there were no adverse physical consequences of the release of radioactivity into the environment, a large portion of the population was profoundly alarmed, and ignorance and misinformation from those in charge created a deep and abiding mistrust.[37]

Love Canal was like the latter because:

In both instances there are real sicknesses to contend with, and the sufferers feel helpless and betrayed by the government's apparent unwillingness to move swiftly to set things right.[38]

Love Canal took its toll on marriages. As early as 1980, 40 percent of the couples involved in the 1978 evacuation were known to be separated or divorced. The typical situation was a wife who wanted to leave for the sake of the children and a husband who didn't want to for financial reasons. The result: the wife left with the children.[39]

What to Do with Love Canal?

Attempts to reinhabit Love Canal began in 1982 when the EPA conducted a two-year, $5.4 million ($8.5 million if EPA's internal costs are added in) study of the area, testing samples of air and other materials. These results were compared with background levels in other cities across the United States. Released in 1982, this extensive study concluded that, outside of the canal-contaminated area, levels of chemicals were comparable to those found in other cities and that no environmental standards were violated. The presence or absence of a substance in a particular sample was to be assessed in a manner that erred on the side of caution to provide that best assurance of protecting public health and the environment. Despite validation by the National Bureau of Standards, the U.S. Department of Health and Human Services, and independent studies, the report was plagued by controversy and distrust and was ultimately rejected.[40]

Science described the controversy that led to the report's rejection:[41]

> Initially, a panel of six federal scientists convened by the Department of Health and Human Services (HHS) agreed that resettlement of the area was acceptable. One month before the report's release, however, the panel withdrew this conclusion and stated that "no definite recommendations or conclusions as to the habitability or the potential human health risks of the Love Canal area can be made." One day before the report was released, the panel reversed itself again and reaffirmed its initial conclusions that the area is habitable.

This chapter of Love Canal wouldn't be complete without an explanation for the waffling. At the same time that EPA had asked HHS to examine the data and predict whether adverse health effects would result from resettlement of the area in question, they also asked the National Bureau of Standards (NBS) to verify the reliability of the data. Although some on the HHS panel deemed EPA's data too jumbled to interpret, the majority concluded that resettlement would not pose a risk to human health.

However, when NBS came out with a critical analysis (saying EPA had failed to account for wide variations in the quality of the information it had received from different laboratories), scientists at HHS became concerned about their credibility and withdrew their initial optimistic conclusion. At exactly this time, three senators demanded an immediate release of the report, including the HHS assessment. The EPA foolishly promised the report's release within one month, placing itself in a difficult position.

The NBS ultimately withdrew its challenges to the report, provided that EPA delineate the problems with laboratory performance. Pressure continued from the senators and from Niagara Falls residents to release the results. Although additional time would have resolved any further uncertainties in the report, the continued pressure ultimately forced its release. But the damage had already been done.

That study rejected, another was ordered. A technical review committee (an expert panel comprising independent scientists from across the country) was assembled to design and conduct this new study. Five years and millions of dollars later, this second study reported *exactly the same conclusions as the first.*

The EPA released the results of this second set of comprehensive environmental monitoring data in May of 1987. Soil and air samples from Love Canal, divided into seven areas based on suspected levels of contamination, were compared to residential neighborhoods in western New York at least half a mile from a known landfill. These comparison neighborhoods, picked by the technical review committee and members of the public, had to have soil similar to that of the Emergency Declaration Area.[42]

All areas were tested for evidence of Love Canal Indicator Chemicals, all of which move easily through soil or water and are long-lasting. This comprehensive study revealed that

> except for residual contamination in certain local storm sewer lines and portions of creeks located near the outfalls of those storm sewers, the occurrence and concentration levels of chemicals found in the Declaration Area were comparable to those found at nearby control sites.
>
> In addition, comparative data from other locations in the United States reveal that the observed occurrence and concentration levels of those chemicals monitored in the residential portions of the Declaration Area and elsewhere were comparable. *Furthermore, comparison of the concentration levels of environmental contaminants found in the residential portions of the Declaration Area with existing EPA standards revealed that no environmental standards were violated.*[43]

The study concluded with confidence that it

> is unlikely that undetected Love Canal–related contamination exists in the residential portions of the Declaration Area, because the targeted substances monitored and the sampling locations selected for monitoring purposes were intentionally directed (based on the best available evidence) to maximize the probability of detecting contaminants that had migrated from the former canal.[44]

Other high points of the study are:

- Hydrogeologic studies demonstrated that there is little potential for migration of contaminants from Love Canal into the Declaration Area.

- The barrier drain system, which was installed around the perimeter of Love Canal in 1978 and 1979, is working as designed to:
  contain the outward migration of contaminants through more permeable overburdened soil;
  to move nearby shallow system groundwater toward the drain.

- Except for some apparently isolated pockets of shallow system groundwater contamination located immediately adjacent to the former canal, no general pattern of contamination was found in the shallow system.

- There was no evidence of Love Canal–related contamination that had migrated preferentially through former swales into the Declaration Area, nor were there higher concentrations of contamination in "wet" area residences than in "dry" area residences.

The findings were used to formulate State Health Commissioner Dr. David Axelrod's "Decision of Habitability." Early in the study process it was decided that if contamination levels in any of the Love Canal neighborhoods were higher than those in the four comparison neighborhoods, that any such area would be declared nonhabitable, without regard to health risks. As a result, two areas east of the canal that showed slightly higher levels of contamination were deemed nonhabitable. About 150 residents in sixty-nine families had never left this area; these people were not told to move as this level of contamination presents no obvious health risk to them. One additional area showed higher levels of contamination, probably not originating from Love Canal but most likely from the deposition of wind-borne material from a nearby landfill. This area was also deemed nonhabitable. Clearly, though, the best available information indicates that these areas do not pose a threat to health. The federal government, in point of fact, has refused to assist in their cleanup, they explain, because the *contamination levels there are insignificant.*[45]

The Love Canal Area Master Plan changed the three areas deemed nonhabitable into an industrial-commercial classification. Area one will be developed into a scenic approach to the city of Niagara Falls. The two areas with remaining residents present an interesting dilemma. The low levels of contamination would be fairly easy to clean up, but very costly (exceeding the cost of the homes). Marketing of abandoned homes would have to wait until remediation was completed, during which time they would continue to deteriorate. Finally, it would be nearly impossible to overcome the label of "nonhabitable," despite the fact that the levels pose no health threat. The commercial-industrial classification, then, was basically by default.

The Love Canal Area Revitalization Agency (LCARA), created by New York State law in 1980 to manage homes near the canal and act in the public's interest, entered the real estate market in July 1990 with the first group of homes to be resold. As of September 1992, fifty-five were under contract or sold, with thirty-four closings and thirty-one new families moved in. Sale prices, averaging $50,000, are approximately 20 percent below comparable markets, lowered by the Love Canal stigma, and compounded by an abandoned and rundown neighborhood.[46]

The Ghost Still Roams[47]

Why, despite a fastidious remedition, clean health reports, and compelling efforts to reinhabit the area, does Love Canal remain a ghost town?

Love Canal's image is ever more tarnished by the media. Consider, for example, the recent Hollywood version of Love Canal, in which a young boy dies from leukemia. The viewer logically concludes that leaking chemicals caused his illness and wonders how many others died from chemical poisoning.

Beyond the severely tarnished image, Love Canal has had to leap formidable legal and financial hurdles.

Opposition to reinhabiting Love Canal neighborhoods has remained strong, vocal, and litigious. Opponents, led by Lois Gibbs (president of the original Love Canal Homeowners Association) and bolstered by the powerful National Resources Defense Council (NRDC), asked for an injunction against LCARA to prevent them from selling homes until they prepared an acceptable Environmental Impact Statement (EIS). New York State's attorney general granted the injunction in 1985 and held it until 1990, when an acceptable EIS was presented by LCARA. Gibbs and NRDC then filed a lawsuit against LCARA for failure to do an adequate EIS, claiming that health risks were not assessed. They lost in the first round but are now appealing the case. NRDC, on behalf of all opponents, is also filing a suit against the EPA, claiming they, too, failed to adequately assess human health risks.

Against tremendous odds, though, buyers are appearing for the homes. But the final impasse is at the bank: lenders refusing to hold mortgages on Love Canal homes, fearful of being held liable for future cleanup of the secured property. "Although Congress has enacted a provision to protect lenders from this liability," writes Alvin L. Arnold in *Real Estate Environmental Law Report,* "courts as well as the EPA have interpreted the provision to create liability for two classes of lenders: (1) those who become owners after foreclosing on property that secures a loan; and (2) those who participate in the management of the property securing the loan." A ray of hope: U.S. Congressmen John LaFalce (from the Niagara Falls area) has recently introduced a bill that would protect lending institutions from such tremendous liability.

As of late 1992, however, home sales were dependent on the potential buyer paying cash or LCARA holding the mortgages.

The Controversy Continues

To be sure, the Love Canal controversy will continue. Twelve years and billions of dollars later, a neighborhood that caused no measurable physical ailments is just beginning to pick up the pieces.

Love Canal, according to former New York Governor Hugh Carey, "is the story of people trying to create an issue where there wasn't one, a perfect example of junk science and politics surfacing and reigning forever." Governor Carey further summarizes the Love Canal saga:

> The media never told the story of all that was being done to remedy the situation, however, because they were intent on creating the unrivaled drama. Inaccuracy was allowed to prevail because so many people and factions sought their own personal gain from Love Canal.

Without a doubt, no one wants another Love Canal; we must strive to manage the benefits of technology safely and appropriately. We must also acknowledge that the heavily industrialized areas of this country are no longer pristine. That doesn't mean we should simply write them off, as the environmentalists are trying to do with Love Canal.

NOTES

1. New York State Department of Health, "Love Canal: Public Health Time Bomb; A Special Report to the Governor and Legislature" (Albany, New York, 1978): p. 2.

2. E. Zuesse, "Love Canal: The Truth Seeps Out." *Reason* (February 1981): p. 20.

3. Ibid.

4. Deed of Love Canal property transfer, April 28, 1953.

5. Zuesse, "Love Canal," p. 19.

6. *Niagara Gazette,* November 22, 1957.

7. M. Brown, *Laying Waste: The Poisoning of America by Toxic Chemicals* (New York: Parthenon, 1980), p. 8.

8. S. Epstein, et al., *Hazardous Waste in America* (San Francisco: Sierra Club, 1982), p. 94.

9. L. Regenstein, *America the Poisoned* (Washington: Acropolis Books, 1982), p. 141.

10. R. Blumenthal, "Fight to Curb 'Love Canals,' " *New York Times,* June 30, 1980, pp. B1, B11.

11. Regenstein, *America the Poisoned,* pp. 138–39.

12. Ibid.

13. A. G. Levine, *Love Canal: Science, Politics, and People* (Lexington: Lexington Books, 1982), p. 149.

14. *Newsday,* May 31, 1980.

15. Personal communication with former Governor Hugh Carey, July 24, 1991.

16. H. Cox, "Love Canal Special Supplement," *The Regulatory Action Network: Washington Watch* (September 1980): p. 1.

17. G. B. Silverman, "Love Canal: A Retrospective," *Environment Reporter* 20 (1989): p. 840.

18. Ibid.

19. Ibid.

20. Cox, "Love Canal Special Supplement," p. 1.

21. Occidental Petroleum Corporation, "The Other Side of the Love Canal" (July 31, 1980): p. 9.

22. New York State Department of Health, "Adverse Pregnancy Outcomes in Love Canal" (April 1980).

23. Occidental Petroleum Corporation, "Other Side," p. 9.

24. Ibid.

25. *Science* (June 19, 1981): p. 19.

26. *New York Times,* June 12, 1981, p. B1.

27. New York State Department of Environmental Conservation, Division of Hazardous Waste Remediation, "1989 Love Canal Annual Report" (February 1989); New York State Department of Environmental Conservation, Division of Hazardous Waste Remediation, "1990 Love Canal Annual Report" (May 1991); New York State Department of Environmental Conservation, Division of Hazardous Waste Remediation, "Status of Remedial Activities," Love Canal Remedial Action Project to Love Canal Technical Review Committee (May 15, 1991).

28. New York Governor's Panel, October 1980.

29. Ibid.

30. Ibid.

31. AMA News Release, "Love Canal Residents Not at Risk, Says CDC," March 16, 1984.

32. J. J. Vianna and A. K. Polan, "Incidence of Low Birth Weight Among Love Canal Residents," *Science* 226 (1984): pp. 1217–19.

33. L.R. Goldman, B. Paigen, M. M. Magnant, and J.H. Highland, "Low Birth Weight, Prematurity and Birth Defects in Children Living Near the Hazardous Waste Site, November 1984" (unpublished).

34. L. R. Goldman, M. M. Magnant, and B. Paigen, "Abnormal Anthropometric Measures in Children Exposed to Environmental Toxins," *Pediatric Research* 18 (1984): p. 183A.

35. Committee on Environmental Epidemiology, National Research Council, *Health Effects from Hazardous Waste Sites* (Chelsea, Michigan: Lewis Publishing, 1991), pp. 184–85, 196–97.

36. S. Wolff, "Love Canal Revisited," *Journal of the American Medical Association* 251 (1984): p. 1464.

37. C. Holden, "Love Canal Residents Under Stress," *Science* 208 (1980): p. 1242.

38. Ibid.

39. Ibid.

40. Love Canal Revitalization Agency, "This is the Love Canal"; J. Deegan, "Looking Back at Love Canal," *EPA Environmental Science Technology* 21 (1987): p. 218; R. J. Smith, "The Risks of Living Near Love Canal," *Science* 217 (1982): pp. 808–11.

41. R. J. Smith, "Risks of Living Near Love Canal," pp. 808–11.

42. EPA, *Environmental Monitoring at Love Canal,* vol. 1 (Washington D.C.: EPA, 1987).

43. Ibid.

44. Ibid.

45. New York State Commissioner of Health, "Decision on Habitability, Love Canal Emergency Declaration Area," September 1988.

46. Personal communication, Love Canal Area Revitalization Agency, September 1992.

47. K. Napier, "Love Canal in the 1990s," *Priorities* (Fall 1991): p. 40.

4

Pesticides: Peddling Poison for Profit?

The Charges

. . . less than 1 percent of the poisons reach their target pest; the rest wind up as contaminants in water residues on produce and poisonous fallout on farm workers. Worldwide, the compounds fatally poison an estimated 10,000 people a year and injure 400,000 more. Uncounted millions more may be at increased risk for cancer, reproductive problems and birth defects due to low-level, chronic exposure . . . the dangers are considered so grave that the Environmental Protection Agency has now catapulted pesticides to the top of its list of problem pollutants—above toxic wastes.

—*Newsweek*[1]

Yet no one has ever proven that pesticides are necessary to the food supply, only that they are beneficial economically to manufacturers and growers.

—*Earthright*[2]

According to the National Coalition Against the Misuse of Pesticides, an advocacy group critical of the lawn-care industry, nine of the pesticides may be carcinogenic, 10 may cause birth defects, three can affect reproduction, nine can damage the liver or kidneys, 20 attack the nervous system, and 29 cause rashes or skin disease.

—*Time*[3]

Cancer, of course, is hardly the only concern. Data on the neurobehavioral effects of long-term, low-level exposure to lawn pesticides are poor or nonexistent.

—*Newsweek*[4]

149

The Facts

- There has never been a documented case of human illness or death in the United States as a result of the standard and accepted use of pesticides.

- Although Americans are exposed to trace levels of pesticides, there is no evidence that such exposure increases the risk of cancer, birth defects, or any other human ailment.

- The much-maligned pesticides aldrin, dieldrin, chlordane, and heptachlor were banned from use in the United States solely because they caused liver tumors in mice. They have not been shown to cause cancer in any other species of animal.

- Carelessness in the production of pesticides (for example, the dumping of kepone wastes in the James River) is a cause for concern and regulations—based on science, not emotion and rhetoric. However, deleterious effects from careless use do not justify the argument for deleterious effects from prudent use of pesticides.

Safety and Utility of Pesticides

Pesticides have been used for centuries to combat pests. Even ancient Romans used burning sulfur to control insects and salt to kill weeds. Modern pesticides vary in their uses and are far more efficient than these crude chemical agents. There are several categories of pesticides; insecticides, herbicides, and fungicides are three of the most widely used. Other important agricultural chemicals include rodenticides, defoliants, plant-growth regulators, antimicrobials, and synergists.

Insecticides control insects that destroy food, clothing, and shelter. Insecticides are invaluable in protecting and preserving public health by controlling insects that carry disease. "One of the outstanding achievements in science and medicine during the past few decades," insecticides are likely to be "essential weapons for protecting man and animals . . . for many decades to come."[5]

Herbicides are used to control weeds, greatly reducing the competition for water and nutrients in croplands. One authority estimates that the use of herbicides yields at least five additional bushels of bread grain per acre, which is a 10–20 percent increased yield in treated acreage,[6] and provides a net increase of fifteen loaves of bread for each person on earth. Herbicides also assist ranchers in providing suitable and productive grazing areas for livestock.

Fungicides help combat plant diseases that have been serious problems for mankind's survival throughout history.[7] If fungicides had been available at the time, the nineteenth-century Irish potato famine probably would have been averted. An estimated one million people died of starvation and another million were forced to emigrate.[8]

STRICT REGULATIONS ENSURE PESTICIDE SAFETY

Pesticide safety is assured by extensive regulations that affect the research, development, distribution, promotion, handling, storage, disposal, and use of pesticide products, all delineated in the Federal Insecticide Fungicide and Rodenticide Act (FIFRA).[9] Early research involves screening new chemical compounds for biological activity and toxicological effect. Outdoor testing for effectiveness is initially performed on small plots. Long-term toxicology studies are conducted to test for cellular or tissue abnormality, illness, cancer, birth defects (teratogenesis) or mutations in laboratory animals. Field studies under actual farming conditions are conducted according to an EPA-granted experimental use permit. Residue levels in crops are determined through field tests and safety of the levels is demonstrated by the toxicity data from animal-feeding studies. The result of all of the above testing and evaluations of the pesticides are then submitted as a registration package to the EPA, which then considers the benefits in comparison to the pesticide's potential acute, chronic, and environmental risks.

Tolerances are levels of agrichemicals allowed to remain in food for human consumption or feed for livestock at the time the crop is harvested. EPA sets tolerances after public review and comment, then the FDA and other agencies enforce these tolerances on food and feed in commerce.

Residue levels in crops are determined through field tests. Safety of the levels is demonstrated by the toxicity data from animal-feeding studies. A no observable adverse effect level (NOAEL) is determined to be the level at which the chemical has no harmful effect on the most sensitive test animal. By dividing the NOAEL by a safety factor of up to 100 or more, an acceptable daily intake (ADI) is established. EPA plans to replace the ADI and implement a "reference dose" (RfD) approach to reach regulatory decisions about the significance of chemical exposures.

FIFRA does allow emergency exemptions for new agricultural pests or diseases for which no EPA-approved pesticide is available for control. An emergency exemption is granted only under highly restricted conditions, including limited time, precisely defined area and rigid use restrictions.

Most farm chemicals and home use pesticides are "general use" products; that is, they can be used safely by anyone who follows label directions. However, some chemicals are classed as "restricted use" pesticides. They are only sold to and used by "certified applicators," persons who satisfy EPA and state training requirements. "Restricted use" pesticides are not considered suitable for use by the general public; that is, the label instructions alone are not considered adequate to assure safe and proper use for restricted use pesticides.

Once the new pesticide is approved by EPA and begins to be used according to the label, further research will continue to uncover other major uses of the product. Each new use of or additional pest controlled by the pesticide requires further review and acceptance by EPA before it can be added to the pesticide label.

Clearly, pesticides are strictly regulated, and approval of a new pesticide is not simple, inexpensive, or fast. Data submitted to EPA in support of a typical new agricultural chemical can represent as much as $25 million of cost and more than seven years of laboratory, field, and environmental testing—an investment that cannot be recovered unless and until EPA approves the pesticide. The review of a registration document by EPA typically requires about three years for new pesticides; thus, the total time involved in development of the new product is about ten years from initial testing to final marketing approval, a considerable period of time.

The development of pesticides operates on a progressive testing system that eliminates large numbers of candidate compounds during the initial years of toxicological testing. The study costs for these rejected substances must be included in the expenses pesticide manufacturers hope eventually to recover through approval of new products. Due to increased risk arising out of increasingly stringent requirements, new pesticide development is now primarily feasible only for the largest companies and for pesticides having wide agricultural markets.

WHAT ABOUT PERSISTENCE?

Most pesticides are nonpersistent and are degraded fairly rapidly (a few weeks or less) by sunlight, soil microorganisms, and moisture, so they do not remain in the environment for extended periods. A few pesticides—for example, some organochlorine insecticides—are considered persistent because they maintain their pesticidal potency for some time after application. This often represents an advantage in that fewer applications are needed. Costs for labor and materials can be lower compared to more frequent applications of rapidly degradable pesticides.

Fundamental to the issue of persistence are the toxicity and utility of the pesticide. For example, the organochlorine insecticides have been widely criticized for their persistence; however, they are generally less toxic than many other insecticides, particularly in their toxicity toward mammals, including humans. The low cost and stability of the organochlorine insecticides such as DDT, lindane, and dieldrin are "precisely the reason why they have been such useful pesticides in the last 35 years and the mainstay of vector-control programs."

Persistence is essential for certain applications where frequent, repeated applications are not desirable. Since termites are relentless destroyers of wood, for example, persistent pesticides are the preferred treatment to protect homes and farm buildings from destruction.

BIOMAGNIFICATION NOT EVEN A CONSIDERATION

A commonly held belief is that some pesticides biomagnify as one proceeds up the food chain as, for example, from algae to planktonic crustaceans to small fish to larger fish to predatory birds or mammals. The consumption of low levels of pesticides within each prey animal was presumed responsible for increased amounts in higher predators. Careful research has revealed that this phenomenon is uncommon in nature and that pesticide concentrations in predators have little to do with biomagnification up the food chain.[10] As one reviewer stated,[11]

> The popular conception of food biomagnification of chemical contaminants is not well substantiated . . . the role of biomagnification has recently been minimized as a significant contribution to the accumulation of residues.

Another reviewer similarly concluded:[12]

> Biomagnification of contaminants is not a dramatic phenomenon in marine and freshwater food webs . . . most of the evidence for the existence or nonexistence of biomagnification within aquatic food webs has come from highly circumstantial and/or marginally relevant data.

Finally, pesticides are designed to prevent biomagnification; hence, biomagnification is not even a theoretical problem.

WILDLIFE PROTECTED

One important result of modern agriculture, including the use of pesticides and chemical fertilizers, is greater productivity per acre. Modern farmers can produce much more than their predecessors and require less acreage to do it. This situation releases land for other uses, including conservation for wildlife habitat and human recreation such as camping, hiking, bird-watching, etc. Under less productive agricultural methods, more land must be utilized for farming—to the detriment of other land uses.

The presumed detrimental effect of pesticides on wildlife (e.g., as expressed in *Silent Spring* by Rachel Carson) has been widely accepted by the public but lacks scientific support. (Reduction in wildlife population is generally due to habitat destruction, overfishing, and similar factors.) In fact, one author stated, "Wildlife populations all over the nation are bigger and healthier than ever, not in spite of pesticides, but in many cases because of them."

He cited surveys by fish and game authorities who reported widespread and increased abundance of waterfowl, deer, and small and big game compared to decades ago before widespread use of pesticides.

PESTICIDE RESIDUES NOT EXCESSIVE

As analytical methods are developed and improved, identification and measurement of smaller and smaller amounts of pesticides, pesticide metabolites, and other trace chemicals become possible. Since the 1950s, analytical detectability has advanced from microgram (10^{-6}g) to nanogram (10^{-9}g) to even picogram (10^{-12}g) amounts. As a result, residues previously reported in the parts-per-million (10^{-6}) range are now measurable in parts-per-billion (10^{-9}) or even parts-per-trillion (10^{-12}) concentrations.

With such incredibly minute quantities now detectable, pesticides and other chemicals can be found almost anywhere in the environment, food, water, or human or animal tissues. This too often results in fears of the "pesticide contamination" of the earth and inspires calls for more restrictions or bans on chemicals . . . a kind of "toxic terror."

The ability to detect, however, has no relation to the biological effects of substances; that is, "residues only matter if they affect organisms." The presence of minute pesticide quantities or other substances rarely presents even the slightest risk to human health. Since any biological effect is related to the size of the residues, the environment is similarly unaffected by minute residues. The extensive testing of and occupational exposure to much higher pesticide levels clearly demonstrate the lack of risk from minuscule amounts of these materials.

Many people are concerned about pesticide residues on our food supply. But the belief that poison in pesticide spray will somehow be transferred to human food has been blown far out of proportion. Agricultural scientists who use pesticides properly are regulated by government codes specifying the amount of residue that may be present in their products. The levels of residue are so small that their presence would have to be multiplied by 100 or more to reach a level that might possibly be harmful to human beings. In 1990 the FDA tested 19,962 food samples. Ninety-nine percent of the domestic samples contained no illegal residues, i.e., less than 1 percent of the samples had residues exceeding tolerances set by the Environmental Protection Agency (EPA).

Sixty percent had no residues at all. In the imported samples, less than 1 percent had over-tolerance residues, 4 percent had residues for which there was no tolerance set, and 64 percent had no detectable residues.[13]

FDA's annual Total Diet Study, then, once again indicated that any residues found were well below the acceptable daily intakes established by the United Nations' Food and Agriculture Organization and World Health Organization.

GROUNDWATER POLLUTION BY PESTICIDES RARE

Groundwater pollution rarely occurs when pesticides are properly applied. Groundwater is particularly critical for agricultural applications; nearly 70 percent of it used annually is for agricultural irrigation. Obviously, farmers have a strong incentive to avoid poisoning their own water sources. Contamination of neighboring groundwater subjects a careless pesticide applicator to civil and criminal penalties plus lawsuits for damages.

Trace amounts of pesticides have been detected in groundwater, but this fundamental question has to be addressed: Are the trace amounts detected toxic to humans or animals or otherwise detrimental to the use of the groundwater? Unfortunately, the "sophistication of present-day analytical methods may have outstripped our ability to interpret what they reveal, our ability to determine the significance of low concentrations of contaminants on the environment and on public health."

What Effects Do Pesticides Have on Human Health?*

Given the widespread utility of pesticides in controlling insects, weeds, plant diseases, rodents, and other nuisances, how can much controversy exist about them? Are these benefits now sufficient to show the value of pesticides? The answer hinges on consideration of the toxicity of pesticides to humans and the effect of pesticides on the environment.

Unlike most other substances, pesticides are designed to kill pests and must be toxic to them to work. A few pesticides are toxic to nearly all animal and plant life, such as fumigants used to eliminate insects and rodents from buildings, vehicles, and grain storage containers. Most modern pesticides, however, are relatively specific because their primary toxic effects are directed only to target species. For instance, under normal conditions of use, phenoxy herbicides kill most broadleaf plants but do not adversely affect grain crops,

---

*Much of this discussion was taken from *Pesticides: Helpful or Harmful?* (New York: American Council on Science and Health, 1988) by Leonard T. Flynn, Ph.D., M.B.A., a regulatory and scientific consultant.

grasses, insects, or rodents.

Toxicity to animals, plants, or humans can be acute or chronic. Acute toxicity refers to the damage a substance can do as a result of a single exposure to relatively large amounts of the material. Chronic toxicity describes the ability of a substance to cause damage as a result of many repeated exposures during a prolonged period of time to relatively low levels of the material. Toxicity can arise from dermal (skin) contact, ingestion (oral), or inhalation. Eye exposure to some chemicals may be potentially hazardous, but eye damage is usually due to the local irritant properties of the substance rather than its systemic toxicity.

The interspecies difference in toxicity explains why a given concentration of an insecticide spray or dust is lethal to insects but harmless to humans. The tremendous difference in body weight between insects and larger animals or humans also provides protection since a larger individual can tolerate greater amounts of a toxicant than can small insects. There is always a need to keep any chemical away from children, who are both smaller and generally more sensitive than adults to toxicants. For example, common table salt can be lethal to small children; the lethal dose for a one-year-old child is about two tablespoonfuls.

To properly estimate human chronic toxicity hazards for pesticides already in use, the best population to study is not laboratory rats or *in vitro* (test-tube) laboratory experiments, but workers who face occupational exposure to the substances, usually in much greater quantities and for longer periods than consumers would ever experience from residues. Based on this information, "if the people receiving the heaviest exposure during the application of a pesticide show no ill-effects, then it is extremely improbable that those absorbing minute traces in food will suffer any ill-effects."

Americans Lobby Against Pesticides

To the extremists, *pesticide* has been a term synonymous with death. Pesticides are feared and misunderstood. Most people, however, don't understand that the pesticides in use today are selective. That is, they only exert their toxic effect on small numbers of species, usually those species whose elimination increases crops and preserves foodstuffs. As with any chemical or drug, pesticides can be dangerous to human life if our exposure to them exceeds safe limits. Indeed, pesticide poisoning has resulted in human illness and environmental harm. Fortunately, though, such instances are rare. Of the approximately 4,500 lethal poisonings in the United States each year only about 25, or 0.6 percent are due to agricultural chemicals.[14]

The general public's fear of man-made chemical carcinogens could well be the result of the poor manner in which the results of scientific studies are presented to the public. This fear and misunderstanding is compounded by sensationalized and inaccurate accounts proliferated by the news media.

In the years since *Silent Spring* was published, and more intensively since the early 1970s, pesticides have been maligned by the "America the poisoned" lobby. Numerous pesticides have been banned because of data that failed, by all scientific standards, to indicate a hazard to humans. Incredibly, some pesticides, such as aldrin and dieldrin, have been banned based solely on laboratory cancer data in one species of animal, oftentimes the mouse. And, as any toxicologist will tell you, mice have a high rate of *naturally* occurring liver tumors; to show that a chemical is a potential carcinogen in humans, tumors should be induced in at least one other species.

But, even more incredible, as in the case of aldrin and dieldrin, there was conclusive evidence that humans who were heavily exposed showed no ill health effects. Let's look more closely at these two pesticides.

Aldrin and Dieldrin—A Cancer Hazard to Humans?

The suspension—and eventual cancellation—of aldrin and dieldrin use was one of the most controversial of the pesticide bannings of the early 1970s. These compounds were at one time major pest-control agents for use on corn. At the peak of their popularity, the compounds (principally aldrin) were used on some 20 percent of U.S. corn acreage.[15] Dieldrin was amply used as a cotton insecticide in the 1950s but never achieved the popularity of aldrin.

Aldrin and dieldrin are usually treated together because they differ by only one oxygen atom (dieldrin has the extra) and aldrin can be metabolized to dieldrin. Both are part of a class of chemicals called chlorinated cyclodienes. Other pesticides in this class are endrin, heptachlor, and chlordane.

Are aldrin and dieldrin hazardous? Interestingly, these pesticides, now banned, are some three times less toxic than the most acutely toxic pesticides still in use today. The aldrin-dieldrin case is one of the few decided back in the early 1970s when the EPA had just taken over, from USDA, the job of regulating pesticides. EPA's decisions turned purely and simply on what was going to be called a carcinogen and what wasn't. Let's review the human evidence, true environmental concerns, and then the laboratory data that actually made the decision *and* set the precedent for other chemical bannings.

Accidental human poisoning by aldrin and dieldrin has sometimes caused temporary liver damage. But, aldrin and dieldrin were not even frequently involved in human poisonings.[16] There was basically little to suggest that aldrin and dieldrin were notoriously bad actors in regard to human poisoning or other health effects. Although aldrin and dieldrin persist in the environment, and had been implicated in some wildlife problems,[17] an EPA advisory committee said in 1972 that these pesticides did not pose an environmental concern. They further said that direct application to soil should be continued because the risk was so minimal.[18]

Numerous studies were conducted on various animal species to evaluate the carcinogenicity of these pesticides. A summary of the results includes

1. Aldrin in mice: Incidence of liver tumors in the animals fed aldrin was well within the normal range, and the tumors that did occur could have occurred by chance.[19]

2. Aldrin in rats: When rats were fed doses of aldrin eight times greater than the doses fed to mice in the above study, there was no statistically significant excess of tumors at any site.[20]

3. Dieldrin in mice: Some studies have produced inconsistent results between males and females, but other studies have actually suggested that dieldrin has a *protective* effect; that is, animals who received dieldrin actually had fewer tumors than the animals who did not.

4. Dieldrin in dogs and monkeys: Such tests were deemed inadequate because the testing period was too short.

How, then, have various scientific bodies evaluated the evidence of carcinogenicity for aldrin and dieldrin? One major review concluded that available data did not meet criteria required to detect carcinogenic activity.[21] A Health, Education and Welfare (HEW) committee later concluded that aldrin and dieldrin could be judged positive for tumor induction on the basis of one or more adequate tests.[22] The International Agency for Research on Cancer concluded that dieldrin was a liver carcinogen in the mouse, but that conflicting results prevented making a judgment on aldrin.[23] The consensus appears to be that dieldrin at least can in some way increase the incidence of liver tumors in mice. This may or may not be true of aldrin. Neither compound appears capable of elevating tumor rates in rats, even when fed at much higher levels than those fed to mice.

However, despite the lack of any condemning evidence aldrin and dieldrin *were condemned;* they were banned. The aldrin-dieldrin case was significant indeed. As we shall see, the decision in their case set an undesirable precedent for dealing with other chemicals. It said, in essence, that if there was any suggestion of excess tumors *regardless of how inappropriate the test system or negative tests in other systems,* then that chemical should be labeled a cancer threat. Neither was there consideration of the level of human exposure.

Let's take a minute and delve further into this issue of how carcinogenic tests in animals should be interpreted.

The crux of the matter is: If a substance elevates the incidence of liver tumors in mice, but not in any other species, what does this mean for it as a human cancer hazard? Scientific opinion has been divided on this, but even back in 1974 the majority view among toxicologists was that a compound that produced *only liver tumors in only mice* should be further evaluated before making pronouncements on whether or not it could pose a cancer risk in humans.

For example, the suspension notice for aldrin-dieldrin cites a 1973 report of the FAO Working Committee on Pesticide Residues; the report states:

> The meeting agreed that there is a serious lack of knowledge regarding the processes involved in the development of liver tumors by mice and that it would be unwise to classify a substance as a carcinogen solely on the basis of evidence of an increased incidence of tumors of a kind that may occur spontaneously with such a high frequency.

In general, it was felt that if exposing mice to a pesticide was associated with an increased risk of developing liver tumors, long-term feeding studies on at least one other species should be required.[24]

The hearing examiner (an administrative law judge) for aldrin and dieldrin, however, chose to disregard the joint statement of these two expert committees, solely on the grounds that, of all the many experts on these committees, one was subsequently retained by manufacturers of aldrin and dieldrin to testify in their behalf. The hearing examiner, instead, chose to base his decision on the relevance of mouse-liver tumors and almost exclusively on the testimony of a single expert, who had based his remarks on a published review with the following conclusion:

> The present review indicates that the induction of liver tumors in the mouse should be considered as valid as the evidence obtained in the rat and/or the hamster at any site. *It does not imply that the chemical which has been tested with negative results in one or more species should be automatically regarded as having a possible carcinogenic effect on man solely on the grounds that it induces liver tumors in the mouse* [emphasis added].[25]

In other words, this expert actually recommended *against* relying solely on mouse-liver data to ban a chemical. By these criteria, aldrin and dieldrin should not have been automatically presumed to pose a cancer risk to man. That the judge did presume them to be carcinogenic was based on his *incorrect* conclusion that tests in rats had not been adequately conducted (in actuality, the rat tests were quite adequate; they indicated no carcinogenicity). Aldrin and dieldrin were suspended and eventually canceled on the basis of "potential carcinogenic risk to humans," all based solely on evidence involving the livers of mice. The suspension actually required a finding of "imminent hazard," something that is usually considered to be quite difficult to show. In the judge's order, sixteen "findings of fact" were listed that referred to the rationale for finding that aldrin and dieldrin posed an "imminent hazard" of cancer to humans (none of these referred to human exposure levels). In the subsequent cancellation orders, these were recast into seventeen points that took on the popular name "EPA's seventeen principles" for assessing cancer hazards. It is crucial to recognize, however, that these principles were so at variance with the views of the general toxicological community that the decision was ridiculed world-wide. (The distinguished British medical journal *Lancet* soon after published an article facetiously titled "17 Points About Cancer of Something."[26]) And finally, most people who came to fear aldrin and dieldrin after the hearings never knew that Dr. Saffiotti, the misinterpreted witness, *disavowed the "principles" and indicated that he did not consider aldrin and dieldrin to be carcinogens in humans.*

Contemporary scientific thinking about the relevance of mouse-liver tumors have not changed much from those expressed nearly twenty years ago in both the World Health Organization expert group report and the review cited by the judge's favorite witness (if the conclusion isn't misread). The mouse-liver tumor is still considered a shaky basis for considering something to be a carcinogen if that is the only tumor seen. In addition, other evidence casts further doubt on past interpretations of mouse liver tumors. Scientists know that tumors that develop in the strains of mice used in cancer bioassays seem to fall into four types (based on microscopic analysis), and only two are caused by carcinogenic agents. Interestingly, the other two types of tumors may occur spontaneously at rates of up to 60 percent and may or may not be influenced by chemicals. (Such tumors can be influenced by chemicals to grow more rapidly or less rapidly, but they must first occur spontaneously.)[27] Clearly, then, we'll never be sure what type of tumor was seen in the old bioassays; only careful reanalysis could ever clarify the issue.

Clearly, if the cancellation of aldrin and dieldrin was based essentially on their posing a cancer hazard to humans (as EPA claims[28]), the decision simply did not accurately reflect scientific understanding of the issues then or now. How such a decision could have been made is perhaps illuminated by a statement in a document on the pitfalls of animal data in hazard evaluation prepared by the Task Force of Past Presidents of the Society of Toxicology:

Confusion between the scientific and societal determinants is certain to occur when a societal determinant of some decision is enunciated in terms that appear scientific but make no sense scientifically. For example, a regulatory philosophy which declares that the finding of a tumor in some animal species as a result of exposure to a given chemical at any dosage must be taken as evidence of the potential carcinogenicity of that chemical in man *stems totally from a social judgment and not at all from hard science* [emphasis added]. Yet, the statement may be such as to constitute unwarranted crossing of the borderline into science for the justification of the social policy decision to regulate under the rubric of potential carcinogenesis.[29]

Unfortunately, it would appear that the regulatory decision on aldrin and dieldrin fell somewhere in that twilight zone between science and policy.

Chlordane and Heptachlor, and the Termites

Chlordane and the chemically similar heptachlor are another classic example of pesticides banned in the 1980s solely on the basis of causing liver tumors in mice.

All uses of heptachlor were canceled or phased out by EPA by 1988 in a consolidated proceeding in which heptachlor and chlordane were considered together.[30] Like that for chlordane and for aldrin-dieldrin, the "evidence" for a presumptive carcinogenic risk to humans was *solely* mouse-liver tumors.

Before the total ban, there was a partial ban in the 1970s, allowing chlordane to be used to termite-proof homes. This exception was allowed largely because nothing else really works as well or lasts as long. The termite-proofing of a home needs to last at least twenty years to provide adequate protection.

As it turns out, chlordane is one of the least active compounds for increasing the frequency of mouse-liver tumors of the five or six chemicals that seem to be useful in termite-proofing. Chlordane is applied as a subsurface injection to protect the foundation of a home, an application method that renders it unlikely that humans will have much, if any, exposure to chlordane.

The chlordane controversy peaked in 1982 when it was learned that some armed forces housing units had measurable levels of the chemical, used to control termites there. Disregarding the fact that these levels *were well below NAS guidelines for permissible exposure to chlordane vapors,* many vented the usual hue and cry to ban this use of chlordane. The canard was that chlordane was a "suspected" carcinogen and so any exposure was intolerable. Since this was based on *mouse-liver data* only, the suspicion would at most be weak. Nonetheless, there was considerable public concern since several million homes nationwide had been termite-proofed with chlordane.

Did these chemicals pose a health risk to humans? A Harvard School of Public Health study on workers who were employed in the manufacture of chlordane and heptachlor from 1946 to 1976 and heavily exposed to the chemicals found "no overall excess of deaths from cancer, even among workers followed twenty or more years after entry into the occupation."[31] Another study done on chlordane-producing workers at the Velsicol plant in Marshall, Illinois, during the same period (and then extended through 1980), similarly concluded, "There is, thus, no evidence of any long-term latent effect on health-related disease in any way to employment at the Velsicol plant in Marshall, Illinois[32] (which manufactured chlorinated hydrocarbon insecticides for thirty-four years).

Unfortunately, a person alarmed by partial or distorted facts often jumps on the bandwagon to ban the chemical that has been represented as dangerous. Fearing cancer and/or other health effects, that person, who has now become an alarmist, frequently pays no attention to facts on the rare occasions that such facts are readily available. Frequently, confusing information complicates the picture to an even greater extent. Unfortunately, a number of scientifically meaningless papers are published, papers that unfortunately carry a lot of political and legal value, and they confuse consumers and policymakers alike. Consider the claim of Peter Infante, D.D.S., of OSHA, who found an alleged association between chlordane exposure and some childhood illnesses, such as blood disorders. Amazingly, Dr. Infante supplied no data on chlordane or heptachlor levels in blood or fat samples of the affected children. He simply assumed that since these products were used in the residences of these children, a causal relationship existed. Subsequent studies discredited his claim that pesticide exposure leads to blood disorders, but the damage—further alarming people—had already been done.

The whole controversy seemed to die down once it was realized that the entry of chlordane vapors into the houses in which it had been found appeared to result from faulty installation of heating/cooling ducts underneath slab foundation houses. Interestingly, what cooled the situation down was not the realization that chlordane did not pose a significant hazard (if any) at the levels found in the military houses, but the collective sigh of relief when millions of homeowners realized, "My home's not one of that type so I don't have a problem."

In 1984 "chlordane, the human health hazard," was once again elevated to the nightly news programs and daily newspaper columns when detectable levels of the pesticide residue were found only in rooms in five Long Island public schools. While the levels found were within the acceptable safety guidelines, a frightened public—thanks to a media that embellished the news—once again became chemophobic, waving the anticorporate/antichemical banner. A sample of the coverage follows:

It is too late to save that home in East Islip. It is too late to save those who have died from pesticide contamination. It might be too late to save those who are now dying. But it is not too late to save our environment. Yet.
　　　　　　　　　　—Patrick Halpin, New York State Assemblyman[33]

I care for my children properly and here's something I have absolutely no control over, and I want to help. I want to help my children grow up healthy. . . .
　　　The chlordane problem surfaced in the schools when pregnant teachers complained of miscarriages and respiratory problems.
　　　　　　　　　　—"Eleven O'Clock WCBS-TV News," New York[34]

Although one should not dismiss the finding of chlordane—or any other chemical for that matter—in a public school, one must thoughtfully consider the necessary facts. Appropriate monitoring to test that dangerous levels of chlordane had not accumulated and cleanup procedures were certainly called for. But based on the large body of knowledge about chlordane toxicity collected after many years and compulsive research, it was evident that Long Island teachers and children were not at any health risk from exposure to the levels of pesticide residue present there.

　　　Now let's turn to some pesticides for which no credible evidence of hazard to humans under normal-use conditions exists, but which have been tarred and feathered anyway.

Malathion versus Medfly

Few people will soon forget the image that stands out as the highlight of summer 1981—the medfly holding the richest state in the United States for ransom. Many in the California agricultural community believe that the medfly infestation would not have reached the extent it did if aerial treatment of the infested areas with malathion had been started sooner. Whether this is an accurate assessment or not, there is no question that the aerial application of malathion (which did eventually eradicate the medfly in California) was personally delayed by the governor of California. The governor gave the go-ahead to spray malathion only when the secretary of the U.S. Department of Agriculture threatened to place California under quarantine. What was it about malathion that concerned the governor sufficiently to get involved in this colossal game of "chicken" with the USDA?

　　　Factually, nothing. Regarding its toxicity in any form, malathion is one of the safest pesticides currently in use. It is practically nontoxic to man, has *not* been found to be carcinogenic, and seems not to create problems in any of a number of public health applications where it finds considerable use (mosquito control is one major use of malathion). The same techniques to which Governor Brown objected had proved safe and effective in medfly outbreaks in Texas and Florida. So why would anyone be concerned about using malathion to get rid of fruit flies?

The trouble seems to trace to a group of environmental activists in the area that was to be sprayed. While these folk may have been well intentioned, their reaction to the prospect of malathion use was irrational. Their basic fears received fuel in the form of an out-of-date (and since discredited) study dug up by a Stanford University professor, a study that suggested that malathion might pose a risk of genetic damage. Despite numerous, more modern studies establishing that malathion was not likely to injure anybody's genes, the opponents of spraying dug in around the professor and his study.

But by repeated stalling tactics, Governor Brown and this band of environmentalists succeeded in unnecessarily frightening hundreds of thousands of Californians, costing the state roughly $100 million and providing the Japanese with a convenient excuse to embargo California fruit, to the benefit of their balance of payments, and to the detriment of ours.

The sequence of events during the medfly crisis provides a classic example of nonscience in action. As a proponent of the "organic" way of life, Brown based his objections to spraying malathion on what he felt was America's increasing addiction to polluting pesticides and chemicals. He expressed concern for the public health threat that the "addiction" poses for future generations. Perhaps one can argue that the governor's goals may have been admirable, but such flagrant disregard of the evidence in this specific case does much to ruin his credibility.

BROWN VERSUS EXPERTS

The California Department of Health Sciences made an extensive study of the recommended malathion bait spray and concluded that it was completely safe. Brown didn't accept this. When new medfly sites were discovered at an alarming rate in 1981, a committee of experts *appointed by Brown* insisted that immediate aerial spraying was necessary. The governor still refused and suggested that malathion spraying would cause cancer. This was contrary to scientific fact. Dr. Bruce Ames, of the University of California and an expert on the relation of chemicals to cancer, was quoted as saying that aerial malathion spraying carries about the same cancer hazard as that posed by spreading a can of diet soda over your whole front lawn.

Although California has countless agricultural experts, Governor Brown put the campaign against the medfly in the hands of an inexperienced young attorney.

The governor finally permitted aerial spraying after other states and Japan embargoed California fruit. By that time, the medfly had spread so far that the state's richest agricultural areas were threatened and extreme pest-control measures were necessary. Farmers wishing to export fruit had to spray very heavily and resort to the use of fumigation chambers. These chambers cost about $100,000 each and used chemicals of a magnitude much more dangerous than the malathion that Brown had found so objectionable.

Fortunately, the USDA and the California courts prevailed before California's citrus agriculture was irrevocably lost to the medfly. The aerial spraying went on, the medfly was eradicated, and as reported in a number of media across the United States, no one was harmed by malathion. In 1992, there are no restrictions on the use of malathion in the United States.

Sevin and the Gypsy Moth

This is yet another case where the opposition of so-called environmentalists is puzzling. Gypsy moths annually destroy millions of acres of prime forest in the United States. Originally a problem in the Northeast, it has now spread to other areas of the United States, endangering forests in those places. What makes the gypsy moth such an environmental problem is the fact that it has few natural enemies (it was imported into the United States) and the caterpillars are voracious. An active infestation can defoliate an area of forest land. Sufficient defoliation can kill many of the trees and other plants affected.

One would think that true environmentalists would welcome a compound that is virtually nontoxic to humans, doesn't cause cancer in animals, and kills the defoliating gypsy moth. However, a policy position against pesticide use outweighs any concerns that environmentalists may have for preserving our forests.

What charge do these opponents of gypsy moth control level at Sevin to keep it from being sprayed? Sevin can cause birth defects!

Carbaryl (generic chemical name for Sevin) has been shown to produce teratogenic effects in beagle dogs. But this effect has been shown in a number of other studies and international scientific reviews to be a peculiarity of the way beagle dogs metabolize carbaryl. *No qualified, competent toxicologist would today claim that Sevin poses a risk of birth defects in humans;* in 1992 the EPA classifies Sevin as having only low teratogenic *potential.* Epidemiological studies of health, with particular emphasis on reproductive health and birth outcomes done in areas in which Sevin has been used against gypsy moths and comparable areas, have revealed absolutely no differences in health or birth outcomes. These studies, conducted by the New Jersey Department of Public Health, were done in response to public concerns fanned by opponents of gypsy moth control, not because there was a credible scientific reason to look for an effect in humans.

Not all environmentalists oppose gypsy moth control per se, although there are many who assert that the gypsy moth problem will go away on its own (it hasn't done so for the last ten or fifteen years). Those environmentalists who go along with some effort to protect trees and land from loss to gypsy moths generally seem to favor the use of a spray containing the bacterium *Bacillus thuringiensis,* also called BT for short. Unlike Sevin, BT does not provide a quick reduction of pest populations since it takes longer for the bacterium to act on the caterpillars than it does for the carbaryl (which kills the caterpillars within minutes). As a result, BT may not be as effective against heavy infestations as is Sevin. Furthermore, BT is not very specific for the gypsy moth, and BT is far more expensive.

While the opponents of Sevin use continue to disinform the public about "hazards," gypsy moths continue to ruin prime woodlands. Millions of pet owners who safely use Sevin-based flea powders and millions of home gardeners who safely use the various Sevin-based garden insecticides sit back and wonder at it all. As with malathion, in 1992 there are no restrictions on the use of Sevin in the United States.

Kepone—The Polluting of the James River

I have made the point that when a pesticide is not used properly or a faulty health hazard evaluation covers up the true toxicity of a compound, both human and ecological poisoning can occur. A classic example of this is the story of the pesticide kepone.

Kepone has never been widely used in this country. In tropical areas outside the United States, including Puerto Rico, kepone has been used to combat the banana root borers that threaten banana crops. Domestically, however, the pesticide has been used only for fire ant and cockroach control, almost exclusively in small traps marketed for residential use. Because of its limited uses, the scientific community has given little attention to kepone over the years. Environmental exposure had been minimal; therefore, little is known about the hazards posed.

Hopewell, Virginia, was the site of the only kepone-producing plant in the country during the mid-1970s. Kepone production had previously been done by the Allied Chemical Corporation, with no record of worker safety violations or history of adverse health effects. Because of the limited use of kepone, Allied decided to cancel production of the product for business reasons in the early 1970s. But shortly thereafter, Allied contracted Life Science Products, a small company run by the two former Allied employees who had developed and patented kepone, to produce kepone for it. Production began in early

1974 and continued for sixteen months at the Hopewell plant, which was a converted gasoline service station.

It wasn't long before many workers began to experience kepone's classic first syndrome, referred to as the shakes. Company doctors and other physicians in town repeatedly failed in properly diagnosing the ailments described by the workers. Most workers were not overly concerned about the shakes, assuming that since everybody seemed to have them, it must not be worth getting upset over. In addition, there was a widely held desire not to "bite the hand that feeds you." The plant provided a major boost to the local economy, and without it many jobs would be lost.

Yunan Chou, M.D., came to Hopewell in 1976 to practice as an internist. He, too, was baffled by the symptoms of one worker he examined. Dr. Chou sent a blood sample from this worker to the CDC in Atlanta, where analysis showed the blood loaded with kepone. State epidemiologists were immediately notified. Upon visiting the plant, the epidemiologists and health officials were horrified. Kepone was literally everywhere—on the floor, on the machines, on workers' clothing. Direct contact with the dust was the norm in the plant. The plant was closed immediately.

About half the plant's one hundred fifty workers, plus an estimated ten family members, suffered from some degree of acute kepone poisoning. Symptoms included liver damage, tremors, blurred vision, skin discoloration, joint and chest pains, stuttering, anxiety, and memory loss. In addition, the Medical College of Virginia reported that fourteen workers were probably sterile as a result of their exposure.

During the time that the workers were exposed to kepone, Life Science was dumping large amounts of untreated waste into the James River. The city of Hopewell had applied for and received a permit for discharge into the waterway. However, industrial wastes were not mentioned in the permit application. The effluent standards were immediately and continually violated during the operation of the plant.

In the aftermath of the Hopewell incident, a new study was begun to try to determine the effects of kepone on man and the environment. The findings as summarized in the 1978 National Academy of Sciences report indicate that kepone "appears to be capable of causing adverse chronic effects [including tumors in mice] in various terrestrial organisms at relatively low levels of exposure."[35] The chemical was found to be lethal to rats, rabbits, and dogs, also causing in these test animals a wide variety of health effects, including liver, skin, and nervous system ailments.

Environmental studies indicate that kepone is stable and persistent. It can leach through soil, making groundwater contamination a potential problem if it is used in vulnerable aquifer recharge zones. Aquatic plants and animals alike were shown to accumulate the chemical, posing a threat to eaters of fish drawn from contaminated waters.

This incident cost Life Science an estimated $25 million. Since the episode left Life Science and its owners bankrupt, there were no fines collected from those mainly responsible for creating the occupational hazard at Hopewell. Allied contributed approximately $8 million to the Medical College of Virginia, which used the funds to study the toxic effects of kepone on the human body. The company was fined for dumping wastes without a permit, an activity that took place before the Life Science debacle and was probably insignificant in comparison. The sum of $6 million went to the state of Virginia and the rest went to compensate the victims of the kepone contamination, both the workers in the plant and the fishermen of the affected James River and Chesapeake Bay.

A study at the Medical College of Virginia produced a means of treating those suffering from kepone poisoning. The compound is, for the most part, stable, and is not excreted from the body. It will therefore remain in the body and accumulate with repeated exposure. But a treatment was developed that enables the system to collect kepone and subsequently excrete the chemical. The body burdens of those afflicted were thus reduced to negligible levels and the observed symptoms disappeared.

Fortunately, the amounts of kepone used in home ant and cockroach traps were less than nontoxic acute doses in test animals. However, in 1977 the USDA reported fifty-six cases of acute kepone poisoning, most of which were children exposed in their homes by contact with the traps.

In 1976 the EPA issued a notice telling of its intent to cancel use of kepone in ant and cockroach traps. Life Science Products had gone bankrupt; Allied Chemical did not object. With the closing of the Hopewell plant, there no longer were any plants manufacturing the product in the country. All uses of kepone were canceled by the EPA in 1977.

Kepone, a chemical that caused human suffering and ecological damage, serves to remind us of what can happen when worker safety is jeopardized and poorly treated wastes are dumped thoughtlessly into our waterways. But that event does not mean that all pesticides, or chemicals for that matter, are hazards. What it does mean is that we need to carefully produce, monitor, and test the products being developed today, using the scientific technology available to prevent future Hopewells while working toward ensuring that the billions of people in the world do not go to bed hungry.

IBT Labs—Scandal Jolts the Pesticide Industry

To say that chemicals used in the manufacture of pesticides are tested and found safe is not something that can be taken for granted. In the late 1970s and early 1980s we learned how the major private laboratory conducting toxicological studies on developing products deceived industry, federal regulators, and the public through negligent study procedures and make-believe results. When the practices of Industrial Bio-Test, Inc. (IBT), a subsidiary of Nalco Chemical Company, became known to the public, shock waves rocked the toxicological testing community. At worst, it could have led to a huge public health hazard. At best, it constituted large-scale scientific fraud.

When in 1976 the Food and Drug Administration (FDA) and later the Justice Department began their investigations, the IBT nightmare emerged from the labs and file cabinets at the Northbrook, Illinois, plant to the desktops of pesticide manufacturers and federal regulators. As a result of the IBT incident, the EPA and the FDA have revised and coordinated the process by which laboratory work is inspected. This should prevent future IBT-type scandals.

In addition, the EPA was saddled with the task of wading through the IBT files to determine what, if any, IBT work was valid.

In 1952 Joseph C. Calandra founded what was to become the biggest commercial lab in the country, IBT. Dr. Calandra was, at the time, a recent graduate of the Northwestern University School of Medicine. His business was a gold mine. Manufacturers were producing countless new chemicals and products, and laboratory study was needed to comply with federal regulations on chemical safety. Many branches of the federal government sought services provided by private labs, and IBT quickly found clients in agencies like the Department of Defense, the FDA, and the National Institute of Drug Abuse.

By the time it folded in the late 1970s, IBT had conducted approximately twenty-two thousand validation studies. Such studies are done with the purpose of clearing a chemical for use in a commercial product, such as a pesticide or pharmaceutical drug. A host of products eventually were marketed whose safety was based solely or in part on IBT studies.

The beginning of the end for IBT occurred in April 1976, when a former FDA investigator, Adrian Gross, turned up for a spot check of the lab's recent testing reports. Upon reviewing IBT's study on the arthritis drug Naprosyn, Dr. Gross became suspicious of foul play. The spring 1983 *Amicus Journal* quotes Gross as saying that "none of the rats had developed cancer. Now, any pathologist knows that rats and mice on these long-term studies develop cancer naturally and will have a certain level of mortality. IBT's study said the rats were all clean."[36]

In the months and years that followed, the seedy operations at IBT were uncovered. Perhaps most indicative of the bogus science coming out of IBT was the use of a room known as the "Swamp." A faulty automatic watering system that was intended to clean cages and fill drinking water bottles turned a large feeding room into a hideous mix of decomposed and dying rodents.

The FDA and the Justice Department gathered evidence for five years, and in May 1981 a federal grand jury indicted four executives from IBT:

Calandra, IBT's ex-president; Dr. Paul Wright, a former toxicology department head; Dr. Moreno Keplinger, a former general manager; and James Plank, Keplinger's former assistant. The charges included fraud for the distribution of phony data and an attempt at covering up the deceptions practiced at IBT.

After much delay, the trial started in Chicago on April 4, 1983. However, on July 11, John A. Nordberg, the federal district judge, granted a mistrial to Calandra because of poor health. The remaining three defendants were convicted on multiple counts of fraud or falsifying data after a six-month trial.

When the IBT story broke, officials at the EPA were quick to recognize the statutory problem—no existing legal framework allowed EPA scientists to carry out sufficient quality-assurance programs. As a result of the newfound necessity to monitor validation studies closely, the EPA in 1977 entered into an interagency agreement with the FDA, which does have the legal right to audit laboratory facilities. Under the new arrangement, EPA staff members can accompany FDA officials when auditing labs. The FDA is responsible for examining the conditions of facilities, quality of staff, and procedures employed for a given study. EPA scientists have access to laboratory records, including all data compiled and reports filed by the lab personnel. The EPA attempts to ensure that validation recommendations are backed up by properly obtained raw data.

Validation studies for new pesticides must be submitted for EPA approval before registration and marketing. The EPA and the Canadian Protection Board of Health and Welfare jointly undertook the tedious process of reviewing IBT studies for validity. In all, 801 studies were identified as significant to regulatory decisions. On July 11, 1983, EPA released the long-awaited results of the review program.

The studies were broken down in a number of ways and the statistical findings get a bit confusing. Of all pesticides tested by IBT, 93 percent have valid non-IBT data available. This leaves twelve pesticides whose data base is solely derived from IBT studies. But of the twelve, seven are not being used in the United States. The IBT data on three of the remaining five pesticides were found to be partially valid, or "supplemental." Six studies on these five products will be replaced.

Of the 801 pesticide studies reviewed, 594 were found invalid. After eliminating the studies that have been replaced (212), are planned to be replaced (38), are no longer required for registration (45), or involve products not in production because of cancellation or nonregistration (140), 159 studies remain for which replacement data neither exist nor are planned.

As a result of the data gap, manufacturers of nineteen pesticides received notices informing them that the registration of the products would be suspended if no agreement for new studies was reached within ninety days. Without registration, sale of the pesticides is illegal. Fifteen more pesticides were designated by the EPA as requiring further review and discussion to determine need for studies.

To assess the impact of any chemical insult on the general population, the exposure to which we are subjected must be looked at. The EPA report stressed that of all the pesticides on the market today, only 65 percent account for approximately 80 percent of the volume of those products used. And of the 65 percent, only one, the herbicide prometon, was supported exclusively by IBT data. Therefore, the EPA concluded ". . . the data bases for the high-volume chemicals to which people are most likely to be exposed are for the most part unaffected by the IBT situation, and where there is an impact, EPA has taken active regulatory steps to obtain replacement data."

Reflecting on this dark chapter in modern science, one gets the feeling that we, as a society, dodged a bullet. The IBT fiasco could have exposed countless people to a vast array of chemicals of unknown toxicity. That this did not happen can be largely attributed to luck. The EPA-FDA audit program, which was born in the aftermath of the IBT negligence, should provide an effective method of ensuring quality control throughout the pesticide testing industry. The existence of such a program, combined with the memory of how a respected, successful laboratory disintegrated into a swamp of lies, should serve to make the registration of future pesticides safer for all of us.

Should We Restrict Lawn-Care Chemicals?*

Americans spent $6.4 billion in 1990 on lawn-care products, up 13 percent from 1989. It is estimated that about 40 percent of the nation's private lawns are treated with pesticides.[37]

Most lawn-care pesticides are "general use" products—the federal Environmental Protection Agency (EPA) considers them safe for use by anyone who follows label directions. However, some types of lawn products are "restricted use" substances. They are only sold to and used by "certified applicators," persons who satisfy EPA and state training requirements. For "restricted use" pesticides the label instructions alone are not considered adequate to assure safe and proper use.

Many lawn-care pesticides have been used for decades on turf and for agricultural purposes, so experience with human exposure has been substantial. Nevertheless, scientists continue to study the toxicity of pesticides and other commercial materials to attempt to determine whether there are any unsuspected chronic effects.

---

*Much of this discussion is taken from *Lawn Care Chemicals: What Consumers Should Know* (New York: American Council on Science and Health, 1987), by Leonard T. Flynn, Ph.D., M.B.A.

Lawn-care professionals handle undiluted pesticides while they mix the solutions for lawn applications, so their potential exposure to the chemicals is much greater than that of the homeowners who hire them or their customers' neighbors. It would seem hard to disguise significant numbers of chronic health effects for such workers from health insurance investigators, occupational safety and health professionals, industrial hygienists, and medical professionals in occupational health—not to mention government regulators. Despite this comforting lack of adverse information, effects possibly related to lawn-care pesticides have recently appeared in the news.

An interesting problem with lawn-care chemicals is that homeowners use three to six times as much pesticide per acre as farmers do, often not reading the warning labels nor taking precaution to protect themselves. It is this improper overuse that most commonly causes problems, not the proper, used-according-to-the-label uses by certified applicators. Interestingly, though, when the EPA noted that geese were dying from the pesticide diazinon, the agency banned it for use on sod farms and golf courses—places where it was probably used properly by certified applicators. EPA did not ban diazinon's far more extensive use on home lawns, where it is often used excessively.[38]

RISK REDUCTION THROUGH LAWN POSTING LAWS?

Despite the rarity of allergic effects from pesticides, several local governments have adopted various requirements for notifying the public about pesticide use. From 1986 to 1988, sign-posting ordinances were adopted in Wauconda, Illinois, and in Montgomery and Prince George's Counties in Maryland. Both ordinances were challenged successfully in court by industry groups. The courts decided that under FIFRA (Federal Insecticide, Fungicide and Rodenticide Act), state or federal statutes specifically preempted the local jurisdictions from enacting pesticide regulations.

Whatever legal arguments ultimately prevail (both decisions were appealed by the local authorities), the fundamental issue is the public's "right to know" about potential hazards and the ability of sensitive individuals to, in effect, give "informed consent" to possible allergic reactions through their awareness that pesticides will be applied nearby. For these purposes the sign-posting ordinances are inferior to a program of direct notification of sensitive persons who request that they be notified of imminent pesticide treatments.

Direct notification is a standard procedure used to notify apiarists (bee-keepers) of impending pesticide applications that might endanger their hives. For example, New Jersey pesticide regulations require at least thirty-six hours advance notification to each apiarist within one-half mile of the application site for a pesticide having a label indicating it is toxic to bees. Apiarists must register with the New Jersey Department of Environmental Protection (NJDEP) prior to March 1 of each year, and the NJDEP may charge five dollars to offset its registry cost. Many other states have similar programs.

Where in effect, notification requirements provide sensitive individuals with the notice and opportunity to exercise informed consent to potential exposure. In contrast, lawn posting does not provide specific information to sensitive individuals and invites spurious complaints of illness from passers-by. The industry concern about such incidents is not without justification; "mass psychogenic illness" has been documented and hysterical reactions to sign postings for application of lawn-care chemicals are not inconceivable.

The sign posting/notification issue really raises an ethical question beyond the scope of strict scientific evaluation: how can society deal with supersensitive individuals? If your neighbor is deathly allergic to paint fumes, may you paint your house? May you allow ragweed to grow on your property and provoke serious asthma attacks next door? Must you get rid of your pet cat if the lady in the apartment across the hall is allergic? Are people compelled to gain "implied consent" and incur significant expense and inconvenience to protect their less hardy neighbors? Is the sensitive person solely responsible for him/herself and parents responsible for their sensitive children?

None of these questions is simple to answer and posting laws will do little to resolve them. In any case, the risk to anyone from lawn-care chemicals is minute compared to other common allergens and irritants that are untouched by the posting laws.

What If We Didn't Have Pesticides?*

Critics of pesticides often state that alternative pest-control methods are vastly superior to the use of chemicals and can easily replace them. This view cannot be supported by the facts.

A place exists for pesticides and for their alternatives. The development of alternate methods to suppress pests requires applying technical knowledge and conducting scientific research with the same diligence as for pesticides. For the foreseeable future, most pesticide alternatives have significant limitations, but we need all options to increase food production, improve public health, and foster a better environment.

---

*Much of this discussion is excerpted from *Pesticides: Helpful or Harmful?* (New York: American Council on Science and Health, 1988), by Leonard T. Flynn, Ph.D., M.B.A.

BIOLOGICAL CONTROLS

Various kinds of biological controls have successfully controlled a few pests. The cottony cushion scale accidentally entered California in 1868, and by 1886 it threatened to ruin the citrus industry. The vedalia ladybird beetle was intentionally introduced from Australia in 1888, and within two years the scale was under control, as it has been ever since.

At about the same time, the European gypsy moth established itself in the eastern United States, where it continued to spread despite the introduction of more than forty-five species of insects to try to control it. Only when DDT insecticide spraying from aircraft became available could the pest be controlled. When spraying was halted by public pressure, the moth spread and forest destruction continued.

Introducing predators to control pests is a limited method because many pests are native to America and flourish here in spite of their enemies. Ladybird beetles eat many aphids in a dense aphid population. They are less effective against scattered numbers of the insects that can infect a whole crop of beets and cause great losses.

Detailed knowledge of the ecological behavior of predators is required before an alien species can be safely introduced, but acquisition of this information is very expensive and may not be transferable from one region to the next. Errors can be costly: the hoped-for friend may turn out to be a pest itself.

Diseases have been used to control pests. Development of new diseases for pest control is slow and expensive. The same regulatory requirements apply to them as for chemical pesticides, and lengthy toxicological testing is required by the EPA. Because it is impossible to test all possible hosts, there is no absolute assurance of target specificity.

Advances in biotechnology may revolutionize pest control in the next ten to twenty years, but at present microbial controls are much less satisfactory than standard chemical pesticides. One reviewer of microbial insecticides believes that unless major biotechnological breakthroughs occur, "there may be no future at all for microbial insecticides as commercial products." Another recent reviewer of viral insecticides for insect control observes similarly that baculovirus products "have provided less than expected results when used as substitutes for chemical pesticides" because they are unpredictable in the field.

GENETIC CONTROLS

Development of resistant crop varieties has contributed enormously to increased productivity of modern agriculture. Wheat resistant to the Hessian fly and alfalfa resistant to the spotted alfalfa aphid have been developed. Wheat varieties able to resist black stem-rust are under constant development by wheat breeders. Unfortunately, the stem-rust also produces its own varieties, and they quickly become dominant because they are the only ones that can propagate on the new wheat. Wheat breeders must meet this recurring challenge to produce additional new wheat varieties.

CULTIVATION PRACTICES

Variations in farming practices assist in pest control. Crop rotation and fallowing help starve out insects that can survive only on one kind of plant. Choosing a suitable date for planting can avoid some pest damage; for example, moderately late plantings of corn suffer less corn rootworm damage than early plantings. Cultivation can assist but is seldom an effective substitute for chemical controls.

INTEGRATED PEST MANAGEMENT

Integrated pest management (IPM) is a carefully planned combination of control measures using sound ecological principles to keep pests below economic injury levels. IPM has been touted as a substitute or replacement for pesticides, but only a few pests can be effectively managed by integrated genetic, biological, and cultivation methods alone. A chemical frequently plays a critical role in successful IPM programs, and pesticides are the only answer to a severe pest outbreak or emergency. The diversities of urban environments within a region and among different regions "are likely to make widespread dissemination of IPM controls for home and garden pests difficult to achieve"; therefore, chemical controls are "likely to be preferred" for such uses. Modern agriculture does not neglect nonchemical methods when they are appropriate because today's farmers cannot afford to waste resources on unnecessary chemicals when less costly nonchemical methods will suffice.

Health Effects of Not Using Pesticides

Nature is not benevolent to humans who abandon science and technology. Even without agrichemicals, there is nothing "natural" about planting fields of crops or raising a herd of domestic animals. Nor is it "natural" for large human populations to live in cities or towns without coexisting vermin and the diseases they transmit. In the United States today, pest-borne diseases and attacks by pests themselves account for one hundred to three hundred deaths annually and "probably 20 times this number of serious disabling illnesses and injuries" plus "several million episodes of illness or injury that are serious enough or painful enough to require medical attention." It's been estimated that one pair of insects could produce 191 quadrillion hungry descendants in one single summer season if all of its offspring lived and reproduced normally. Without the active and deliberate intervention of man, nature would rapidly eradicate the world's food-producing capacity and unleash plagues of long-forgotten virulence. In short, humans would suffer and die.

In prosperous modern America, small-scale experiments in food production without agrichemicals can be an interesting and occasionally useful diversion. To meet the desperate food needs in poorer countries, however, such practices can be catastrophic.

Without insecticides, increasing numbers of mosquitoes would spread malaria, yellow fever, and encephalitis. Without rodenticides, a growing rat population could threaten another epidemic of plague, the "Black Death" that killed one-fourth of the population in medieval Europe and occurred as outbreaks in major U.S. cities during this century. Without herbicides, brush would replace grass in rangeland, provoking drought, erosion, and starvation for domestic animals. Without fungicides, roots and seeds would rot in the ground, and another "potato famine" could occur. Without disinfectants, hospitals would find it impossible to sanitize their facilities and thus contain infectious diseases.

Yes, a "world without pesticides" would not be a pleasant place to live. Pesticides provide three important benefits: increased food and fiber production, health protection, and environmental enhancement. They enable us to have an abundant supply of nourishing food at reasonable prices. Pesticides are our first line of defense to avoid food shortages, and they also protect our health by stopping pest-transmitted diseases and sanitizing our food handling and health facilities. Properly used, pesticides improve the environment for desirable plants, domestic animals, and human survival.

Banning Useful Pesticides is Threatening Life and Health: The African Example*

Africa's drought is a tragic legacy of recent decades. Portraits of grotesquely gaunt villagers left to die will endure in memory. During the closing months of the last decade, however, the rains finally came. Even though the soil had become moist, the crops of much of the farmland of the African Sahel were ruined before the harvest. The specter of famine still looms over the land.

---

*Much of this discussion is from an article by Thomas R. DeGregori, Ph.D., and Faith Solovey, printed in *Priorities* (Summer 1989).

TECHNOLOGY FEARS

The cause of Africa's crop destruction is locust infestations. The cure for this blight is the adequate use of effective pesticides. Although this cure, dieldrin, has been invented, it cannot be used. The countries of the African Sahel lack the means to battle locusts and are dependent upon foreign assistance. The United States and other aid donors are prohibited by law and by public opinion from providing the pesticides that can win the fight against locusts. These pesticides are prohibited because of the highly organized, well-intentioned acts of misinformed technophobes in the United States and other developed aid-donor countries. What is even sadder is that there already are large quantities of dieldrin in Africa, but there is no equipment to spread it. The result is that the children of Africa are the latest victims of our technology fears.

THE DAY OF THE LOCUST

Locusts start out, innocently enough, as grasshoppers. Their metamorphosis from grasshoppers into locusts reads like a story line for a science fiction movie. The 1988 "Hunger Report" of the House of Representatives Select Committee on Hunger describes this frightening phenomenon:

> For years at a time, locusts are solitary brown grasshoppers with short wings and long hind legs. They are rather harmless, traveling by night and eating scrub plants by day. In this quiescent form, only a few thousand will occupy an area of 500 square miles. However, when conditions are suitable—i.e., heavy rains and damp soil suitable for egg laying—a transformation occurs. Their wings lengthen and hind legs shorten, their color changes to a dirty yellow. The insect becomes hyperactive, reproduces rapidly, and swarms. In this stage, the destructive capacity is staggering: a square kilometer of swarm— 150 million locusts—can eat 100 tons of food a day. This is enough food to feed 500 people a year.

KILLING FIELDS

There are basically two different kinds of pesticides used to battle locusts. The most effective kinds are chlorinated hydrocarbons or DDT-type compounds, such as dieldrin. This pesticide, which is sprayed over strips of land in advance of the locust swarm, provides a two-pronged attack. It kills the locusts as they pass over the sprayed area and eliminates larvae in their breeding grounds before they become a threat.

The other types of pesticides commonly used against locust infestation are the organophosphates, such as malathion. Once locust swarms are located, they are sprayed directly with malathion, which is about ten times more costly to use than dieldrin. Malathion is very expensive because it works against the swarm only if the target area is sprayed repeatedly.

All evidence points to dieldrin as the obvious solution to Africa's locust-infestation problem. Yet no African country has the means to use dieldrin to save its crops. In the United States, it's illegal to provide DDT-type compounds or the funds to acquire and use them. Most other countries trying to help the African nations are stymied, too. Regardless of the requests or needs of the African nations they assist, these countries are hamstrung by legal prohibition, public pressure, or both.

FEAST OR FAMINE?

African countries have had to make do with more costly, less effective pesticides, such as malathion, that are approved by law virtually worldwide. Malathion is certainly better than nothing. In fact, it's helping to win isolated battles against infestation. However, these victories are fleeting.

Prohibition of dieldrin continues to reduce the food supply in locust-infested areas of Africa. Throughout the continent, there are farming communities whose dreams of improved harvests have been shattered by insect attacks that could have been successfully avoided or counterattacked with dieldrin as part of a program of integrated pest management.

Instead of relative plenty, there is hunger. The victims will once again be society's most vulnerable—the very young and the very old. In Africa's poor areas, hungry people become sick people. And, more often than not, they don't survive.

The ban on DDT-type compounds was initiated by well-intentioned people whose purpose was to protect the environment and human life. Instead, the laws they helped establish are aiding in the destruction of the environment and human lives. Sadly, this destruction can be measured in millions of lives lost.

It is time to embrace the benefits offered by modern science and technology. A critical examination of Africa's life-and-death battle against infestation emphasizes the dire need for the most effective pesticide, dieldrin. Dieldrin's continued ban holds hostage the health and welfare of the people who live in locust-infested areas of Africa. For them, the lawful use of dieldrin cannot come too soon.

Conclusion

With the development of increased scientific knowledge plus the use of modern pesticides and fertilizers, the past forty years have brought more progress in agricultural production than in all previous recorded history. Nevertheless, public "chemophobia"—the unreasonable fear of chemicals—has led to bans on useful products and has jeopardized this progress. Despite the enormous improvements in living standards, it seems "mankind still finds new things to make himself miserable." The news media and other groups too often "sensationalize dangers," and fail to provide a "meaningful perspective" on pesticides and pest-control issues.[39]

The environmental and health fears of pesticide opponents appear groundless. For example, insufficient data are available to estimate the pesticide-related cancer burden for the general population, but it must be considerably smaller than that associated with other environmental factors such as smoking, radon, and asbestos.[40] In contrast, the concerns of pesticide users that their livelihoods may be jeopardized by bans or other severe limitations do not seem unjustified based on recent events.

Ideally, the main thrust of regulation, science, and politics should be to improve the methods of pest management. None of our pest-control systems is perfect, and because the pests keep evolving, our present techniques may be even less effective in the future. Research and development on a wide variety of fronts must continue in order to stay even and in hopes of pulling ahead. This means encouraging research to develop better pest-control tools, including safe and more effective pesticides. Prudence on all sides—environmentalists, industry, researchers, and regulators—would be welcome.

Science and scientists must not be brushed aside by hysteria and the restrictive political decrees that follow. We must not forget that "despite the fears and real problems they create, pesticides clearly are responsible for part of the physical well-being enjoyed by most people in the United States and the western world."[41]

NOTES

1. S. Beglet, "Silent Spring Revisited," *Newsweek,* July 14, 1986, p. 72.

2. H. Patricia Hynes, *Earthright* (Rocklin: Prima Publishing and Communications, 1990), p. 18.

3. J. Skow, "Can Lawns Be Justified?" *Time,* June 3, 1991, p. 63.

4. S. Begley and M. Hager, "Please Don't Eat the Daisies," *Newsweek,* May 16, 1988, p. 77.

5. E. F. Knipling, *Basic Principles of Insect Population and Management,* USDA Handbook no. 512 (Washington, D.C.: U.S. Department of Agriculture, 1979), p. 74.

6. K. C. Barrons, *Are Pesticides Really Necessary?* (Regnery: Gateway, Inc., 1981), p. 122.

7. G. L. Carefoot and E. A. Sprott, *Famine On the Wind: Ma's Battle Against*

Plant Disease (Rand McNally, 1967).

8. G. W. Ware, *Pesticide Theory and Application* (W. W. Freeman, 1983), p. 9.

9. 40 CFR parts 152–80.

10. J. G. Edwards, "The Myth of Food-Chain Biomagnification," *Agrichemical Age* (April 1980): pp. 10, 32–33.

11. G. R. Biddinger and S. P. Gloss, "The Importance of Trophic Transfer in the Bioaccumulation of Chemical Contaminants in Aquatic Ecosystems," *Residue Reviews* 91 (1984): p. 133.

12. S. H. Kay, "Potential for Biomagnification of Contaminants Within Marine and Freshwater Food Webs," U.S. Army Corps of Engineers Technical Report D-84-7, November 1984, p. 73.

13. Food and Drug Administration Pesticide Program, "Residues in Foods 1990," *Journal of the Association of Official Analytical Chemists* 74 (1991).

14. American Council on Science and Health, *Pesticides: Helpful or Harmful?* (New York: American Council on Science and Health, 1988).

15. U.S. Environmental Protection Agency, "Consolidated Aldrin/Dieldrin Hearing: Notice of Intention to Suspend and Findings of Imminent Hazard," *Federal Register* 39 (1974): pp. 37246–72.

16. W. B. Deichmann, "The Chronic Toxicity of Organochlorine Pesticides in Man," in *Environmental Problems in Medicine,* ed. W. D. McKee (Springfield: Charles Thomas Publishers, 1974); H. C. Hodge, A. M. Boyce, W. B. Dhmann, H. F. Kraybill, "Toxicology and No-Effect Levels of Aldrin and Dieldrin," *Toxicology and Applied Pharmacology* 10 (1967): pp. 613–75.

17. Secretary's Commission on Pesticides, U.S. Department of Health, Education and Welfare, "Report of the Secretary's Commission on Pesticides and Their Relationship to Environmental Health" (Washington, D.C.: U.S. Government Printing Office, 1969).

18. U.S. EPA, "Consolidated Aldrin/Dieldrin Hearing" (1974).

19. National Toxicology Program, "Second Annual Report on Carcinogens," NTP-91-43 (Washington, D.C.: U.S. Government Printing Office, 1981); J. M. Ward, "Background Variations of Tumor Incidence in Rodent Populations," in *Safety Evaluation and Regulation of Chemicals,* ed. F. Homburger (New York: S. Karger, 1983).

20. National Toxicology Program, "Second Annual Report on Carcinogens" (1981); Ward, "Background Variations of Tumor Incidence" (1983).

21. Hodge, et al., "Toxicology and No-Effect Levels" (1967).

22. Secretary's Commission on Pesticides, U.S. Department of Health, Education and Welfare, "Report" (1969).

23. IARC, "Aldrin/Dieldrin," *Monographs on the Evaluation of Carcinogenic Risk of Chemicals to Man* (Lyon, France: International Agency for Research on Cancer, 1974), vol. 5, pp. 125 ff.

24. U.S. EPA, "Consolidated Aldrin/Dieldrin Hearing" (1974).

25. Ibid.

26. Editorial Board, "17 Points About Cancer of Something," March 13, 1976.

27. F. F. Becker, "Morphological Classification of Mouse Liver Tumors Based on Biological Characteristics," *Cancer Research* 42 (1982): pp. 3918–23.

28. U.S. EPA, "Consolidated Aldrin/Dieldrin Hearing" (1974).

29. Task Force of Past Presidents (approved by past presidents of Society of Toxicology), "Animal Data in Hazard Evaluation: Paths and Pitfalls," *Fundamentals in Applied Toxicology* (1982): pp. 101–107.

30. U.S. Environmental Protection Agency, "Consolidated Chlordane, Heptachlor Hearings: Notice of Intent of Cancel," *Federal Register* (1974): p. 41298.

31. H. Wang and B. MacMahon, "Mortality of Workers Employed in the Manufacture of Chlordane and Heptachlor," *Journal of Occupational Medicine* 21 (1979): pp. 744–48.

32. Shindell and Associates, "Report of an Epidemiological Study of the Employees of Velsicol Chemical Corporation Plant, Marshall, IL, January 1946–December 1979" (July 1980).

33. Pest Control Technology.

34. "Eleven O'Clock News" (New York: WCBS-TV, January 15, 1984).

35. National Academy of Science, *Kepone/Mirex/Hexachlorocyclopentadiene: An Environmental Assessment* (Washington, D.C.: National Academy Press, 1978).

36. K. Schneider, "Faking It," *Amicus Journal* 4 (1983): pp. 14–26.

37. P. Elmer-DeWitt, "Can Lawns Be Justified?," *Time,* June 3, 1991, p. 63.

38. Ibid., p. 64.

39. R. Snetsinger, *The Ratcatcher's Child: The History of the Pest Control Industry* (Franzak and Foster Co., 1982), pp. 28–88.

40. S. R. Baker and C. F. Wilkinson, *The Effect of Pesticides on Human Health* (Princeton: Princeton Scientific Publishing, 1990), p. 22.

41. B. L. Bohmont, *The New Pesticide User's Guide* (Reston Publishing Co.; Prentice Hall, 1983), pp. 3–4.

5

Food Safety:
Are There Carcinogens in Our Diet?

The Charges

Our nation's children are being harmed by the very fruits and vegetables we tell them will make them grow up healthy and strong. These staples of children's diets routinely, and lawfully, contain dangerous amounts of pesticides, which pose an increased risk of cancer, neurobehavioral damage and other health problems.

—Intolerable Risk: Pesticides in Our Children's Food[1]

The most common American foods contain pesticide residues that constitute nearly 80% of the estimated dietary cancer risk for man, according to a National Academy of Sciences report released in May.

—Audubon[2]

Although a few [natural] additives, preservatives and emulsifiers are useful, most are either unnecessary or used in excess. Worse, most have not been adequately tested, especially in the combinations in which they are consumed.

—Design for a Livable Planet[3]

The problem is that to begin with it may cause cancer, we don't know at this point. The FDA has done studies but it's not done on all of the foods that you might eat. Furthermore, there are nutrient losses. Look at all these good vegetables, but when you irradiate them, what happens to the nutrients? Do they stay there? Not as much. Customers will be getting a bum deal when they have irradiated food.

—Ellen Haas, executive director of Public Voice for Food and Health Policy[4]

Irradiation is believed by many scientists and consumer groups to threaten public health because it depletes the nutritional value of our diet, masks the bacterial contamination of rotting food, and exposes the consumer to cesium 137, cobalt 60, and other carcinogens.

— *Design for a Livable Planet*[5]

The Facts

- There is no evidence that current levels of pesticide residues in food are causing any acute or chronic adverse health effects in the U.S. population.[6]

- The results of Food and Drug Administration (FDA) Total Diet Studies, which identify the levels of pesticide residues actually consumed by various age/sex population subgroups, show that total dietary intake is usually less than 1 percent of the acceptable daily intake for both domestic and imported products.[7]

- The perception that the food supply is unsafe is not supported by scientific data; the American food supply is the safest in the world. Current allocation of resources devoted to food safety is not commensurate with actual risks but more with risks as perceived by the public.[8]

- When food is irradiated under conditions of FDA approval, no new chemical (radiolytic) products have been detected.

- The vast, overwhelming, and unprecedented body of scientific data has convinced the World Health Organization, the U.N. Food and Agriculture Organization, and the super-cautious U.S. Food and Drug Administration that irradiated food is safe, nutritious, and wholesome.

- The U.S. Department of Agriculture estimates that the American consumer will receive approximately $2 in benefits (reduced spoilage, less illness) for each $1 spent on irradiating food.

Alar on apples. Antibiotics in animal feed. Hormones in milk. And, of course, ubiquitous food additives. If we listen to the press, we are convinced that we are being poisoned through our very sustenance. Starting with the apple bin, let's head down the grocery store aisles to assess the safety of our food supply.

The Alar Apple Scam—Lessons Learned*

On February 26, 1989, Americans sitting down to get their usual fill of scandal and wrongdoing on "60 Minutes" ended up getting more than they bargained for: a silent killer in their midst, perhaps right at their very dinner table. "The most potent cancer-causing agent in our food supply," intoned reporter Ed Bradley, "is a substance sprayed on apples to keep them on the trees longer and make them look better."

The story went on to cite the findings of "a number of scientific experts," who argued that eating those apples over a lifetime could cause thousands of cancers. And the individuals at greatest risk turned out to be society's weakest, most vulnerable members: children. So confident of the report's findings was Mr. Bradley that he went on to give them his personal endorsement as the "most careful study yet on the effect of [the apple spray] daminozide and seven other cancer causing pesticides on the food children eat."

So began the great apple scare of 1989. The results were not long in coming. Washington's regulatory apparatus cranked up to prevent the looming baby slaughter. The apple industry turned into apple sauce as apple prices plummeted and sales fell off. Hysterical parents fretted over lunch box contents, in one case sending state troopers to flag down a school bus after a mother realized she had sent her child off to school toting the forbidden fruit. School administrators expelled the apple summarily. Taxpayers got stuck with the bill for apple leftovers.

In fact, daminozide, better known as Alar, isn't a pesticide, Mr. Bradley's remarks about daminozide and "seven other cancer-causing pesticides" notwithstanding. It is a growth regulator that allows the fruit more time to ripen on the tree before it falls to the ground, making it more appealing to consumers with a taste for redder, riper apples. Nor do trace amounts of Alar necessarily cause cancer. Indeed, scientific experts not consulted by Mr. Bradley dismissed health concerns about eating apples. Shortly after the "60 Minutes" program ran, a major scientific group called on consumers to eat more fruits and vegetables, not less. But its message was lost amid the talk shows and headlines trumpeting news about poisons in the vegetable patch—just as David Fenton might have predicted.

Mr. Fenton, a public relations consultant, is the man who orchestrated the apple scare, with staggering success from the point of view of the environmental group that hired him. Just how he was able to do so is worth recalling because, ultimately, the events of the Alar scare say more about media manipulation than about the danger of apples.

---

*Most of the discussion of the great Alar apple scam is based on a report by Kenneth Smith, "Alar: One Year Later. A Media Analysis of a Hypothetical Health Risk."[9]

Preparations for the "60 Minutes" episode actually stretch back to October 1988, when the Natural Resources Defense Council (NRDC) first sought the help of Mr. Fenton, a longtime political activist. The environmental group wanted to publicize the alleged hazards of eating apples sprayed with Alar, but knew the public had heard it all before. One group or another had been complaining about Alar for years. Although some firms did not stop using Alar after Ralph Nader first attacked it, the general public yawned and continued buying apples. The NRDC took a slightly different tack on the risks of Alar—charging it threatened children in particular—but still feared the issue was a sleeper. What to do?

The message isn't the problem, explained Mr. Fenton. The medium is. "Usually public interest groups release similar reports by holding a news conference and the result is a few print stories," he wrote after the campaign was well under way. Television coverage is rarely sought or achieved. The intensity of exposure created by design for the NRDC pesticide story is uncommon in the nonprofit world.

"Our goal was to create so many repetitions of NRDC's message that average American consumers (not just the policy elite in Washington) could not avoid hearing it—from many different media outlets within a short period of time. The idea was for the 'story' to achieve a life of its own, and continue for weeks and months *to effect policy and consumer habits* . . . [emphasis added]."

In other words, the goal was to target the electronic media for the story. That's where most people get their news. Use the print media to echo the story in subsequent headlines and news accounts. To achieve that end, Mr. Fenton sketched out a scenario that started with an exclusive expose on "60 Minutes," continued with a news conference the next day, and with various talk-show appearances and magazine cover stories in the weeks that followed. Key to the plan was a news embargo that would allow reporters to digest complex scientific data and prepare eye-catching film footage to accompany their reports without the risk that some other news outlet would scoop them and render their own accounts dated.

The plan worked, as the *Washington Post* reported, sort of. *Newsweek* magazine reporters got an early draft of the NRDC report and wanted to do a story in January, which Fenton feared would jeopardize the key agreement to give "60 Minutes" first rights to the story. So the NRDC sent no less than actress Meryl Streep, who was sympathetic to the cause, to strong-arm magazine officials into holding the story. It ran anyway, but only after the organization warned scientists who had reviewed the report not to speak to *Newsweek* reporters about it. The incident shows how far Mr. Fenton and the NRDC would go to manipulate the news.

The credentials of the experts involved with the report should have been a third clue. Robin M. Whyatt, one of the two principal authors of the NRDC report, had only a master's degree in public health, when a doctoral degree is considered a minimum standard to prepare such a document. A contributing NRDC author, Janet Hathaway, had degrees in both philosophy and law, but none at all in science. In an interview, Ms. Hathaway explained that the report concerned not just science but public policy, specifically, pesticide regulation. Anyone, of course, can write about public policy. Ms. Hathaway is as qualified as anyone else. But her contribution suggests that the NRDC was as interested in promoting a political agenda as reporting on science.

The credentials of some other experts involved with the report are also suspect, as a federal district judge made clear in a memo he handed down in November 1988, about the same time Mr. Fenton began meeting with the NRDC. Plaintiffs in a case involving alleged PCB contamination claimed that a railroad yard had exposed them to excessive amounts of PCBs and a higher risk of cancer. In support of their case, they cited the findings of Dr. Ian C. T. Nesbit, a self-styled "professional environment scientist," and Dr. William S. Nicholson of the Mount Sinai School of Medicine in New York. But Judge R. F. Kelly, noting that Dr. Nesbit had received his doctorate in physics, dismissed his findings, saying he could "see nothing in Dr. Nesbit's curriculum vitae that would qualify him to testify as an expert" on trace exposure of chemicals to man. Dr. Nesbit was on the so-called peer review committee that gave its blessing to NRDC's report on the hazards of trace exposure to Alar. Judge Kelly went on to downplay Dr. Nicholson's report linking PCBs to cancer because it "has not been peer-reviewed or accepted by anyone in particular." It was Dr. Nicholson who performed the carcinogenic risk assessments of Alar for the NRDC.

These warning signs notwithstanding, other publications subsequently obtained copies of the document and wrote stories in advance of the "60 Minutes" episode. The *New York Times* ran an Associated Press story on Saturday, February 25, and the *Washington Post* its own story the next day. But neither had the impact of the "60 Minutes" episode, which is why Mr. Fenton and the NRDC snubbed print reporters in favor of television journalists in the first place.

From the first sensational sentence in his report, Mr. Bradley did not disappoint them. Although short on science, the episode was long on the sort of theater that could captivate the program's roughly forty million viewers. There were villains in the form of killer apples. There were victims. "Go to a cancer ward at any children's hospital in this country. See these bald, wasting away kids," said Rep. Jerry Sikorsky, a remarkable leap to cause and effect that Mr. Bradley never challenged. And finally there were heroes, like journalists who gave nervous bureaucrats the Perry Mason treatment for not banning Alar, or environmental groups that disinterestedly try to save children from profiteering pesticide peddlers.

Mr. Bradley got to the point quickly during the show, demanding to know why the Environmental Protection Agency (EPA) allowed foods with what he called a "perilously high" cancer risk to remain on supermarket shelves.

Bradley: But you see, a lot of these chemicals . . . got on the market when we didn't know that they were cancer-causing agents.

EPA Acting Administrator Jack Moore: Yes, you're correct.

Bradley: And they're on the market now. We know that they do cause cancer.

Moore: Correct.

Bradley: But you say we can't take them off because they're already on the market, and they went on the market when we didn't know they caused cancer.

Moore: Correct.

Bradley: That's crazy!

Moore: We ought to change the statute.

Bradley: Is it fair to say, then, Mr. Moore, that there are laws on the books that are putting all of us—particularly our children—at risk?

Moore: Could be. Could be.

On the whole, the show left viewers with a clear message. Eating apples or apple products under the circumstances, said the episode's closing speaker, is "supermarket roulette." A big red apple with a skull and crossbones shown during the show helped drive the message home.

With all the apocalyptic rhetoric, Mr. Bradley didn't have room for some information that his viewers might have found useful, such as the fact that Alar's carcinogen label was based on high-dose exposure of the chemical to rodents, not humans. The NRDC then extrapolated the number of tumors caused in rodents to humans, a highly controversial technique in the scientific community. Mr. Bradley did not mention that controversy. Nor did laboratory animals come up in discussion except in passing. He did not mention that scientific advisors to the Environmental Protection Agency had earlier panned the data on which the NRDC had based its report, saying they were too flawed to mandate an Alar ban. Less than a month before the "60 Minutes" show aired, the EPA itself had reported that new findings still were not compelling enough to warrant an immediate ban.

No scientists critical of the NRDC study appeared on the show, although we at the American Council on Science and Health had offered to provide scientists to criticize the NRDC claims. Nor did any lay person ask how Alar could produce "bald, wasting away kids" when the NRDC itself had based its risk calculations on lifetime exposure. Since the NRDC had never submitted its findings to a scientific journal for peer review, impartial experts never got the chance to ask either. This science-by-press-release went straight from the copier to the airwaves.

NRDC attorney Janet Hathaway got a chance to wave the skull and crossbones again the next morning on NBC's "Today" show. The segment began with ominous words from a reporter: "If parents of preschoolers find out the true amounts of pesticides on vegetables, then parents may join their children in trying to hide vegetables under the table." Short of under-the-table disposal, what was a parent supposed to do?

> *Reporter:* I've got to ask you to help out. I talked to a young mother this morning who said she was going to throw out all the apple juice in her refrigerator. Can you tell us if there is anything that is safe or at least less unsafe?

> *Hathaway:* Well, I think that every parent has a real dilemma that they're facing. And I feel quite angry about the situation because there is no way for the consumer, his or herself, to decide what is going to be safer for their children. . . . It's not just apple juice alone that is a problem. Virtually every fruit and fruit juice is treated with pesticides. And there is no way for a consumer simply by looking at a product to know which was and was not treated.

Some twelve camera crews and more than seventy journalists were waiting later that morning when Mr. Fenton held a press conference in Washington. He also arranged press conferences in twelve other cities to take place at the same time. The story made headlines across the country in the days that followed, just as Mr. Fenton hoped. "Preschoolers Face 'Intolerable Risk,' Group Says," reported the *Los Angeles Times.* "Fear: Are we poisoning our children?" wondered *USA Today.* "Watch those vegetables, Ma," warned *Time* magazine. "Will pesticides on food kill us?" asked the *Miami Herald.*

The media barrage didn't stop there. Actress Meryl Streep joined with broadcaster Tom Brokaw's wife to form Mothers and Others for Pesticide Limits, which Mr. Fenton used to set off another round of news stories. Formation of "Mothers" was important, said Mr. Fenton, because it ensured "that the media would have two stories, not one, about this [NRDC] project.

Thereby, more repetition of NRDC's message was guaranteed." So it was. *USA Today* again gave the issue front-page coverage. Five national talk shows, including "Donahue" and the "Today" show, gave Ms. Streep air time.

Like a sandwich-board prophet of doom, Mr. Donahue proclaimed to the show's ten million viewers that the end was near. "Don't look now," he fairly shouted as the program began, "but we're poisoning our kids. I wouldn't lie to ya." NRDC representatives on the show did nothing to discourage such thinking, and no critic of the report appeared with them. Once again ACSH had offered scientists in advance of the program to put the Alar scare into perspective, but Donahue executives rejected the offer. Ms. Streep and the others urged concerned listeners to buy Mothers and Others' book on pesticides, conveniently advertised by Mr. Donahue, and to write their lawmakers. But the audience didn't seem much interested in the postal service approach to food safety. Not, at any rate, when kids were being poisoned by fruits and vegetables and—you heard it on "Donahue" first—killer candy:

Question: What should we be feeding our children?

Donahue: Yeah. What do you feed your kids?

Hathaway: Well, fruits and vegetables are still nutritious foods. And we don't want to say to people that a candy bar is better for your children than fruit and vegetables because *we didn't study candy bars, and they probably have pesticide residues as well* [emphasis added]. The thing about it is there's no reason why we should be feeding our kids cancer-causing chemicals in our fruits and vegetables. . . . All we can do right now is make a situation that's bad better. Because it's bad today. . . .

Ms. Streep's group went on to make public service announcements showing the actress washing her produce in detergent. "This isn't my idea," she told *People* magazine. "I saw a USDA agent on "Donahue" telling people to do this." She concluded, "I just want to be able to go and shop with a clear conscience."

Women's magazines with a combined circulation of seventeen million chipped in with gloomy headlines of their own. *Family Circle* warned of "Forbidden Fruit." *Woman's Day* pointed out "Fruits and vegetables that can poison your kids." *Redbook* detailed a "Shocking Report: The foods that are poisoning your children": it cited a devoted mom who "doesn't realize . . . that the very foods she thinks are good for her children could in fact be threatening their lives."

When yet a second food scare took off over tainted Chilean grapes, Mr. Fenton and the NRDC got an unexpected bonus. News media covering this new case of poisoned products also made mention of the Alar issue. *Time* magazine couldn't help wondering on its cover: "Is Anything Safe?"

NRDC officials delighted in the coverage. In a letter to Mr. Fenton dated March 10, 1989, NRDC Executive Director John H. Adams wrote, "I want you to know how pleased we are with the job you've done so far on the publicity and media campaign. . . . Your advice and hard work were crucial factors in making our report a powerful news story."

Growers, meanwhile, suffered the consequences almost immediately. International Apple Institute Chairman John Rice, a seventh-generation Pennsylvania grower, told *USA Today* that his sales fell 30 percent in the week after Mr. Bradley's attack—even though he didn't use Alar. Apple prices plunged 35 percent in Virginia. Said one grower in the business since 1963, "This is the biggest setback that has faced the apple industry in my memory." A Winchester, Virginia, cooperative serving twenty-five small farmers for thirty years was forced out of business. Said its former president, "Business dropped 100 percent. It killed us."

As producers scrambled to repair the damage, members of the "prestige" papers took a second, harder look at the NRDC report and offered evidence that the group is not the last word on food safety. On March 1, 1989, just days after its own coverage of the NRDC report, the *Washington Post* gave front-page space to the National Research Council study urging consumers to eat more, not less, fruits and vegetables. The 1,400-page report, compiled over a three-year period by nineteen scientists who examined almost six thousand studies along the way, found "no evidence that pesticides or natural toxins in food contribute significantly to cancer risk in the United States," according to the *Post*. On March 3, a *Post* reporter sketched out Fenton's media management for all to see—albeit on page A17. The *Chicago Tribune* took note of Mr. Fenton's manipulations under the front-page headline, "How 'media stampede' spread apple panic." The story cited a "barrage of media reports that failed to give a balanced account."

A month after its initial report, the *Los Angeles Times* followed up with a lengthy profile of the NRDC, contrasting its tactics with the more conservative approach of Ellen Silbergeld, a "highly respected" scientist with the Environmental Defense Fund. She had earlier refused to allow her group to publish a study on contamination of breast milk for fear of setting off a panic. Overall, she said, "the benefits of [nursing a baby] outweigh the risks." (The *Los Angeles Times* pointed out that the NRDC didn't even have an economist on its staff to weigh costs and benefits.) At any rate, Ms. Silbergeld's own review of the NRDC data led her to conclude that there wasn't enough information to draw conclusions.

The *Times* account also raised doubts about the NRDC's claims that it never wanted consumers to stop eating apples, but only to lobby for tougher pesticide regulations. The story quoted an NRDC staffer as saying "don't eat them" unless the apples are certified Alar-free. It went on to cite still another

NRDC official's praise of school boards' decisions to remove apples from school menus.

New York Times health writer Jane Brody devoted a column to concerns that "chemophobia" would drain limited regulatory funds and threaten, not enhance, America's health. She also cited a food toxicologist who pointed out that stomach cancer, "the one cancer you'd think would be diet-related," has plummeted since pesticides came into wide use. The *Washington Post* quoted scientists expressing concern that a complicated issue "was allowed to be decided not by officials charged with protecting the public, on the basis of hard evidence, but by a frightened public acting on incomplete and often erroneous reports." Editorial writers and political columnists picked up on the issue. Writing in the *Wall Street Journal,* columnist Hodding Carter III took a swipe at the media for helping to generate a scare without solid scientific evidence, then standing back to say, in effect, "Oops, so sorry. We only report the news, we don't make it."

Both the *Washington Times* and the *Wall Street Journal* spotlighted tenuous assumptions in the NRDC methodology. In view of the high dose Alar exposure to rodents, said the *Times,* "you'd have to drink 19,000 quarts of apple juice every day of your life even to come close to the 'risk' levels from Alar." Rats don't equal humans, said the *Wall Street Journal.* Two months before the NRDC report, the science magazine *Nature* published an article by researchers from Carnegie Mellon, Case Western Reserve, and the University of Washington raising questions about the usefulness of these rodent bioassay studies. "Extrapolating from one species to another," they wrote, "is fraught with uncertainty." Indeed, they pointed out that "rats and mice are more similar biologically to each other than either is to humans."

Stung by the growing criticism, Mr. Bradley decided to air a second episode, this time giving critics a chance to appear. On May 14, Dr. Bruce Ames, chairman of the Biochemistry Department at the University of California at Berkeley, said fears about Alar were overblown (as I did in this same segment). But he only got a chance to do so after Mr. Bradley had first impugned our motives.

He introduced me by saying "[she] readily admits her organization is subsidized by food-processing companies and pesticide manufacturers, including Uniroyal, which makes Alar." Likewise Dr. Ames was appearing, said Mr. Bradley, "at the urging of the agricultural chemical industry. Dr. Ames *says* [emphasis added] he is completely independent and does no consulting for industry." (Read: We have no assurance of Dr. Ames's independence other than his own word, which is dubious given that industry cited him as an expert.) As for the EPA scientific advisory panel that had criticized the data that the NRDC used to bolster its case, Mr. Bradley accused its members of being industry-influenced too. "Where are the people who are exclusively there to protect the consumers?" wondered Senator Joe Lieberman of Connecticut on the segment. "Why is this panel so dominated by scientists who also are working for the chemical industry?" Given Mr. Bradley's shoot-the-messenger treatment, the public could be forgiven for believing that no independent defenders of Alar existed, that only those scientists on the industry dole believed Alar to be innocent of the cancer-causing charges.

Mr. Bradley's selective skepticism did not extend to detailing his own financial interest in ensuring enough hair-raising stories to keep "60 Minutes" high in the ratings. Nor did it extend to the NRDC or Mr. Fenton, although there was no small amount of evidence that both stood to gain from a scare. For his part, Mr. Fenton got $26,000, high-profit exposure, and lots of kudos from the NRDC that he could use as future references—not bad for a few months work. As for the group itself, Mr. Fenton readily acknowledged in an interview with *Propaganda Review:* "The campaign was designed so that revenue would flow back to NRDC from the public. The group sold a book about pesticides through a 900 number on the 'Donahue' show and to date 90,000 copies have been sold." In a May 22 memo to his own interested parties, Mr. Fenton notes that a "modest investment by NRDC repaid itself manyfold in tremendous media exposure [and substantial, immediate revenue]. . . ." The *Los Angeles Times* noted that NRDC staffers were "overwhelmed" by calls in the wake of the report "and that they expect fund-raising to improve as a result."

Mr. Bradley, interestingly, never mentioned David Fenton at all. He never suggested that this report had come to public attention by any other than routine means. He made no mention of the fact that science ordinarily does not operate by press release or movie-star testimony. He did not tell viewers about the National Research Council report urging people to eat more fruits and vegetables or about the falling incidence of stomach cancer, as columnist Brody did. He simply closed by saying that whoever was right, the EPA had rendered the issue moot by at last proposing a ban on Alar.

So ultimately Mr. Fenton's strategy, carried out by Bradley, Streep, and company, worked as planned. "NRDC and their hired PR council did a superb job of playing the news media like a Stradivarius," Jack Bonner, head of a Washington public relations firm, told the *Washington Post Magazine.* Repeated exposure in the media, particularly the electronic variety, did give the story a life of its own.

"Usually, it takes a significant natural disaster to create this much sustained news attention for an environmental problem," wrote Mr. Fenton in his May 22 memo. By the time journalists were able to put his media-made disaster in better perspective, it was too late. The public had already adopted a better-safe-than-sorry approach. "There may not be any risk, but who knows?" said one shopper who had thrown away unopened cans of apple sauce, as quoted in the *Boston Globe* on March 19. "Why take the chance if you don't have to?"

In the end, the apple industry and taxpayers paid a heavy price for the scare. In a speech to the Virginia Horticultural Society in January 1990, the Apple Institute's Mr. Rice estimated the economic damage to the growers at no less than $250 million, $40 million in the state of Washington alone. Apple processors, he said, lost another $125 million. Said the manager of a seventy-eight-year-old California apple cooperative forced into bankruptcy, " '60 Minutes' and Alar were the final straws." Media General News Service detailed the plight of the Winchester grower forced to sell to developers part of a farm in family hands since 1912—even though he didn't use Alar. In the wake of the scare, the family "took an unexpected $60,000 loss." The *New York Times* described the "severe economic loss" experienced by one New York grower, who had to hire more pickers, raising production costs, while getting less for his apples. Instead of being able to sell them for eating at $10 a bushel, he had to sell apples picked off the ground to a cider mill at $2 a bushel.

Taxpayers felt the bite when the U.S. Agriculture Department announced an emergency purchase of $15 million worth of leftover apples. What purchases of higher-priced organic produce cost consumers is uncertain.

New Hampshire grower Stephen Woods, president of the New England Fruit Growers Council on the Environment, says the scare may have another, ironic cost. Some growers in his region, he explained in an interview, had found Alar a useful alternative to potent pesticides. Insects attacking an apple tree's leaves late in the growing season can cause trees to drop their apples before they are ripe. But Alar helped trees hold their fruit despite the insect infestation, eliminating the need for late-season pesticides. Thanks to the scare, growers relying on Alar rather than pesticides "got creamed," said Mr. Woods. "The real tragedy of this whole thing," he said, "is that the benefits of Alar never really got considered. They just got tossed out the window."

Just why they got tossed out has less to do with the alleged dangers than with the way the media work, or don't work. Writing in the January/February *American Enterprise* magazine, Virginia Commonwealth University communications Professor Ted J. Smith took note of a "special calling" increasingly evident among journalists: "The role of the press is not merely to serve society by providing an accurate account of the conflict of ideas, but to save and perfect it. The watchdog function, once considered remedial and subsidiary, becomes paramount: The primary duty of the journalist is to focus attention on problems and deficiencies, failures and threats. . . ."

In 1992, apple growers continue to ponder their losses, trying to pick up the pieces. The following series of correspondence I had with apple grower Herbert G. Slenker of Ohio's Slenker Orchards summarizes what the public should know about Alar, as well as the far-reaching effects of banning Alar on the fruit and vegetable growing industry overall:

Mr. Slenker's October 14, 1992 letter to me:

Dear Dr. Whelan,

As fruit growers, we have been confronted with the loss of many pesticides essential for growing a consistent quantity of good quality fruit. Their loss has primarily been the result of tests in which extremely heavy doses of those pesticides have been fed to mice or rats.

There seems to be a wide divergence of opinion among investigators as to the value or reliability of such tests. As far as I have been able to determine, no one has taken steps to prove whether such tests are valid or erroneous. An opinion is a poor substitute for knowledge.

If cancer is caused by a high dose of a pesticide rather than the chemical toxicity of that material, then a chemically inert material may possibly cause similar conditions. If that should be true, it would be strong evidence that a massive dose of a pesticide fed to mice would not be a reliable indicator of the carcinogenic effect of that material at a more reasonable dosage.

We know that small amounts of iodine in our salt prevent thyroid problems, but large quantities are very toxic. A small quantity of boron is an essential micronutrient for animals, but a large quantity, again, is very toxic. These two instances indicate that extrapolating a high dosage to a small quantity could give a completely false answer.

If we are to continue to produce fruits and vegetables in sufficient quantity to feed the American people, we must get the high-dose monkey off our back so that we have the essential pesticides available to produce that food.

My response:

. . . The media are now saying that apple farmers do not miss Alar and are doing very well without it. They use that evidence to justify the decision to withdraw Alar, despite the fact that everyone now knows that the risks to human health of Alar were purely hypothetical.

Is it true that Alar was not useful? Are some apple farmers suffering from not having access to it? Would they like it back?

Mr. Slenker's October 29 response to me:

In regard to the media statements that Alar is not missed or is not useful, evidence in our orchard refutes that statement. The McIntosh cultivar is very susceptible to dropping from the tree as soon as it ripens. Alar delays or reduces the normal abscission of the fruit, thereby extending the harvest season so the apples can be picked before they drop. We estimate that we lost 35 to 40 percent of our McIntosh crop. Red Delicious are also susceptible to dropping but to a lesser degree. We estimate that we lost 15 percent of our Red Delicious. The Jonathan cultivar is quite resistant to dropping as well as are other cultivars we grow. Because of variations in the various cultivars, we used Alar only on McIntosh and Red Delicious.

It is inconceivable to me that any grower would ever say that Alar was not useful. However, many have been able to get around the drop problem simply by harvesting before the apples get ripe. That is one reason why it is difficult to buy apples in a store that taste good.

An even greater loss has been that of EBDC (ethylene bis-dithio-carbamate). It has been our standard fungicide for the last 30 years, more or less. During that time, diseases have never built up resistance to it. It is compatible with more other pesticides and has never caused any injury to our trees.

Captan is the only residual fungicide we have left that is effective, and it has many faults. Under certain climatic conditions on some cultivars, captan may cause leaf spotting, which reduces the photosynthetic efficiency of the leaves. It is not compatible with some oils or emulsions and may cause chemical damage if applied with such materials or too close to them. The EPA has imposed a questionable four-day reentry period for employees after Captan has been applied to the orchard. That fouls up an orderly work schedule.

Disease resistance is beginning with some of the newer irradicative types of fungicides and we don't know how much longer they will be effective.

Of even more concern to me than the previously mentioned problems, is the fact that American companies have almost completely halted research on minor use pesticides for fruits and vegetables.

Living things have the ability to adapt to their environment, no matter how hostile it may be. European Red Mites produce anywhere from three to six generations per year. Such rapid reproduction accelerates the buildup of resistance to miticides that are used to control them. Miticides that are highly effective, when first introduced, may fail within five years. This is indicative of what may happen with other species over a longer period of time. We are always going to need new and different types of pesticides. Without research we won't have them.

Environmentalists tell us the mites can be controlled with predators, which is true. But the Apple Maggot, the larva of a fly that lays her eggs on small apples, has no natural predators. After the eggs hatch, the larva eats its way through the apple. As the larva proceeds to eat, apple goes into one end of the larva and feces comes out the other end, leaving a little brown streak all through the fruit. Appetizing? The only way Apple Maggot can be controlled is with pesticides, which also kill the predators of mites and other pests.

In the late summer 1991, California growers lost most of their cantaloupe crop to an invasion of White Flies that became resistant to present pesticides. That is just the tip of the iceberg. What happened to cantaloupe can happen to any fruit or vegetable. Irresponsible and unjust government regulations have discouraged chemical companies from continuing research on pesticides. In time, crop losses will probably occur for most other fruits and vegetables.

Unfortunately, most people didn't bother to learn the facts about Alar. Alar is a registered trademark of the Uniroyal Chemical Company, Inc. The active ingredient in the Alar formulation is a growth regulator generically known as daminozide. Daminozide had been studied by university research groups interested in hydrazine derivatives and compounds capable of generating hydrazine derivatives when metabolized. Many hydrazine derivatives are well known carcinogens.

Daminozide can be broken down to 1,1-(unsymmetrical)dimethylhydrazine (UDMH); Alar as manufactured in fact contains trace levels of UDMH. The Natural Resources Defense Council had been for years attempting to convince the EPA that Alar contained enough UDMH to cause human cancer. The EPA scientific board disagreed.

In 1978, the results of what should have been the definitive carcinogen bioassay of daminozide were published by the National Cancer Institute. NCI concluded that daminozide as tested was a carcinogen, but it was such a weak carcinogen that the EPA could not use the NCI data for risk assessment. Furthermore, the NCI study—following a well-established tradition—tested the ingredient to which humans were exposed, namely daminozide, and did not measure the appearance of UDMH as a breakdown product. Uniroyal sponsored several carcinogen bioassays of Alar designed according to EPA guidelines. They were negative. The EPA, under pressure from the Natural Resources Defense Council, ignored these data.

In an unusual move, the EPA called on Uniroyal to conduct carcinogenicity tests on UDMH in the absence of daminozide. Uniroyal agreed to do so; UDMH doses were set according to EPA guidelines at the MTD (maximum tolerated dose). The EPA, still under pressure from the Natural Resources Defense Council, which for reasons unknown seemed to have continuous timely access to Uniroyal's proprietary files at the EPA, then decided to insist on an even higher dose level of UDMH, a dose level so toxic that Uniroyal scientists complained the study would be compromised by premature deaths. Not surprisingly, this dose level of UDMH was carcinogenic to mice and provided the data for the EPA's mathematical modeling.

Even with the deck stacked against Alar, the results of the quantitative risk assessment using UDMH data were no reason for alarm. The EPA calculated that seventy years of exposure to Alar at the maximum permissible level would lead to one chance in 5×10^5 of contracting cancer. Since Alar had only been on the market twenty years, the EPA had fifty years to make a decision about banning Alar before anyone would be at risk. (This is an absurd number to anyone who knows anything about agricultural chemicals: in much less than seventy years new and better products would be developed). The EPA indicated to Uniroyal that it wanted Alar removed from the market, but that it did not consider Alar an "imminent hazard." If the EPA had considered Alar an imminent hazard, it was obligated to compensate farmers, distributors, and manufacturers for losses they might incur during the removal of Alar. After all, the EPA had approved Alar for specific registered uses. There was no evidence that Alar was being used improperly. The process of removing from the market a chemical not considered an imminent hazard takes about two years. Farmers are permitted some continued uses during this period. The product is phased out, rather than recalled abruptly.

The Natural Resources Defense Council, however, perceived Alar as an "intolerable risk to children" and launched its publicity blitz to discredit Uniroyal and the EPA. The result was a unilateral, de facto, "imminent hazard" designation by a third party. The adverse publicity, threat of a congressional ban, and the pleas of apple growers who were being clobbered financially by the panic, led Uniroyal to voluntarily withdraw Alar's registrations for use on edible products.

Subsequent studies by Cabral have indicated that daminozide is not an animal carcinogen. In fact, it possesses some anticarcinogenic properties that deserve investigation. It will be ironic indeed, if daminozide turns out to be a useful cancer chemotherapeutic agent.

Back in 1989, the British government said, based on the high-dose mouse studies, that there "was no risk to health," considering the small quanities of Alar and its byproduct UDMH (unsymmetrical dimethyl hydrazine) detected in food. The chairman of the Parliament-appointed group said that the British view differed from the EPA's because "we tend to be a bit more cautious" about the science: "We don't always make the assumption that the animal data are transferable to man, particularly in the absence of pharmacokinetics that make it clear that the compound is handled in the same way at massive doses as it is at low doses."[10]

The British were not alone in their views. A United Nations panel concluded in 1989 that Alar was "not oncogenic in mice" and that UDMH raised no special concern. This group, which includes seven members from the World Health Organization and seven from the Food and Agriculture Organization, confident of its opinion, set a high tolerance for Alar residues in food. They recommended that governments permit an acceptable daily intake of up to 0.5 mg/kg of body weight.[11]

The EPA has come closer to this European approach with its late-1991 toxicological analysis of Alar and UDMH. This analysis found Alar and UDMH to be only half as potent as the agency estimated during the Alar crisis in 1989. Those earlier estimates were based on doses that were 266,000 times normal human ingestion. Now, EPA is saying its risk estimates are based on doses over one half million times normal human ingestion.[12]

This latest downgrading of Alar's toxicity gives both fuel and credence to current legal and congressional matters concerning Alar. Apple growers in Washington State have filed a $200-million lawsuit, which began working its way through the courts in early 1992. The growers charge that CBS, NRDC, and its media advisers knowingly hyped the risks of the chemical to get attention. EPA's latest toxicological risk assessment is expected to be important evidence for the apple growers.[13]

The Alar fiasco is also expected to have far-reaching effects on Congress. Congress is expected to consider a variety of bills that would overthrow the infamous Delaney amendment (see later discussion on Delaney). That amendment forbids the marketing of any product that is judged carcinogenic and shows up in processed food—Alar was one such product that fell into the grips of Delaney. New legislation would permit products to be kept in use if the health risks are deemed negligible—as appears to be the case now with Alar.[14]

Several recognized scientists, as well as the respected *Science* editorial page, commented on the Alar fiasco on its third anniversary:

> . . . a clearly dubious report about possible carcinogenicity by a special interest group was hyped by a news organization without the most simple checks on its reliability or documentation. This caused panic among consumers and losses of millions of dollars by apple growers. Confronted with the inadequacy of the data, a spokesman for the public interest group recently suggested that it was excusable because people are eating more apples than ever before. That is like an embezzler justifying embezzlement by saying the banking industry continues to survive.
>
> —*Science,* November 1, 1991

> When used in the approved regulated fashion, as it was, Alar does not pose a risk to the public's health. In matters of health, good science, not misplaced fears, must drive public policy.
>
> —Ralph R. Reed, M.D., American Medical Association

> A chemical is currently tested for cancer by feeding massive doses to laboratory animals. These doses are much higher, sometimes hundreds of thousands of times higher, than humans will be exposed to. . . . The calculated cancer risk values are theoretical worst-case numbers which bear absolutely no relationship to real risk. Unfortunately, these numbers take on a life of their own and are used to convince people that pesticides in food are dangerous to their health.
>
> —Joseph D. Rosen, Ph.D., Cook College, Rutgers University

> There are two kinds of environmentalists . . . scientific environmentalists who rely upon science as the basis for decision-making and others who rely upon ideology rather than science. It's imperative that the media insist upon outstanding science and nothing less as the basis for decision-making in environmental protection. Those who exaggerate the effects of environmental pollutants do not act in the interest of human health and environmental protection. . . . The Alar controversy is a classic case of poor science poorly applied to a societal decision resulting in a poor final decision.
>
> —Alan A. Moghissi, Ph.D., University of Maryland

As a pediatric surgeon, as well as the nation's former Surgeon General, I care deeply about the health of children, and if Alar ever posed a health hazard I would have said so then and would say so now. But the truth is that Alar never did pose a health hazard.

The American food supply is not only the most abundant in the world, but it is also the safest. Paradoxically—it has achieved that position in the world market just because of chemicals like Alar that have made it possible.

—C. Everett Koop, M.D., Chairman, National Safe Kids Campaign,
Former U.S. Surgeon General

The risk of eating an apple treated with Alar is less than the risk of eating a peanut butter sandwich or a well done hamburger.

—Richard Adamson, M.D., National Cancer Institute

Finally, what are the lessons learned from the Alar scare? Consumers and journalists who want to do more than carry baggage for political activists should remember the following key points:[15]

- Beware of science being "used" as a front to achieve political objectives. Peer-reviewed, mainstream science, the type worthy of reporting to readers or viewers, does not operate by media manipulations or "exclusivity agreements," by FAX, leaks, or press releases. It does not use Hollywood personalities, public relations firms, or a "left wing legal activist group," as the *Wall Street Journal* described the Natural Resources Defense Council (NRDC), the group that gave us the Alar apple scare. Solid science is found in reputable journals where it undergoes peer review prior to publication. Such publication does not guarantee 100 percent accuracy or that future findings will not change, but only that it represents sound science at the time. Science advances by reviewed discoveries, a point frequently overlooked by some activists, journalists, and consumers.

- Check with other reliable sources at colleges and universities. Don't rely on activists, government regulators, or industry spokespersons to provide an illusion of objectivity. If you want scientific information, call scientists. They have the expertise.

- If a purported scientific topic requires "60 Minutes," "20/20," the "Donahue Show," or a partisan political group such as the NRDC to gain public attention, beware! The question is not whether the press should have done a better job in presenting NRDC's "Intolerable Risk" study, but whether the media should have reported this study at all.

Ethylene Dibromide

In January 1984, millions of Americans nearly went berserk over news reports that minute traces of the pesticide ethylene dibromide (EDB)[16] had been detected in samples of cereals, baking mixes, citrus, and other food products. The tocsin about this alleged toxin proclaimed that now even those amber waves of grain posed the ultimate health threat—cancer.

Substantial amounts of food were destroyed, EDB, for all practical purposes, was banned, and other agricultural chemicals were phased in to take its place. And then it appeared to be all over, leaving only another bad taste about the quality of our food supply, the ultimate vulnerability of American consumers, and the insensitivity of the food industry that with equanimity will poison for profit.

But the EDB saga did not end with the ban. In retrospect, it is now clear that while the setting of standards for safe use of EDB was totally legitimate, the fears that EDB posed a human health risk were purely hypothetical, indistinguishable in the maze of other trivial and significant risk factors we encounter every day. The decision to ban the pesticide was based not on scientific data, but on political pressures that resulted from a spectacular media hype; and that the alternatives that are now in use are both less effective and in some cases significantly more hazardous than EDB.

In the context of the recent similar histrionics about Alar, PCBs, and other alleged bad actors that have now been sentenced to the graveyard of chemicals, a close scrutiny of the EDB saga confirms a disturbing and destructive pattern that, if it continues, will be this country's most threatening albatross in the remaining years of this century, the primary threat to economic growth, societal affluence, and, ironically, our current unprecedented state of good health.

BACKGROUND

Ethylene dibromide has been used for some fifty years as a gasoline additive and as a soil fumigant for controlling rod worms. Prior to the ban, it protected stored wheat, corn, and other grains against destruction by insects and contamination by molds and fungi, killed fruit flies on quarantined fruit supplies, and kept milling machinery free of insects. Because of the widespread use of EDB and other pesticides, we in America have escaped the negative health consequences of eating uncontrolled amounts of insect fragments, insect excrement, and mold toxins in our food. Beyond that, safe storage of grain products over prolonged periods has ensured stability in our food supplies despite variations in harvest yield from year to year.

DOES EDB CAUSE CANCER?

There is no doubt that under some specific conditions, EDB causes cancer in laboratory animals.

Three long-term, high-dose studies of EDB in rats and mice all found a higher incidence of cancer with increasing dose.

There was, however, no data indicating EDB was carcinogenic to humans. There was considerable information on its effects on workers engaged in EDB manufacturing, some of whom were exposed to doses five to ten thousand times higher than consumers for upwards of sixteen years. The incidence of cancer among these workers, however, was *not* significantly different from that expected in an unexposed population.

At the time of the EDB ban, the EPA estimated that the average consumer took in five to ten micrograms of EDB per day, which many scientists thought was unrealistically inflated. Even so, ten micrograms is an extremely small amount. By comparison, we daily ingest 140,000 micrograms of saffrole, a carcinogenic substance found in pepper. Ten micrograms per person per day of EDB is on a proportional body-weight basis, less than a quarter-millionth as much as the rats were given in the cancer tests. That means a person would have had to eat at least 250,000 times as much food as he or she normally does every day, or some four hundred tons daily over a lifetime to equal the cancer-producing dose given to lab animals. Such an immense difference in the doses experienced by test animals and humans is in itself enough to justify skepticism about the reality of the hazard faced by consumers.

Against the background of natural dietary carcinogens the risk from ten micrograms of EDB per day was insignificant and meaningless. Aflatoxin, for example, is a potent carcinogen naturally found in grains and other foods. Far more potent than EDB, it is allowed by the FDA at a level of twenty parts per billion in grain and other foods, which means that consumers can legally be exposed to as much as 667 times the carcinogenic hazard from aflatoxin as they would ever have gotten from EDB at the residue levels set by EPA.

In summary, the EDB saga is a case where an effective, useful, and health-promoting substance was banned on the basis of laboratory evidence, and was replaced with chemicals that offered no safety advantage to the consumer and posed *greater* threats to agricultural workers. And this happened in the context of disruption, chaos, and enormous expense, all of which have been passed on to every American citizen. We are thus left with the question, Why? How could such a travesty of science occur in our educated, technologically advanced society?

Both EDB mania and the Alar fiasco were brewed from five major ingredients: affluence, the scapegoat phenomenon, agricultural naiveté, chemical naiveté, and the power of the environmental movement.

Affluence

The Alar and EDB phenomena could happen only in a highly affluent society. We tend to forget that the preoccupation of most of the world is not with traces of pesticides or additives, but with getting enough food to live a healthy life. Only where food is abundant do we have the luxury of throwing out perfectly wholesome products, and not feeling the immediate economic and health effects of such action.

Historically, we have observed that although technological abundance may initially elicit feelings of happiness and gratitude (for example, with the arrival of sanitary water, sewage disposal, and pasteurized milk, people acted positively because they saw the direct beneficial effects), the romance soon fades and is replaced by discontent and suspicion. Jean Jacques Rousseau (1712–78) set the stage for the Enlightenment with his comments about how civilization made men evil, and why life "in the state of nature" was superior to forms of sophisticated living. So perhaps a portion of EDB and Alar phobia can be explained by our relative complacency, which translates into the feeling that we are so rich and healthy we need something to worry and complain about.

Perhaps this complacency, almost a boredom with our general good shape, can explain the ironic fact that the growth of chemical phobia and concern about "cancer-causing agents" being spewed into our environment by industry, is occurring at the very time we are living longer than ever and experiencing, with one exception (lung cancer), a stabilization or decline in cancer mortality. (More irony: the cancer site where mortality has most declined in the past forty years is cancer of the stomach, the site allegedly affected by pesticide residues.)

Scapegoat Phenomenon

In primitive societies it was common for people to believe in malevolent witchcraft based on a type of scapegoat psychology, one that relieved themselves of any potential guilt or complicity in a tragic occurrence. For example, Polish American anthropologist Bronislaw Malinowski noted that an African mother frequently assuaged her guilt at the death of a child by ascribing the death to a spell cast on the child's food by a jealous neighbor. Similarly we Americans have found that it is easier to cast blame elsewhere than to be introspective about our own role in disease causation.

During the early part of this century, we in this country made great strides by having our government, and others, "do something" to improve our health; hence, immunizations, chlorination of water, and other things. And we saw dramatic, positive effects, with little or no effort by us. Today, however, the more we learn about chronic diseases such as heart disease and cancer, the more we realize that the government, or anyone else, can't help us, since so many of the major risk factors (cigarette smoking, medicating elevated blood pressure, being overweight, etc.) lie within our own control. Given that (1) we know that the cause of 30 percent of cancer deaths in this country is cigarette smoking, and that a great deal of personal willpower is needed for most smokers to quit smoking; and (2) we don't know the causes of most of the remaining 70 percent of cancers—the banning of EDB and Alar might have been accepted as a type of psychological gratification, that "something" was being done in the "war on cancer," and that something didn't involve our own behavior modification.

Agricultural Naiveté

Most of us have had very little contact with farms and agricultural science. Our urban centers are so far from the farm heartlands of the country that we are removed from the whole process, and perhaps take too much for granted. And perhaps too many of us simply assume that God meant our food to be bug-free.

The reality is that we compete with insects for food. Losses on a global basis have been estimated to be as great as 45 percent. Pesticides of varying toxicity must be used selectively to kill pests such as insects and their larvae, fungi, root worms, slugs, weeds, rats, mice, and other organisms. Pesticides are an indispensable tool in reducing these depredations. It would be a sad state of affairs if we had to experience widespread food shortages and contaminations before Americans once again become grateful that high-tech agricultural chemicals exist.

Chemical Naiveté

For most consumers, chemistry, like agriculture, is an unknown, and the unfamiliar is always a likely target of exaggerated and unrealistic fears.

The naiveté about chemicals is primarily twofold. First, American consumers have been brainwashed into believing that what is natural is safe, and what is synthetic is suspect. Thus EDB immediately had the odds stacked against it: after all, it *sounded* like a concoction fresh from the test tube of a greedy alchemist.

Second, American consumers believe that even minute traces of a potentially dangerous chemical must be removed. In fact, we have long known that natural foods have plentiful supplies of natural toxins, otherwise known as poisons. Shrimp and other shellfish contain arsenic; potatoes are a complex mixture of some 150 volatile chemicals, including solanine, arsenic, tannins, and nitrate; and lima beans contain that classic suicide potion hydrogen cyanide. Only relatively recently, however, have we become aware of the large number of carcinogens in natural foods. In a classic paper on this subject, published in the September 1983 issue of *Science,* Dr. Bruce Ames, chairman of the Department of Biochemistry at the University of California, Berkeley, noted that "the traces of the carcinogen EDB now allowed in food is insignificant compared with the level and risk of many cancer-causing agents found in every meal, most of which are natural and traditional." He explained that plants synthesize toxic chemicals—"nature's pesticides"—in large amounts to defend against insects and other predators. And, according to Dr. Ames, "the amount of nature's pesticides we are ingesting is at least 10,000 times the level of man-made pesticides. Nature's pesticides, in fact, are found in levels of parts per hundred or parts per thousand, while man-made pesticides are present at parts per million or parts per billion. The man-made pesticide residues currently allowed in our diet don't represent, in my opinion, any significant cancer hazard to the public."

In other words, in their naiveté about chemistry, consumers fell for the EDB and Alar scares, thinking that these carcinogens were unique and therefore somehow had to be eliminated. In this context, banning EDB and Alar is like removing a few grains of sand from a beach.

The bannings of EDB and Alar are classic examples of what is often known as the "exorcist approach" to carcinogen regulation—the belief that even a minute trace of a potentially dangerous chemical must be removed to ensure safety. Given the myriad of natural toxins and carcinogens around us, this is absurd. Indeed, this hypothetical problem of trace levels would not even present itself were it not for the dramatic advancement in technologies that allow us to detect minute traces of just about anything. As Heinz R. Fagels writes in his book *The Cosmic Code,* "In your last breath it is almost certain that you have inhaled at least one atom from the dying breath of Julius Caesar as he lamented 'Et tu, Brute!' "

But with the announcement that minute traces of EDB and Alar were on food, the chemically naive consumer was not interested in what we knew—but fixated on the question, What if? as in, What if these low levels even caused one case of cancer, particularly in me? It's not worth the risk, so ban it. Unfortunately, the consumer was fully unaware and uninformed about the potentially adverse health consequences of the ban itself. The cases of EDB and Alar are classic examples of how ignorance triggers an anxiety of the unknown, with the unknown being actually scarier than the real thing.

Power and Organization of the Environmental Movement

The so-called environmental movement, in this case dominated by the Natural Resources Defense Council, Inc. (NRDC), can take the major credit for the banning of both EDB and Alar. The NRDC, with offices in New York, Washington, San Francisco, Denver, and Natick, Massachusetts, and a budget of more than $14 million per year, lists as its number one goal "the protection of human health and the environment," and had designated itself as the self-appointed guardian of the Environmental Protection Agency. As the NRDC's name implies, litigation is its primary tool for developing and implementing federal regulations related to air and water quality.

NRDC and other environmentalists have scored two major victories with EDB and Alar. But a quick analysis of their success here leaves a number of unsettling questions:

- Why would a group whose mandate was the "protection of human health and the environment" focus its big guns on a chemical that, relative to other naturally occurring chemicals, posed little or no hazard to human health?

- Why isn't the NRDC at least as concerned about table pepper or afla-toxin on peanuts, which, on the basis of animal experiments, are a hundred to thousands of times more carcinogenic than EDB and Alar?

- Why is it that a group interested in the "protection of human health and the environment" concentrated its environmental efforts on hypothetical causes of cancer like EDB and Alar and ignored proven ones like inhalation of tobacco smoke?

- How could a group sincerely dedicated to the "protection of human health and the environment" demand the banning of one chemical (EDB) when it knew full well that the alternatives either had not been tested for carcinogenicity or had already been proved to pose a much greater risk to workers.

Looking at the leadership role of the NRDC in the banning of EDB and Alar leaves one swirling in inconsistencies and loose ends. What are the real motivations and intentions of such a group?

What About Other Pesticides?

The Food and Drug Administration's 1989 report "Residues in Foods"[18] agreed with reports from the previous two years, all finding that levels of pesticide residues in the U.S. food supply are generally well below established safety standards. Of the domestic samples studied, less than 1 percent had residues that were over EPA tolerances, and less than 1 percent had residues for which there was no established tolerance for that particular pesticide/commodity. Among the import surveillance samples, less than 1 percent had residues that were over tolerance, and 3 percent had residues for which there was no tolerance.

The 1989 Institute of Food Technologists' report on food safety says that current evidence indicates that any health risk associated with pesticide residues "is negligible and is orders of magnitude less than that of foodborne diseases such as Salmonella and Shigella."[18] Indeed, it is estimated that up to about 6 million cases of food- and water-borne disease causing some 9,000 deaths may occur in the United States each year, at an economic cost of between $1 billion and $10 billion per year.[19]

Other studies indicate that by far the largest intake of pesticides is of those produced in nature. The Food and Drug Administration (FDA) assays food for the 200 compounds thought to be of greatest significance. The FDA found that the average human intake is approximately 0.09 milligrams per day of man-made chemicals, but 1.5 grams of naturally occurring pesticides. That means that 99.99 percent of pesticides consumed in food are actually naturally occurring.[20]

The Office of Pesticides and Toxic Substances in the EPA issued a 1991 statement in response to the frequently asked question, "How safe is the food supply, and are our children at special risk from pesticide residues in their food?"

> The food supply of the U.S. is among the safest in the world. Although many of the foods we consume do contain low levels of pesticide residues as a result of the legal use of pesticides, numerous safeguards are built into EPA's pesticide regulatory process to ensure that the public (including infants and children) are protected from risks posed by eating pesticide-treated foods. . . . In establishing or reviewing any pesticide tolerance (the legal maximum residue level that may remain on a treated food), EPA does evaluate the risks which might be posed to a variety of subpopulations, including infants and children. . . . In summary, EPA gives special consideration to the food consumption patterns of children and infants in evaluating pesticide risks and setting pesticide tolerances, to ensure that children are fully protected. The Agency is continually evaluating its own pesticide risk assessment procedures and assumptions, and will implement any changes needed to protect children better.
>
> Office of Pesticides & Toxic Substances
> Environmental Protection Agency
> April 30, 1991

The Circle of Poison: Shipping Pesticides Overseas

The term "circle of poison" is a catchy phrase used to describe the fact that some pesticides that are not registered for use in the United States are used in foreign countries and can enter the United States in the form of residues on agricultural commodities. This is supposed to form a circle of poison around the United States.

This concept is simply naive. Certainly some pesticides that might be inappropriate for use under U.S. conditions are used in other countries (we do not intend to get into whether or not the United States should, or even has any right to, impose its regulatory policies on the sovereignty of other nations), where their use is under the control of the relevant national or local authorities.

The fact that some pesticides are not approved in the United States might simply be a function of the fact that they are not needed in this country. North Americans, for instance, have little need for pesticides used on banana and coffee crops. The registration process is expensive and time-consuming. Chemical companies would not elect to register a pesticide in the United States unless they intended to sell it here. But unregistered does not mean untested. Although the chemicals may not be registered in the United States, they are registered in the country of use.

These pesticides can leave residues that appear on agricultural exports from these countries to the United States. The residues, however, do not pose a credible health risk to U.S. consumers of such products since the residues are controlled by tolerances set by the FDA in cooperation with the Codex Alimentarius Commission of the FAO, an international body for setting safety standards.

It is also claimed that some of these foreign-use pesticides were banned in the United States as carcinogens, based on evidence of mouse-liver tumors *alone*— weak evidence at best for nearly 50 percent of the compounds so banned. The fact also remains that one can still set a residue tolerance that will be amply protective of health for these compounds. There seems, in summary, to be no credible basis to assert that the use in foreign countries of pesticides that are banned in the United States poses a health threat to the American public.

Are Food Additives Adding Cancer?

There are many categories of food additives; the four main categories are coloring agents, antioxidants (preservatives), flavorants, and emulsifiers. Some of the many other food additives include agents for maturing, bleaching, stabilizing, thickening, anticaking, leavening, curing, and a variety of other purposes.

Food colors, manufactured in the laboratory since the mid-1800s, are perhaps the most controversial food additive. Food technologists can produce such pure dyes that so resemble their counterparts found in nature that it is virtually impossible to distinguish between the two.

Unlike coloring agents from "natural" sources, synthetic dyes require certification. This means that each batch of dye must be inspected and approved as it comes from the manufacturer before it can be used in food.

In the history of food dyes, the most widely used food coloring was amaranth, better known as Red No. 2. It was used in soft drinks, ice cream, baked goods, candy, and other foods. This food dye had been used extensively in the United States since the turn of the century without any reported risk to human health. In spite of this long history of safe use, Red No. 2 was called into question in 1972 after Russian scientists suggested it might cause cancer or other health problems in animals. Although American researchers had some difficulty evaluating these studies—the relative purity of Russian Red No. 2 wasn't known—damaging doubts had been raised. The FDA spent two years doing additional intensive testing on Red No. 2 and again concluded that it was safe for use in human food. As described at that time by *Food Chemical News,* the "tests of Red 2 for carcinogenicity boiled down to two categories: one positive test and dozens of negative tests."

Although Red No. 2 had been tested more extensively than any other food-coloring agent, some consumer activists still complained. Its tongue-twisting name (trisodium salt of 1- [4 Sulfo-1-naphthylazo]-2-naphthol-3, 6-disulfonic acid) made Red No. 2 a natural target for anyone suffering from "chemical phobia." In the end, the prevailing fear of cancer won out and Red No. 2 was banned in 1976. Then, as now, the law didn't require proof that a dye was unsafe for humans.

Red No. 3 has come under similar regulatory scrutiny. In early 1990, the FDA banned the provisional uses of Red No. 3 (which accounted for about 20 percent of all uses), after male rats who were fed very high doses of the dye developed thyroid tumors. Interestingly, the action does not affect the permanently approved uses, such as in fruit juices, gelatin desserts, and fruit-cocktail cherries. In announcing the ban on provisional uses, the FDA reassured consumers that the risk associated with using such items is so small as to be negligible. Consumers were encouraged, in fact, to use up existing supplies of products containing Red No. 3. In their January 29, 1990 press release the FDA said:

> Under the so-called Delaney Clause of the 1960 Color Additive amendments to the Food, Drug and Cosmetics Act, products shown to have carcinogenic effect in laboratory tests, no matter how small, cannot be approved for use by FDA. The decision to ban the uses of Red No. 3, therefore, is *not based on risk but on the legal mandate of the Delaney Clause* [emphasis added].

The scientifically unnecessary but politically motivated partial ban on Red No. 3 forced the FDA to take a critical look at food-safety regulation, largely driven by the Delaney clause. The January 29, 1990 FDA press release said that:

> [HHS] Secretary Sullivan noted that the National Academy of Sciences has recommended that the Delaney Clause be replaced by a "negligible risk" standard, especially to reflect significant technological advances since 1960 in the detection of low levels of carcinogenic substances. The Administration is concerned about the rigidity of the Delaney Clause and has proposed a change on a similar risk assessment issue involving pesticides in foods as part of its food safety initiative announced last fall.

Let's back up for a minute and talk about the Delaney Clause and why it doesn't work.[21] The Delaney Clause was passed in 1958, amending the Federal Food, Drug and Cosmetic Act of 1938. It stated, "No additive shall be deemed safe if it is found to induce cancer when ingested by man or animal, or, if it is found, after tests which are appropriate for the evaluation of food additives, to induce cancer in man or animal."

But proponents of the Delaney amendments were as shortsighted as they were impassioned with the idea of preventing cancer. To this day, society feels the tremendous impact of the clause, which bans a substance without regard to the dose or species used in testing. The Delaney clause has not calmed, but fueled food-related fears. Some experts believe that this "anti-cancer" clause has been the primary impetus for today's panic-in-the-pantry phenomenon.

WHY DOESN'T DELANEY WORK?

The Delaney clause has never been the answer to preventing cancer for the following reason.

1. There is no room for scientific judgment. The Delaney clause calls for a total ban of any substance that causes, or is even suspected of causing, cancer in man or animals—regardless of dose or testing protocol. In the infamous Alar-treated apple fiasco, for example, Alar was forced off the market in a flurry of panic when the Natural Resources Defense Council blew the dust off one old, scientifically unsound study. Mice in that study were fed levels of Alar over 500,000 times normal human ingestion.

2. It doesn't allow for benefit vs. risk analysis. A classic example is DDT, which was instrumental in reducing morbidity and mortality from malaria. But when DDT-fed mice developed tumors, DDT was banned, causing malaria deaths to soar.

3. Delaney is wrought with inconsistency. Delaney ignores the fact that foods contain far more naturally occurring than man-made carcinogens. Al-

though we don't advocate banning foods containing natural carcinogens, the inconsistency defies scientific reason. Other inconsistencies arise when some substances "slip through" on a technicality. An example is acrylonitrile, used to manufacture plastic beverage bottles. Regulated as a food additive, one of its subcomponents is an animal carcinogen. This subcomponent, however, escapes Delaney because it is not an additive itself, only a constituent of an additive. Consumers should be assured that concentrations, as judged by the FDA, are safe. The point is that other substances with even less significant carcinogenic risk have been banned because they fall within the realm of Delaney. This happened with cosmetic dyes Red No. 19 and Orange No. 17, both banned because they caused cancer in laboratory animals. Although the FDA knew that carcinogen levels were far less than those in acrylonitrile, strict interpretation of the Delaney clause held the ban.

4. Delaney doesn't take into account the uncertainty in the extrapolation of animal test results to human health effects. Scientists know that animal species vary widely in their response to chemicals, making it impossible to extrapolate with any certainty. Cancer can be over- or underestimated, depending on the species of test animal used. Furthermore, studies at the molecular and metabolic level, which could show why a chemical that may induce cancer in animals would not do so in humans, must be ignored with strict adherence to Delaney.

5. Substances banned by Delaney may be replaced by considerably less safe products. When the courts banned Red Dye No. 19 and Orange Dye No. 17, they did so hesitatingly, saying: "The primary goal of the (FDA) Act is human safety, but literal application of the Delaney Clause may in some instances increase risk" because "Manufacturers . . . [may] substitute other coloring agents that were safe with respect to the risk of cancer but more dangerous in other respects."

6. The Delaney clause causes regulatory inconsistencies. Pesticide residues in foods are regulated according to two sections of the federal Food, Drug and Cosmetic Act. One sets tolerances for residues in raw foods, the other for residues that concentrate in processed foods and/or are applied during or after food processing. The Delaney clause applies only to the latter and absolutely prohibits any level of a pesticide with any evidence of carcinogenicity. The National Academy of Sciences calls this the "Delaney Paradox" because a pesticide residue that is legal on a raw food could render a processed food unacceptable under the law.

7. The Delaney clause never anticipated scientists' exquisite ability to detect levels of a carcinogen (or any other substance) in a food (or other medium). When the Delaney clause was enacted, scientists could barely measure substances in parts per million. Today, they can detect parts per trillion with instruments a million times more sensitive than those in 1958. As a result, although more impurities are found, their significance may be nil.

WHY CONSUMERS LIKE DELANEY

Consumers embrace Delaney, despite its problems, because of fears that have been initiated and perpetuated by a media that releases only limited or selective coverage of relevant scientific issues. For example, while consumers heard that Alar caused cancer, they were never notified of the phenomenally high doses that rodents had to consume to produce the tumors nor of the questionable study protocol. People only remembered that it causes cancer.

Most consumers want assurance of absolute safety, especially when it comes to cancer. Although more Americans die of heart disease than cancer, Americans rate cancer as the most feared disease. Says former FDA Commissioner Frank E. Young, M.D., Ph.D., "We may be much more willing to accept risks in activities over which we have some control, such as driving or skiing, than things over which we have little control, such as industrial pollution and food additives."

As far back as 1972, then FDA Commissioner C. C. Edwards, M.D., said about consumers finding comfort in Delaney: "This 'all or nothing' philosophy of the Delaney clause sounds eminently reasonable to the consumer—who wants absolute assurance that no harm will come from anything he or she eats."

However, Dr. Edwards continued, "We must regulate in the certain knowledge that absolute safety is impossible and that science is nearly always incomplete." Dr. Young echoed this thought fifteen years later: "We must consider that safety can never be absolute or guaranteed." Fred R. Shank, Ph.D., director of the FDA's Center for Food Safety and Applied Nutrition, also agreed when he said in 1991, "FDA is keenly aware that absolute safety can never be guaranteed." Dr. Young also drew on a phrase of the Hippocratic Oath: "Above all, do no harm," commenting, "The Delaney clause . . . is based on the same principle. But the corollary, in both law and medicine, is to be able to make distinctions between actions that cause harm and those that don't—and concentrate our remedial efforts on the former."

The prevailing thought at the FDA spanning two decades, then, is that it makes no sense to simply ask, "Is a carcinogen present?" One must ask the more significant question, "What real risk does it pose to human health?"

A WORKABLE SOLUTION WITH A PROVEN TRACK RECORD

Former FDA Commissioner Young proposed a more reasonable version of Delaney: "To apply the law in a reasonable way, we as a Federal agency have to be aware of the difference between insignificant and significant risk. . . . We need to find a 'threshold of risk' . . . that we can use as Federal regulators. . . . We need to take into account the advances in science that have given us tools that were missing in 1958 to make reasonable assessments of safety."

De minimis non curat lex, Latin for "the law does not concern itself with trifles," could effectively temper the Delaney clause, precluding the strict interpretation that defies scientific logic. The EPA and the Occupational Safety and Health Administration already use this concept. Determining a *de minimis* dose, or one clearly without public health threat, embodies risk evaluation, balances risk against benefits and uses scientific reason. And, according to Dr. Young, helps federal agencies, "who must apply reasonable standards as they apply laws that were never meant to be enforced without an eye to reason. *De minimis,* then, introduces limited flexibility to laws when no legal purpose or public benefit will be gained by applying the law literally.

A *de minimis* dose is set with a very wide margin of safety to protect human health, yet not waste precious resources on negligible risks. Dr. Young comments: "Public health law must be consistent with real life. No activity is completely safe, no action without risk. We must spend our resources and time on real human risks."

Regulatory agencies have defined one in a million as an acceptable level of risk. This number is not an actual risk, however, only a very conservative theoretical risk which depends on the assumptions behind the assessment method. The EPA, for example, doesn't expect one person in a million to develop cancer from eating Alar-treated apples. For the FDA to use the one-in-a-million risk figure, it is confident that the risk to humans is virtually nonexistent.

De minimis boils down to acknowledging the wisdom in the adage, "The dose makes the poison."

FDA's attempts to use *de minimis* have met with mixed results. The agency attempted to invoke the *de minimis* concept to clear the aforementioned cosmetic dyes. Unfortunately, this FDA action was successfully challenged in court by the Public Citizen Litigation Group. However, the FDA was successful in applying *de minimis* to methylene chloride, a substance used to decaffeinate coffee, leaving a small residue.

But perhaps the most disappointing failed attempt was in the summer of 1992 when the EPA attempted to use the negligible risk policy for four pesticides leaving trace residues on foods. The U.S. Court of Appeals for the Ninth Circuit rejected EPA's announced policy that residues of pesticides could remain on foods so long as the concentration was so low it represented only a negligible risk. Their decision basically upheld the strict interpretation of Delaney. The EPA issued a response to the court's decision:

> While the Court directs EPA to revoke the tolerances at issue in this case, the undisputed court record shows the dietary risks of the four pesticides involved are trivial. . . . EPA is disappointed in this decision. The literal interpretation imposed by the Court will hinder EPA's ability to make decisions that will

best ensure the overall safety and affordability of the food supply. . . . The Court's decision makes even more urgent the need for Congress to act immediately on the Administration's 1989 proposal to replace the outdated Delaney Clause with a uniform negligible risk standard for pesticides in the diet.

. . . EPA intends to assess the potential impacts of the Court's decision, which may have broad impacts upon pesticide users and consumers. Because the Agency believes that a strict interpretation of the Delaney Clause is not the most effective way to improve the safety of the food supply, the Agency intends to continue to call for legislation by Congress to replace the Delaney Clause with a uniform negligible risk standard. Regardless of the ultimate outcome of this decision, the Agency intends to regulate pesticides conservatively—in other words, to err on the side of safety when there is uncertainty about the extent of risk in order to protect public health.

EPA Statement, July 9, 1992[22]

In summary, are additives safe? As you stew over the safety of chemicals added to food, remember:

1. All foods are made up of chemicals. Just because the label on a milk carton reads "contains lactose, casein, lactoalbumin, calcium, phosphorus, and more than one hundred other chemicals," don't feel that you need to serve it in a test tube.

2. Food additives, especially those introduced in the last twenty-five years, have survived rigorous testing procedures. For example, before a food additive can be used, it has endured years of testing. All additives must be tested for acute, short-term, and long-term toxicity. Acute toxicity tests reveal what, if any, immediate effect a chemical has (on a variety of laboratory animals). In short-term toxicity tests (usually lasting about ninety days), varying amounts of the chemical are fed to animals. The animals are monitored for changes in general appearance, behavior, growth pattern, and, at autopsy, abnormalities in internal tissues and organs. Finally, long-term toxicity studies look for effects on fertility, reproduction, and the occurrence of cancer. Only those additives that survive all three rounds may be submitted to the FDA, as a "petition for approval." These extensive procedures cost upwards of $100,000.

   The petition for approval includes all testing information, foods of intended use, amounts to be used in food, and labeling directions. An additive doesn't have a chance of approval if it poses even a minuscule threat to human health. To better understand how rigorous is the testing process, note that certain "natural" substances, such as vitamin A, would never survive the testing process.

3. Keep in mind that additives (not including common additives such as sugar and salt) make up less than 1 percent of the food we eat each year. In light of this, it seems logical to worry less about additives and more about the safety of the other 99 percent. Of course, if some additive or food is shown to represent a hazard to human health, then even "a little bit" may be too much to accept in our food supply. But we monitor our food constantly and have found no such hazard or any suggestion that various food chemicals are "stored up" to cause trouble later on.

4. Remember that allowed levels of food additives leave a generous margin of safety to protect human health. Strict regulations set allowed amounts at just one-hundredth of the level at which no adverse effects were shown in animals. This is a hundred-fold margin of safety. As a matter of fact, the laws are so strict (as we'll see in later chapters) that some products have been removed from supermarket shelves before being given a full and fair trial. The FDA's motto is: guilty until proven innocent.

5. There is no evidence linking food additives to any form of human disease or illness. The American Cancer Society published its "Guidelines on Diet, Nutrition and Cancer" in late 1991, concluding that, "Knowledge about the possible cancer risks or benefits of food additives is insufficient at this time to warrant a recommendation for or against their use."[23] The only type of cancer that has shown a dramatic increase since the 1940s, when additives began growing in popularity, is lung cancer. And there is no link between additives and lung cancer. In addition, heart disease, still our biggest killer, hasn't been linked to the use of additives.

6. Consumers are in far greater danger from improper food preparation and storage than from food additives. Both pale in comparison to the known health effects of overeating.

So why are some people afraid of chemical food preservatives? I'll tell you why. It's a lack of education and insight. It's just another manifestation of an irrational fear of chemicals known as "chemophobia." The emphasis is on "irrational," because chemophobes worry about traces of these chemical substances—and selectively at that—because nobody fears salt, acids, or nutrients, all of which are chemicals. The fear must be irrational because the presence of chemical preservatives in our food supply has caused no disease or death in our population. On the contrary, when chemical preservatives are not present in our food, death and disease appear.

The Centers for Disease Control estimate that about 250 million Americans every year suffer from bouts with food poisoning bacteria, and about 5,000 victims die.[24] We cannot say that with heavier use of chemical preservatives those numbers would be lower, but we can be certain that without chemical preservatives more people would get sick and far more would die.

The Beef Over DES

DES (short for the tongue-twisting diethylstilbesterol) is a synthetic (manu-factured in the laboratory) form of estrogen. It's been in use since the 1940s as a medication, since 1954 as a growth stimulant in cattle, and in 1973 was approved for emergency use as a "morning after" contraceptive pill.

When DES is used as a growth stimulant in cattle, a five-hundred-pound animal reaches a marketable weight of a thousand pounds in thirty-four days less time *and* with five hundred pounds less feed than an animal not receiving DES. DES also has desirable effects on meat quality. It increases protein and moisture by 7 percent, thereby decreasing the percentage of fat in that meat. Prior to its 1972 banning, DES was fed to 75 percent of the 30 million cattle slaughtered each year in the United States.

It was no secret in 1954 when DES was first used in cattle that it didn't have a clear record. Since 1940, experts have known that DES, like all types of estrogen, causes cancer in test animals—breast cancer in mice and rats and testicular cancer in mice. When the Delaney Clause was adopted in 1958, experts in the cattle industry together with government officials searched the fine print of Delaney to allow the continued use of DES. They were successful, finding that DES could be used as long as no residue was found in the meat.

As early as 1959, though, residues were found in chickens, resulting in the immediate banning of DES use in poultry. But its use in beef remained legal as long as no residue could be found. As a precautionary measure, cattle farmers were required to stop using DES in their animals forty-eight hours before slaughter.

Cattle farmers continued to use DES in beef cattle during the 1960s. The testing methods had improved to the capability of detecting ten parts per billion of a substance in another substance (which is about the same as five drops per 25,000 gallons of water). DES was still immune from Delaney's grasp because either it wasn't found at all in beef, or was at levels below this testing ability.

RARE VAGINAL CANCER CAUSES ALARM

In 1971 Boston gynecologist Dr. Arthur Herbst, of the prestigious Massachusetts General Hospital, reported a link between young women with an extremely rare form of vaginal cancer (adenocarcinoma) and their mother's use of DES during pregnancy (DES was used to decrease their risk of miscarriage).

Needless to say, a red flag about the safety of DES use in cattle immediately went up after Herbst's findings were published in the *New England Journal of Medicine*. By the end of 1971, the pressure was on and DES use in animals was severely criticized. Cattle raisers were told to withdraw the drug seven days before slaughter, and residue testing continued.

By 1972 a highly sensitive form of radioactive tracer technique became available, and DES residues were found in the livers of about 2.5 percent of randomly selected animals. Senator Edward Kennedy held a subcommittee meeting on DES in July 1972, further alarming the public with the words: "We are here today because DES, a known cancer-causing agent, is appearing on thousands of American dinner tables. . . ."

Americans were up in arms. They didn't want any cancer-causing hormones in their hamburgers. The "us versus them" attitude surfaced once again. Critics of DES described it as a means of "saving cattlemen some $90 million yearly." (Of course, they didn't stop to think that it wasn't cattlemen at all who were saving money, but they themselves in lower-priced beef products.)

INCONSISTENCIES IN THE BANNING OF DES

In the ruckus over their meatloaf, consumers failed to seek out essential facts.

First, DES is not the only source of estrogen in the food supply. Milk, eggs, and even honey contain estrogen. It's been estimated that one egg provides a thousand times the amount of estrogen found in a serving of liver from a *DES-treated animal.* Birth control pills, which many women use almost daily, contain far more synthetic estrogen than does a serving of DES-tainted liver.

Second, and even more basically, is the fact that a woman's body regularly produces estrogen (men also produce some estrogen, but not as much as women). The prestigious British journal *Nature* estimated that it would take five hundred pounds of liver containing two parts per billion of DES to equal the amount of estrogen produced each day by a woman during her reproductive years.

Third, the women who were treated with estrogen to prevent miscarriage received up to 125 mg a day during pregnancy. To get that amount of estrogen, you would have to eat 62.5 tons of beef liver (containing two parts per billion of DES) at one sitting. Any woman who has used DES as a "morning after" birth control method would have to eat 500 tons of liver containing DES residues to equal the estrogen in just one pill (again, at one sitting).

Fourth, DES was condemned in spite of the fact that there was no evidence that the tiny traces of DES in beef liver were harmful to man or animals.

Fifth, all present evidence points to the fact that there is a "no-effect" level for DES and other estrogens. The no-effect level is that level of a substance that doesn't cause tumors or other health problems. This "no-effect" principle has been demonstrated in mice. And the fact that all of us, male and female, have natural levels of estrogen and yet don't all develop cancer suggests that the same principle holds true for humans.

It was indeed alarming to find out that massive doses of DES given to women during pregnancy could contribute to the development of cancer in some of their daughters. As alarming as it was, however, this observation shouldn't have been applied to the tiny traces of estrogen in food, *especially* in light of our own natural estrogen production.

But hysteria and politics teamed up and in August 1972, FDA Commissioner Charles C. Edwards announced that he had "no choice" but to discontinue approval for DES in animal feed. His ruling still allowed slow-release DES implants in animals' ears. But less than a year later, the FDA banned these implants after 0.04 to 0.12 parts per billion of DES were found in beef liver from animals so treated.

In protest, the manufacturers of DES requested an FDA hearing. Hearing refused, they appealed. Finally, in January 1974, the United States Court of Appeals ruled that the FDA's orders were invalid and that the manufacturers of DES could resume marketing their products until the FDA had held a hearing. The court took action because

> The FDA chose to act summarily, without a hearing, without making known to petitioners the nature of the "new evidence" or of the underlying tests, and without giving the petitioners an opportunity to controvert the new evidence.

In late 1979, DES manufacturers and cattle farmers lost a hard-fought court fight and DES was banned from livestock use. This led to widespread illegal use of DES, described in a 1980 issue of the *Kansas City Star* as "the biggest veterinary drug scandal in U.S. history."

No More Cookouts?[25]

In 1963, Italian researchers found small amounts of benzo(a)pyrene (BaP), an animal carcinogen, in charcoal-broiled meat. The carcinogen might have resulted from smoke that was generated when fat from the meat dripped into the underlying coals. Barbecue lovers who heard of these findings were understandably concerned.

Unfortunately, large-scale human studies of cancer risk due to BaP are difficult to perform. For one thing, a person's recollection of his dietary past is bound to be inaccurate. Second, BaP is also present in other human exposures, such as automobile exhaust and industrial smoke. These obstacles make it nearly impossible to quantify a person's exposure to BaP, leaving the relationship between charcoal-broiled meat and cancer in humans unproven.

Please Pass the Bacon . . .[26]

Nitrates have been used for centuries to cure meat, fish, and poultry. These preservatives prevent the growth of the bacterium that causes botulism, an extremely serious form of food poisoning. But in the 1960s, scientists discovered that nitrites could combine with amines, chemicals naturally found in foods, to form nitrosamines—substances shown to cause cancer in animals.

Some human studies have shown a relationship between nitrite intake and digestive cancers. But many of these studies examined small populations in underdeveloped countries, where meat treatment differs from that in the United States. In addition, the methods used to determine nitrite intake among study subjects are also debatable.

Like BaP, nitrosamines are ubiquitous in our environment, making it difficult to quantify a person's exposure. For example, nitrosamines exist in cigarette smoke, beer, whiskey, and the air inside new cars.

The International Agency for Research on Cancer recently concluded that human evidence linking nitrites to cancer is inadequate. Bacon, as are all foods, is safe when used in a moderate, varied, balanced diet.

Nonetheless, to protect human health with a generous margin of safety, the FDA set and then lowered the permissible levels of nitrate in foods. Allowed levels vary with the specific meat product: for example, cured meats such as bologna and salami, which aren't usually heated, may have higher levels than bacon, where the cooking process can convert nitrates to nitrites. As an added safety measure, manufacturers add vitamin C to nitrate-containing products, which effectively blocks the formation of nitrosamines.

But let's put the whole issue of nitrates and nitrites into proper perspective. Their use greatly reduces our chance of falling victim to botulism—a risk with *proven* serious consequences. And it's estimated that cigarette smoking contributes up to ten times as many nitrosamines as food, water, and other sources in the environment combined!

Antibiotics in Animal Feed: A Threat to Human Health?[27]

Antibiotics are used in two different ways in the raising of livestock and poultry. High doses (therapeutic levels, defined roughly as above 200 grams per ton of feed or equivalent intakes through water) are used to treat diseases, just as they are in human medicine. Lower, subtherapeutic doses are used for other purposes that do not have a parallel in current human medical practice except for low-level long-term prophylactic treatment for acne. They are routinely included at levels below 100 grams/ton in livestock and poultry feeds because they increase the rate of weight gain in growing young animals or birds, increase the amount of meat that can be produced from a given amount of feed (feed efficiency), and help to prevent bacterial diseases. Specific levels that are considered therapeutic vary with disease organism and drug and may change over time.

Feeding antibiotics to farm animals poses a theoretical risk of increasing the prevalence of antibiotic-resistant bacteria that might cause human diseases that in turn could not be treated successfully with the same drugs.

All of the steps necessary to produce this type of health hazard can occur. There is a lack of direct evidence, however, to indicate the extent to which they do occur in practice.

Some scientists claim that a disease "time bomb" may soon explode as a result of more than thirty years of antibiotic use in animal agriculture. If this were true, smaller "time bombs" would be expected to explode first in those populations most heavily exposed to antibiotic-resistant bacteria from farm animals: the animals themselves, livestock producers, and slaughterhouse workers. The effectiveness of the drugs as animal-growth promotants would also be expected to decrease. Since these events have not occurred, a major hazard to the health of the general human population does not appear to be imminent.

Food activists have generated recent headlines that focus attention on the possible dangers of trace levels of antibacterial substances in cows' milk, one of our most sacrosanct foods. Properly so, these critics stop short of recommending that consumers, especially infants and children, discontinue milk consumption.

How did this sophomoric attempt to undermine consumer confidence in our milk supply begin? In late December 1988 the *Wall Street Journal* (*WSJ*) and the Nader-affiliated Center for Science in the Public Interest (CSPI) scared American consumers with two separate surveys in an article headlined, "Milk Is Found Tainted with a Range of Drugs Farmers Give Cattle." The subtitle "Residues in 38% of Samples" provided little or no comfort or reassurance on the safety of our milk supply.

Unfortunately, the *WSJ* and CSPI based their alarming survey on *screening* assays and failed to perform the required *confirmatory* assay. These screening assays merely indicate that some residues of a drug class *may* be present. The word "may" is highlighted because crude screening assays often indicate the presence of a substance that cannot be confirmed by specific tests—giving rise to so-called "false positives." The Food and Drug Administration then conducted a nationwide sampling and testing program using the same *screening* tests the

WSJ and CSPI used. The key difference was that the FDA performed *confirmatory* assays to measure the presence of specific animal drug residues. In February 1990, the FDA presented its results with the following statement[28] (slightly paraphrased):

> A nationwide survey of milk has found no residues of any antibiotics, including sulfa drugs. These findings, based on the most current analytical methods, contradict earlier conclusions reached after publication of an unconfirmed screening test sponsored by a national newspaper.

The facts are clear—the nation's milk supply is safe when properly assayed. It is not contaminated by antibiotics, unauthorized drugs, or any other substances harmful to health. The millions of routine samples assayed regularly by federal and state regulatory authorities, dairy processors, and farmers attest to this basic fact—our milk is safe!

To put this issue in proper perspective, Professor Thomas H. Jukes, University of California at Berkeley, wrote (slightly paraphrased): "In the *WSJ* survey, sulfa drugs were found in the range of 5–10 milligrams per ton of milk. A dose of sulfa drugs is about 2,000 milligrams per day for an adult. To obtain such a therapeutic level, a daily intake of 200 tons [200,000 quarts] of milk per day would be required!"[29]

Our advice to the *WSJ* and CSPI is to stop trying to scare consumers and get the facts straight before publishing such stories.

Pseudoscientists Milk Publicity[30]

Will radical international and domestic agitators succeed in thwarting a major advance in biotechnology—the use of bovine somatotropin (BST) to increase milk production in U.S. dairy cows?

The answer to this question is still uncertain as critics, principally from Europe and far removed from mainstream science, oppose this development in major U.S. dairy states such as Wisconsin. As typically happens with critics of technology, they are using arguments unrelated to human safety and efficacy. According to these opponents, BST represents an economic threat to the family farm. They also claim that BST use can "overstress" dairy cows, an "animal rights" charge unsupported by scientific evidence.

Bovine somatotropin is a naturally occurring peptide hormone, composed of approximately 190 amino acids. Produced by the pituitary gland, it regulates milk production in dairy cows. The fact that BST supplementation makes dairy cows more productive has been known for decades, but until recently, BST could not be produced economically. Now, thanks to a biotechnology breakthrough, dairy farmers can obtain more milk from the same cows by supplementing their natural BST.

Proponents of BST state that it will be the first major use of a biotechnology product related to milk production, resulting in a 10–20 percent increase in milk production. Since BST works within a day or so, milk producers can respond quickly to demand fluctuations without having to increase herd size.

There is no known ill health effect from consuming milk produced with BST supplementation. BST is naturally present in trace amounts in milk and is readily digested by humans as a typical protein. Moreover, tests show that cows receiving BST supplement have no higher BST levels in their milk than those not receiving the supplement.

As for the allegation that BST will harm cows, a dairy scientist who reviewed more than 150 published scientific papers reported recently that none made any reference to metabolic "overstress" or "burnout."

Food "Chemicals" in Perspective: Natural Toxins in Food

As previously alluded to, naturally occurring carcinogenic substances in food are far more abundant and numerous than man-made carcinogens in food. Not only are there large numbers of naturally occurring food carcinogens, but there are also many more produced during cooking and by the actions of microorganisms.[31]

Consider, for example, a typical holiday dinner menu[32] (see Table 1). The mushroom soup, for example, contains hydrazines, which are potent animal carcinogens. The main entree, roast turkey with stuffing and cranberry sauce, contains heterocyclic amines and malonaldehyde (mutagens), eugenol (animal carcinogen), and furan derivatives.

We must emphasize the toxicological adage, "Only the dose makes the poison."[33] A toxic dose of caffeine requires ninety-six cups of coffee, and 3.8 tons of turkey would be needed to deliver a toxic dose of malonaldehyde—all at one sitting. Eating a mere fifty to eighty pounds of cinnamon or black pepper could cause cancer from the safrole contained within, though you might sneeze yourself to death first.

Three conclusions can be reached. First, the best way to minimize the potential hazard posed by naturally occurring carcinogens would be to eat a wide variety of foods, since this would minimize the chance that any single carcinogen would be eaten in a quantity that would overwhelm the body's natural ability to handle a small amount of a hazardous substance with relative safety. Certainly, it would be unrealistic to attempt to remove from our food supply every known trace of naturally occurring cancer-causing agents or to avoid all exposure to them, just as it would be unrealistic to seek "zero exposure" to sunlight (a skin car-

Table 1

A HOLIDAY DINNER MENU

What's on the plate   *What's in it*

APPETIZERS

CREAM OF MUSHROOM SOUP	Hydrazines
FRESH VEGETABLE TRAY	
CARROTS	Carotatoxin, myristicin, isoflavones, nitrate
RADISHES	Glucosinolates, nitrate
CHERRY TOMATOES	Hydrogen peroxide, nitrate, quercetin glycoside, tomatine
CELERY	Nitrate, psoralens

ENTRÉES

ROAST TURKEY	Heterocyclic amines, malonaldehyde
BREAD STUFFING (with onions, celery, black pepper, and mushrooms)	Benzo(a)pyrene, di- and tri-sulfide ethyl carbamate, furan derivatives, dihydrazines, psoralens, safrole
CRANBERRY SAUCE	Eugenol, furan derivatives

CHOICE OF VEGETABLE

LIMA BEANS	Cyanogenetic glycosides
BROCCOLI SPEARS	Allyl isothiocyanate, glucosinolates, goitrin, nitrate
BAKED POTATO	Amylase inhibitors, arsenic, chaconine, isoflavones, nitrate, oxalic acid, solanine
SWEET POTATO	Cyanogenetic glycosides, furan derivatives, nitrate
ROLLS	Amylase inhibitors, benzo(a)pyrene, ethyl carbamate, furan derivatives, diacetyl

DESSERTS

PUMPKIN PIE	Myristicin, nitrate, safrole
APPLE PIE	Acetaldehyde, isoflavones, phlorizin, quercetin glycoside, safrole

BEVERAGES

COFFEE	Benzo(a)pyrene, caffeine, chlorogenic acid, hydrogen peroxide, methylglyoxal, tannins
TEA	Benzo(a)pyrene, caffeine, quercetin glycosides, tannins
RED WINE	Alcohol, ethyl carbamate, methylglyoxal, tannins, tyramine
WATER	Nitrate

ASSORTED NUTS

MIXED NUTS	Aflatoxins

cinogen) or to medical radiation (which would mean giving up the benefits of X-rays and therapeutic radiology for treating cancer). In any case, there is at this point no evidence that low-level exposure to natural or man-made chemicals in the U.S. food supply poses a significant risk of cancer.

Second, although scientists are just now scratching the surface in identifying natural carcinogens and the hazards they pose to humans, it is already evident that we should reject the presumption, if not superstition, that "natural" is safe and "man-made" suspect. There is no scientific evidence to support this belief.

Third, the increasing body of evidence documenting the carcinogenicity of common, everyday substances in nature (at least under laboratory conditions) highlights the contradiction that we have created in our past regulatory approach to carcinogens. The contradiction consists of the huge discrepancy in the weight we have hitherto placed on man-made carcinogens by trying to purge our land of them and natural carcinogens that we have simply ignored, even though our means of assessing cancer hazards indicates that the latter hazard is far greater than the former. Our new regulatory emphasis should be on the potency of a chemical carcinogen and the level of human exposure to it rather than on the chemical's natural vs. artificial origin. There is a need to distinguish between functional and unnecessary substances when setting these regulatory priorities. These priorities must distinguish between the risks that really matter and the multitude of tiny ones that don't. We must gain a renewed appreciation in the context of carcinogens for the scientifically sound and time-honored principle, the most basic tenet of toxicology, that "only the dose makes the poison."

Preserving Food—Understanding Food Irradiation[34]

Over the centuries, great efforts have been devoted to finding ways to preserve food and protect it from microorganisms, insects, and other pests. Drying was one of the first techniques developed. Fermenting, salting, and smoking also have long histories. Later inventions, including freezing, refrigeration, canning, and the use of preservatives and pesticides, have further increased the quality, quantity, and safety of our food supply by protecting it against contamination and spoilage.

Radiation used on food is called "ionizing radiation" because it produces electrically charged particles. Ionizing radiation can be produced from radioactive isotopes of cobalt or cesium, or from devices that produce controlled amounts of beta rays, gamma rays, or X-rays. (Beta rays are streams or beams of electrons accelerated by a machine to energies of up to 10 MeV. Gamma rays are electromagnetic radiation of very short wavelength, similar to "short" X-rays. Gamma rays are emitted by radioactive isotopes of cobalt and cesium as they disintegrate spontaneously. X-rays are ionizing electromagnetic radiation of a wide variety of short wavelengths. They are usually produced by a machine in which a beam of fast electrons in a vacuum bombards a metallic target.) These ionizing radiations have a higher energy than other, nonionizing radiations such as light, microwaves, and radio waves.

This process does not make the food radioactive. The doses and energy levels of radiation approved for the treatment of foods simply do not have enough energy to induce radioactivity in food. Neither does the process generate radioactive wastes. The process simply involves exposing food to a source of radiation. It does not create any new radioactive material. Of course, when radioactive isotopes of cobalt or cesium are used as the radiation source, they must be disposed of properly after they are used. But using these materials for food irradiation does not make their eventual disposal more difficult.

Irradiation has several uses in food processing, most of which prolong the useful life of foods. Food irradiation can be used in the following ways:

1. To reduce the number of disease-causing organisms in fresh meat, poultry, and fish. Irradiation kills bacteria and renders harmless disease-causing parasites, such as those that cause trichinosis. The United States is one of the few technologically developed countries that still has a problem with trichinosis transmitted by commercial pork. Although the disease is rare, it can be very serious.

2. To delay mold growth in fresh fruits, thereby prolonging shelf life.

3. To kill insects or prevent them from reproducing, thereby reducing food losses. Irradiation could partially replace post-harvest fumigants used for this purpose.

4. To extend shelf life of many fruits and vegetables by delaying ripening and inhibiting sprouting.

5. To sterilize meat, poultry, fish, shellfish, some vegetables, baked goods, and prepared foods, allowing the treated product to be stored at room temperature without spoilage, and rendering it safe for hospital patients who require microbiologically sterile diets.

Food irradiation is hardly new. Indeed, the armed forces have used it since the 1950s. The U.S. Army has sponsored extensive research on radiation sterilization, with the goal of producing better quality meals for troops in the field. Some of the army's earliest experimental radiation-sterilized foods, produced in the 1950s and early 1960s, were less than successful in terms of flavor, aroma, and texture—although the products were undoubtedly safe. However, improvements have been made in the irradiation procedure since then, and the radiation-sterilized meat and poultry products produced by current methods have been rated by experts as superior to their canned counterparts in texture, appearance, and in some cases, flavor and vitamin retention.

The U.S. Army has reaffirmed its interest in using irradiated food in the field. As part of its post–Persian Gulf War review, General William Tuttle, Jr., the commanding officer of the U.S. Army Materiel Command, has notified the U.S. Department of Agriculture that the army wishes to incorporate irradiated foods into the military subsistence system. General Tuttle indicates that the army is planning a program for securing FDA approvals to extend the current approval of fresh poultry to other fresh meats and fish, to inhibit pests in fruits, and, most importantly, to obtain approval for radiation-sterilized meats, poultry, and fish. General Tuttle stresses that the need of the soldier in the field to have maximum access to meals that are nutritious and morale-enhancing has prompted a renewed military interest in irradiated foods.

Irradiation would facilitate the interstate and international shipment of fruits and vegetables. Many states and countries prohibit the importation of foods suspected of contamination with live insects, fearing the introduction of a pest problem along with the produce. During the 1981 Mediterranean fruit fly (medfly) infestation in California and Florida, the reluctance of buyers in other states and countries to accept produce that might be contaminated with live medflies led to substantial economic losses. Irradiation would be very useful in situations of this type by allowing produce to be shipped to uninfested areas without the risk of spreading the insect infestation.

There is not one knowledgeable, credible, responsible scientist or physician who opposes irradiated food. Critics often use irradiated food as a front on which they promote their antinuclear and political ideologies. There is no link between irradiated food and nuclear weapons production when cobalt 60 (the preferred source) is used.

Despite its proven safety and efficacy, consumers have reacted with a level of hysteria sufficient to push legislators into unnecessary and factually unfounded legislation, such as in New Jersey.[35] Antinuclear activists have succeeded in lobbying two state legislators to sponsor a bill not to delay, but to permanently ban the sale and distribution of irradiated food in the state.

The sponsors of this bill are operating on at least two very serious fallacies. First, the sponsors, probably having little or no scientific background, believe that scientific issues can be resolved legislatively. This type of "resolution" completely ignores the scientific procedure of collecting additional evidence, subjecting it to peer review, and arriving at a position by consensus.

The second major fallacy concerns the so-called "controversy" over irradiated food. Valid scientific controversy over this issue no longer exists. Food irradiation has been approved by thirty-seven countries including the United States. Twenty-four countries have successfully adopted this technology since 1958, and the number is growing by two to three countries per year.

The Big Green: Proposition 128

So what difference does it make if Alar gets a lot of print? Who cares if lots of our resources are devoted to getting it out of our food supply? What is the harm in some hype about pesticides as long as it sounds the alarm about good health? Why not spend a little extra money to be sure our kids are safe?

Why? Because it is a moral outrage and a political fraud to ask the American people to invest their money and emotions in something that gives no return in improved health, nor peace of mind, and yet causes serious economic damage in the process. We need to be deeply concerned about the welfare of our families when public health policy is set not by scientists but by political operatives and special interest groups with an ax to grind and agendas to fulfill. But most important of all, spending money on improperly identified problems wastes precious resources that could be spent fighting the real killers.

Look at the so-called "Big Green" initiative that went before the people of California in the fall of 1990. It was an environmental wish list to help cure a bundle of ills, from the allegedly depleting ozone layer to "unsafe" foods. Big Green was also proof that a hippo is a mouse built to government specifications: Specifically, it mandated that any pesticide, *in any amount,* causing cancer in laboratory animals would be banned, regardless of risks or benefits associated with its use.

What also made Big Green notable was the vocal support of many of America's most famous personalities. Predictably, there was not a scientist nor a cancer expert among them. Scaring the public was the order of the day: Oliver Stone, the director of *Platoon,* claimed that Americans are "choking to death." Jack Lemmon said swimmers are contracting "mysterious diseases." Other stars warned of "deadly fruit." An ad for Big Green declared that "Scientists are unable to find uncontaminated fish in California waters. Cancer in children is up by 20 percent since 1950." And we were told, "20,000 Americans will develop cancer and 3,000 will die because of pesticide exposure this year."

There is absolutely no scientific evidence to support any of these charges. State officials and many distinguished scientists have repeatedly said so. But it doesn't make any difference. Big Green and other environmental initiatives since then are political debates, not scientific exercises. Fact and reality aren't important. As Big Green campaign spokesman Bob Mulholland, confided: "In a political debate, science doesn't matter much. It's really how you feel about the issue."

Today, people are regularly asked to make judgments about public health policy based on negative advertising and media hype. And when it comes to environmental and health issues, everything is supposedly black and white: You are either for the environment and against greedy industrial polluters, or you are in the enemy camp. And Ed Bradley, Meryl Streep, Oliver Stone, and the others don't have to worry about growing apples or vegetables, or whether new regulations will drive small businesses into bankruptcy.

Nor do they have to worry about the fact that Big Green would have drastically lowered all crop production in the nation's largest agricultural state by an estimated 40 percent. It would have sent the cost of food skyrocketing—with many prices 50 percent higher—for millions of people. Clearly this would have increased the risks of poverty and disease for the people who are the least able to pay in society—the poor and the elderly. Big Green would have undermined the very economic expansion that is needed to ensure financing of sound environmental and public programs.

Fortunately, Big Green did not pass. It was defeated by nearly two to one. Voters didn't care for the idea that they couldn't vote separately on some of the provisions. They realized that a "czar" with authority and autonomy that supersedes all levels of state government is a dangerous abuse of the traditional American system of checks and balances. It may well be that the tide is beginning to turn against the inverted priorities this initiative promoted.[36]

Conclusions

Our food supply is safe. As concluded by the 1989 food-safety workshop convened by the Institute of Food Technologists' Office of Scientific Public Affairs and representing eighteen scientific societies and over 100,000 scientists, "the perception that the food supply is unsafe is not supported by scientific data. . . . Current state and federal legislation provides sufficient authority to protect consumers [and] further legislation is not required."[37]

It is a misperception that pesticide residues in food are a major threat to health. Dr. Richard Adamson of the National Cancer Institute assured me that "I am unaware of [any] evidence that suggests regulated and approved pesticide residues in food contribute to the toll of human cancer in the United States."[38] Indeed, the IFT[39] also concludes that "the health effects from pesticide residues may be relatively insignificant when compared to those associated with naturally-occurring chemicals in foods."

Back in 1985, Cornell University held a symposium entitled "The American Food Supply: Are We At Risk?" They, too, concluded that the major risks in the food supply, in order of priority, are food-borne disease, malnutrition, environmental contaminants (natural and man-made but not pesticides), naturally occurring toxicants, and, finally, pesticides and food additives.[40]

Exhibit "A"

OUR FOOD SUPPLY IS SAFE!*

To date, 1989 will be remembered as the year that an epidemic of fear spread throughout the nation and caused Americans to doubt the safety of their food supply. We, members of America's scientific community, sympathize with consumers' concerns but condemn efforts of certain environmental groups to exaggerate risk and cause needless anxiety. We wish to set the record straight.

THERE IS NO SCIENTIFIC EVIDENCE THAT RESIDUES IN FOOD FROM REGULATED AND APPROVED USE OF PESTICIDES HAVE EVER BEEN THE CAUSE OF ILLNESS OR DEATH IN EITHER ADULTS OR CHILDREN.

The Government has *strict* standards for food safety. It sets tolerance levels for pesticide residues in food. The standards currently in place are *stringent and effective.* The Food and Drug Administration recently reported that the overwhelming percentage of tested foods has no residue.

THERE IS NO SCIENTIFIC MERIT TO CHARGES THAT PESTICIDE RESIDUES IN OUR PRODUCE CAUSE CANCER IN HUMAN BEINGS.

These charges are based exclusively on studies that expose rats and mice to enormous doses of chemicals. Humans would have to eat tons of produce every day for many years to ingest similar amounts. As a recent article in *Nature,* a highly respected international scientific journal, pointed out: "Extrapolating from one species to another is fraught with uncertainty." *Mice are not little men.*

AMERICA'S FOOD SUPPLY IS THE SAFEST AND MOST PLENTIFUL IN THE WORLD. PESTICIDES DESERVE MUCH OF THE CREDIT.

If Americans really want to go "back to nature," they will have to coexist with vermin and insects and the diseases they bring. Dismantling the agricultural system will reduce the food supply, forcing consumers to pay the cost.

---

*The American Council on Science and Health placed this ad in the *New York Times, Washington Post,* and *USA Today* in the spring of 1989 to assure Americans about the safety of our food supply.

IT IS DANGEROUS TO FOCUS ON UNSUBSTANTIATED CLAIMS WHEN REAL RISKS TO OUR HEALTH ABOUND.

Our country faces major hurdles in its attempt to conquer premature, preventable death. From AIDS to cigarette smoking to hard drugs, there are mammoth health challenges facing us. Why then are we becoming obsessed with irrational allegations that find so little support in the scientific community? Why aren't we focusing on the real problems?

LET'S COUNT OUR BLESSINGS AND REJECT UNFOUNDED ATTACKS ON THE SAFETY OF OUR FOOD SUPPLY.

Blaine L. Blad, Ph.D.
University of Nebraska
Edward E. Burns, Ph.D.
Texas A & M University
Ogbourne D. Butler, Ph.D.
Texas A & M University
Elwood F. Caldwell, Ph.D.
University of Minnesota
Ernest E. Campaigne, Ph.D.
Indiana University
C. Jelleff Carr, Ph.D.
Columbia, Maryland
Robert G. Cassens, Ph.D.
University of Wisconsin
F. M. Clydesdale, Ph.D.
University of Massachusetts
Donald G. Cochran, Ph.D.
Virginia Polytechnic Institute
Julius M. Coon, M.D.
Thomas Jefferson University
Bernard D. Davis, M.D.
Harvard Medical School
Thomas R. DeGregori, Ph.D.
University of Houston
Robert M. Devlin, Ph.D.
University of Massachusetts
James E. Enstrom, Ph.D.
University of California, Los Angeles
Lloyd J. Filet, Jr., M.D., Ph.D.
University of Iowa Hospitals and Clinics

Kenneth D. Fisher, Ph.D.
  Fed. of Amer. Societies for Exp. Biology
Leonard T. Flynn, Ph.D., M.B.A.
  Morganville, New Jersey
F. J. Francis, Ph.D.
  University of Massachusetts
Glenn W. Froning, Ph.D.
  University of Nebraska, Lincoln
Leonard J. Goldwater, M.D.
  Chapel Hill, North Carolina
Helen A. Guthrie, Ph.D.
  Pennsylvania State University
Wayland Jackson Hayes, Jr., M.D., Ph.D.
  Vanderbilt University
Virgil Hayes, Ph.D.
  University of Kentucky
William E. Hazeltine, Ph.D.
  Butte County Mosquito Abatement District
Agnes Heinz, Ph.D.
  American Council on Science and Health
Victor Herbert, M.D., J.D.
  Bronx Veterans Administration Medical Center
John Higginson, M.D., F.R.C.P.
  Institute For Health Policy Analysis
Joseph H. Hotchkiss, Ph.D.
  Cornell University
William T. Jarvis, Ph.D.
  National Council Against Health Fraud
Kathryn Kolasa, Ph.D., R.D.
  Greenville, North Carolina
Manfred Kroger, Ph.D.
  Pennsylvania State University
James A. Lowell, Ph.D.
  Pina Community College
Howard D. Maccabee, Ph.D., M.D.
  Radiation Oncology Center
Roger P. Maickel, Ph.D.
  Purdue University
Judith A. Marlett, P.D.
  University of Wisconsin, Madison
Margaret N. Maxey, Ph.D.
  University of Texas, Austin

John McKetta, P.E., Ph.D.
University of Texas, Austin
W. J. Miller, Ph.D.
University of Georgia
A. Alan Moghissi, Ph.D.
Institute of Regulator Science, Virginia
Eric W. Mood, LL.D., M.P.H.
Yale University
Richard Oksas, M.P.H., Pharm. D.
South Bay Free Clinic, California
Robert E. Olson, M.D., Ph.D.
State University of New York at Stony Brook State
Jane M. Orient, M.D.
Tucson, Arizona
M. Alice Ottoboni, Ph.D.
Berkeley, California
Albert M. Pearson, Ph.D.
Michigan State University
R. T. Ravenholt, M.D.
World Health Surveys
Edward G. Remmers, Sc.D.
American Council on Science and Health
David B. Roll, Ph.D.
University of Utah
Edward Runge Ph.D.
Texan A & M University
Paul D. Saltman, Ph.D.
University of California, San Diego
Wallace I. Sampson, M.D.
Stanford University
Herbert P. Sarett, Ph.D.
Sarasota, Florida
Lowell D. Satterlee, Ph.D.
Pennsylvania State University
Sarah Short, Ph.D., R.D.
Syracuse University
Frederick J. Stare, M.D., Ph.D.
Harvard School of Public Health
James H. Steele, D.V.M., M.P.H.
University of Texas
Stephen S. Sternberg, M.D.
Memorial Sloan-Kettering Institute

Martha Barnes Stone, Ph.D.
Kansas State University
Stephen L. Taylor, Ph.D.
University of Wisconsin
William A. Toscano, Jr., Ph.D.
Harvard School of Public Health
Murray M. Tuckerman, Ph.D.
Temple University
Robert P. Upchurch, Ph.D.
University of Arizona
W. E. Wardowski, Ph.D.
University of Florida
Elizabeth M. Whelan, Sc.D., M.P.H.
American Council on Science and Health
Panaylotis Michael Zavos, Ph.D.
University of Kentucky

NOTES

1. Natural Resources Defense Council, *Intolerable Risk: Pesticides in Our Children's Food* (1989).

2. "Death on Your Dinner Table,"*Audubon* (September 1987).

3. J. Naar, *Design for a Livable Planet* (New York: Harper and Row, 1990).

4. E. Haas, "Public Voice for Food and Health Policy," "Donahue" show #06246.

5. Naar, *Design for a Livable Planet,* p. 174.

6. S. R. Baker, and C. F. Wilkinson, *The Effect of Pesticides on Human Health,* vol. 18 (Princeton: Princeton Scientific Publishing, 1990), p. 2.

7. Ibid., p. 14.

8. Institute of Food Technologists (IFT), *Assessing the Optimal System for Ensuring Food Safety: A Scientific Consensus* (Chicago: Institute of Food Technologists, 1989).

9. K. Smith, *Alar: One Year Later. A Media Analysis of a Hypothetical Health Risk* (New York: American Council on Science and Health, March 1990).

10. E. Marshall, "A is for Apple, Alar, and . . . Alarmist?" *Science* 254 (1991): pp. 20–22.

11. Ibid., p. 22.

12. Ibid., p. 20.

13. Ibid.

14. Ibid.

15. E. Remmers, "Will We Use Mainstream Science to Defuse the Next Food Scare?"*Priorities* (Fall 1990): pp. 16–17.

16. American Council on Science and Health, *Ethylene Dibromide* (New York:

American Council on Science and Health, 1984).

17. Food and Drug Administration, *Residues in Foods: Report from the FDA* (Washington: Food and Drug Administration, 1989).

18. IFT, "Assessing the Optimal System," p. 18.

19. Baker and Wilkinson, *Effect of Pesticides,* p. 28.

20. B. N. Ames and L. S. Gold, "Dietary Carcinogens, Environmental Pollution, and Cancer: Some Misconceptions,"*Medical Oncology and Tumor Pharmacotherapeutics* 7 (1990): p. 71.

21. This discussion of Delaney is based largely on an article by Kristine Napier, "Freeing Society from Trifling Matters: Reworking the Delaney Clause," *Priorities* (Spring 1992).

22. Environmental Protection Agency, "Note to Correspondents," Statement responding to court decision on *NRDC et al.* v. *EPA,* July 9, 1992.

23. S. Weinhouse, D. G. Bal, R. Adamson, and J. Dwyer, "American Cancer Society Guidelines on Diet, Nutrition and Cancer," *Ca—A Cancer Journal for Clinicians* 41 (1991): pp. 334–38.

24. M. Kroger, "And Now a Positive Word About Food Preservatives," *Priorities* (Fall 1990): p. 23.

25. R. Zaloum, "Whatever Happened To . . . ?" *Priorities* (Winter 1990): p. 34.

26. Ibid.

27. American Council on Science and Health, *Antibiotics in Animal Feed: A Threat to Human Health?* (New York: American Council on Science and Health, 1985).

28. Ibid.

29. E. G. Remmers, "A Tempest in a Milkbottle?" *Priorities* (Summer 1990): pp. 13–14.

30. E. G. Remmers, "Pseudoscientists Milk Publicity," *Priorities* (Summer 1990): pp. 8–9.

31. National Cancer Institute, Office of Cancer Communications, "Heterocyclic Aromatic Amines in Cooked Meats," March 25, 1991.

32. American Council on Science and Health.

33. A. Ottoboni,*The Dose Makes the Poison* (New York: Vincente Books, 1974).

34. American Council on Science and Health.

35. E. Remmers, "Irradiated Food: Facing Pseudoscience and Toxic Terrorism in New Jersey," *Priorities* (Fall 1991).

36. E. D. Miller, "The Big Green Initiative," *Priorities* (Fall 1990): pp. 45–46.

37. IFT, "Assessing the Optimal System," p. 2.

38. Personal communication with Dr. Richard Adamson, National Cancer Institute.

39. IFT, "Assessing the Optimal System," p. 18.

40. V. O. Wodicka, "Prioritizing Risks Associated with the Food Supply," in *The American Food Supply: Are We at Risk?* (Ithaca, N.Y.: Cornell University, 1985), Proceedings of Symposium II, Institute for Comparative and Environmental Toxicology.

6

PCBs: Mad Dogs of the Environment?

The Charges

PCBs are among the most widespread—and most poisonous—chemicals ever produced. . . . Since the tiniest doses . . . have caused birth defects, loss of hair and death in test animals, the presence virtually everywhere of these chemicals has grave implications for the American people, and for much of the world's population.

—*America the Poisoned*[1]

PCBs are believed to cause cancer, still births, bone and joint deformities, skin rashes and liver damage.

—*Science News*[2]

As liquid or vapor, they are easily absorbed into the body through the skin and lungs, and they remain in body tissue indefinitely. As with radiation, which requires only one particle to cause health damage, one PCB molecule may be enough to do damage, potentially causing vomiting, fatigue, the skin disease chloracne, liver damage or cancer.

—*When Technology Wounds*[3]

At that moment, sitting side by side with my scientist friend, I experienced pure panic. My arms and legs got limp, and my gut felt as if it were going to dissolve. I realized that PCBs and DDE and other poisons are swimming around in my body fluids just as they do in sewers and polluted streams. Worse, they are in the milk I am so conscientiously feeding to my helpless infant daughter.

—*Parents*[4]

The Facts

- Between 1940 and the early 1970s, the state-of-the-art mode for disposing of PCBs, as well as some isolated accidents, led to much PCB contamination of rivers, streams, and fish in the United States.

- PCBs have been found in human fat tissue and in mother's milk. Although this is an understandable source of concern, no evidence exists that the mere presence of the trace levels causes adverse effects.

- Contamination did occur, but there is no evidence of a substantial adverse effect on human health from PCB exposure in the United States.

- No evidence exists that PCBs cause cancer in humans. Indeed, the evidence from studies of highly exposed PCB workers indicates that the substance does not have a carcinogenic effect on man.

- There is no evidence that PCBs caused human death or disease in the United States, but it is likely that PCBs saved lives in their function of minimizing the risks of fires by replacing combustible insulating fluids.

- Efforts to clean up PCBs from the environment are desirable, but should be based on common sense, science, and economic realities.

PCBs gained widespread notoriety in the early 1970s as a cancer-causing agent, not because of scientific evidence, but because they were a pawn for passage of the the Toxic Substances Control Act. PCBs continue to suffer from a tainted reputation, and from the press not reporting the scientific evidence that clears the scarlet letter from its reputation. What was acceptable science in the early 1970s must yield to the science of today, which has advanced and given us the scientific insight to understand much more at a far more intricate level.

Background

PCBs, chemicals consisting of two chemically bonded benzene rings and one or more chlorine atoms, are a family of some 209 chemical compounds, ranging in characteristics from light, oily fluids to heavier, greasy, or waxy substances. PCBs were discovered over a hundred years ago and their production and use began in 1929. Because of their remarkable insulating capacity and their nonflammable nature, they soon gained widespread use as coolants and lubricants in transformers and other electrical equipment where these properties are essential. PCBs replaced combustible insulating fluids and thereby reduced the risk of fires in office buildings, hospitals, factories, and schools. In fact, some city codes required that transformers in some locations be of the PCB type. Not only did they make capacitors flame resistant, but they also allowed these capacitors to be made smaller, thus lowering equipment costs. Insurance companies required PCB equipment in many locations.

For several decades, PCBs were routinely used in the manufacture of a wide variety of common products, such as plastics, adhesives, paints and varnishes, carbonless copy paper, newsprint, fluorescent light ballasts, and caulking compounds. Between 1929 and 1977, it is estimated, about 1.2 billion pounds of PCBs were produced in the United States.

How Did PCBs Get into the Environment?

Three practices thought acceptable and hazard-free in the past have led to PCB release into the environment: (1) Industries using PCBs in their processes and products discharged their PCB-containing wastes into rivers and streams, sometimes under permit. (2) Other PCB-containing wastes were often disposed of in open landfills. (3) PCBs were in the condensate at compressor stations along natural gas pipelines. Thus, an ever increasing amount of PCBs became part of our environment. These practices, though permitted by law then, were inappropriate and potentially hazardous procedures.

When used in transformers and electrical capacitors, PCB compartments were sealed so that the chemical would remain in place for the life of the equipment. On occasion, seals leaked or the external structure was damaged, resulting in PCB leakage.

Current Status of PCBs

The Toxic Substances Control Act (TSCA) was passed in 1976 and called for a ban on the manufacture, processing, distribution, and use of PCBs in all products in which the PCBs were not totally enclosed. In May 1979, when TSCA was being implemented, the EPA established some exceptions to the general ban, among them oils and other items containing fewer than 50 ppm PCBs.

Current regulations require that capacitors in areas where public exposure might occur (such as utility poles in backyards) had to be out of service by 1988,[5] and that by October 1990 PCB transformers within thirty meters of commercial or public access buildings should have been replaced or provided with enhanced electrical protection.[6] In addition, a regular inspection and maintenance program for certain PCB-containing equipment is required.

Causes for Concern

The PCB regulation of the 1970s was based on three red flags:

1. The belief that PCBs are generally persistent in the environment and resistant to biodegradation, which is nature's usual way of dealing with environmental organic chemical contaminants;

2. The 1968 Yusho human poisoning incident in Japan, which produced chloracne and other symptoms;

3. The 1975 study by the Centers for Disease Control finding that high-dosage feeding with Aroclor 1260, a mixture containing highly chlorinated PCBs, caused liver cancer in rats.

Let's look at each of these separately.

FIRST RED FLAG: ENVIRONMENTAL ACCUMULATION

Concern about the presence of PCBs in our environment began around 1966 when Swedish researchers reported an environmental accumulation of PCBs. Study results confirmed suspicions that the rate of biodegradation (natural breakdown) was slower, particularly for some compounds, than the rate of environmental acquisition.

SECOND RED FLAG: THE YUSHO DISEASE EPISODE

PCBs again caught the public eye in 1968, when thirteen hundred people on the island of Kyushu, Japan, became ill from consuming rice oil contaminated with a PCB heat-transfer agent. The victims developed a severe and persistent form of chloracne (a severe skin rash) after eating the rice oil, which contained 2,000–3,000 ppm of a Japanese brand of PCB. The disease soon progressed to more than just skin disorders. Victims reported fatigue, nausea, and swelling of arms and legs, and some developed liver disorders. Some babies born to exposed mothers were smaller than usual. By 1973 about twelve hundred cases of "Yusho disease" had been reported as a result of this accident. By 1977, 1,665 cases had been recognized, based on symptoms of ocular disturbances, skin lesions, and primarily subjective neurological symptoms. During the eleven years following exposure, fifty-one Yusho patients died, with the cause of death known in thirty-one cases.[7] Eleven of the deaths (or 35.4 percent) traced to cancer. Only 21.1 percent would be expected in a control population. The media were quick to report that a toxic chemical was linked to liver cancer among Japanese exposed to PCBs.

Interestingly, in the years after the Japanese poisoning incident, it became increasingly likely that PCBs were not the cause of the illness.[8] Indeed, the heat-transfer fluid that contaminated the rice oil contained only 50 percent PCBs. Furthermore, due to mechanical problems—a combination of high temperature and some air in the heat exchanger—about one-half of the original PCB fluid had been converted into quaterphenyls. In addition, some of the original PCB fluid had been converted to polychlorinated dibenzofurans, substances far more toxic than PCBs.

It is very clear, then, that it is impossible to relate the illness caused by the Yusho incident to PCB exposure in this country. Most researchers who have studied the Yusho tragedy agree that it had little relevance to potential health effects from PCB exposure in this country, as reflected by the following statements:

> The scientific community assumes now that most of the effects observed in [the Yusho] outbreak [were] caused by ingestion of the polychlorinated dibenzofurans.
>
> National Institutes of Health[9]

> Recent studies indicate that the major etiologic agents in Yusho were polychlorinated dibenzofurans rather than polychlorinated biphenyls. . . . Thus a discussion of the human health effects of polychlorinated biphenyls should not use "Yusho" as an example. Industrial exposure data more accurately reflect human health effects.
>
> EPA[10]

Despite convincing evidence that PCBs were not guilty in Yusho, the Yusho episode fueled the rising concern over PCBs. Beginning around 1970, PCBs became the most prominent chemical material used to promote the Toxic Substances Control Act (TSCA) under consideration by Congress.[11] PCBs were chosen as the paradigm of toxic substances by TSCA and received a considerable amount of sensational press. This press coverage mounted in 1975–76 when enactment of TSCA seemed more likely. A story in the *New York Times* at that time referred to PCBs as "a class of chemicals . . . linked to cancer and birth defects, water pollution and wildlife contamination" and noted that some House members believed "banning PCBs was a moral responsibility to the people."[12] That *New York Times* piece began PCBs' reputation as a "cancer-causing agent," despite the lack of scientific evidence to justify such a reputation.

THIRD RED FLAG: THE 1975 FINDING
THAT PCBS CAUSED CANCER IN RATS

This study used only one PCB variety, a PCB mixture that is 60 percent chlorinated, and was the first study to show that this type of PCB caused liver cancer in rats.[13] Two additional studies of 60 percent chlorinated PCBs, Aroclor 1260 and Clophen A60, confirmed this specific carcinogenic response.[14]

Further research, however, yielded two important qualifiers about PCBs' carcinogenic potential:

1. An early reevaluation of those initial carcinogenicity tests clearly reveals that even the class of PCBs labeled most carcinogenic should be downgraded.[15] The expert pathologists who reevaluated the rat-liver lesions unequivocally agreed that the number of animals with benign or malignant liver tumors was less than originally reported. This more accurate appraisal comes from scientists' greater understanding of how the liver reacts when exposed to chemical substances, as described in the dioxin chapter (chapter 9).

2. The second qualifier is that additional studies on other PCB mixtures, i.e., those with less than 60 percent chlorination, failed to produce cancer in laboratory animals. Two such studies involved PCB mixtures that were 54 percent[16] and 42 percent[17] chlorinated. Scientists now understand, then, that only certain PCB mixtures, namely, those that are at least 60 percent chlorinated, may cause some cancer in rats.

But the government has failed to account for this significant downgrading of PCBs' toxicity, continuing to regulate them as if they are all 60 percent chlorinated and also according to the 1975 assessment of carcinogenicity. But at most 12 percent of all PCBs ever sold in this country by the sole domestic supplier from 1957 to the end of production were of the 60 percent chlorinated variety. Not only are the lower chlorinated varieties less carcinogenic, they are also less persistent in the environment.[18]

Philip H. Abelson, deputy editor of *Science,* described the government's failure to account for this updated information in its regulatory decision making.[19] Abelson reports that John A. Moore, a former EPA official and current president of the Institute for the Evaluation of Health Risks said of its reassessment:[20]

These reassessment results indicate that the following two traditional EPA policy positions be reconsidered: 1) an assumption that all PCB formulations are probably human carcinogens; 2) the assumption that all PCB formulations have the same quantitative potency to cause cancer.

Both of these positions were initially established years ago when our knowledge base from which to determine the cancer potential of PCBs was meager. They represent the use of conservative default assumptions. However, since then new data and knowledge have accrued that have not been effectively incorporated into the PCB risk assessment. *Data, when available, should have priority over default assumptions* [emphasis added].

According to Moore, a revised PCB cancer risk assessment should reflect the following:[21]

> *Develop separate risk assessments for each of the major PCB formulations.* While the results from studies of mixtures with 60 percent chlorination consistently report a high incidence of liver tumors, studies in rats which were fed mixtures with 54 percent or 42 percent chlorination did not detect statistically significant elevations of liver tumors. It is not proper to continue a policy which does not consider data, developed subsequent to the initial judgment, that demonstrates that other formulations are either not carcinogens or at best, weak carcinogens. (There is precedent for such action; several years ago the Science Advisory Panel, which advises the State of California on cancer designations under Proposition 65, voted to recommend Aroclor 1260 as a carcinogen rather than all PCBs. This, however, was later overturned and once again all varieties are regulated according to the most toxic variety.)
>
> *Utilize all available data when calculating cancer potency for PCB mixtures that have 60 percent chlorination.* When one compares the consensus pathology diagnoses across four studies, in three different laboratories, there appears to be no scientific basis for continuing the practice of selecting only part of the available data for deriving potency estimates. Using the approach, the current EPA value of 7.7 would be replaced with a value of approximately 1.9.

Moore continues with several crucial points:

> I am not asking you to focus on an issue that is only of arcane scientific interest. The current cancer policy is clearly overstating the cancer risks associated with many exposures to PCBs in the environment. In a number of instances it is driving regulatory decisions that, by any standard are a major economic impact for, at best, trivial public health gain. As an illustration, mixtures with 60 percent or greater chlorination comprised about 12 percent of total PCB sales in this country; yet current policy calculates *all* PCB exposure as if it were equivalent to Aroclor 1260. While PCBs in the environment undergo changes in composition none develops into the chemical "fingerprint" that identifies Aroclor 1260. Therefore, 88 percent of the PCB that was used is being treated as if it were a potent carcinogen when the data indicate that these lower chlorinated mixtures are either of markedly diminished potency or not carcinogenic at all.

Finally, Moore concludes by citing the government's desire to deal with real risks:

> A request to develop a risk assessment utilizing all pertinent data, I believe, is consistent with the Agency's stated goals of focusing on risks which represent true public health or environmental concern and of reducing the uncertainties in risk assessment by applying sound scientific knowledge.

Next, let's look at the effects of PCBs on humans, which further confirm that PCBs are not to be feared.

Do PCBs Cause Disease in Humans?

A number of attempts have been made to assess the effects of PCBs on human health. As with any chemical, if PCBs cause human disease, including cancer, it would seem logical that signs and symptoms would appear first in groups that are heavily exposed. We have the tremendous advantage of over fifty years passing since the first workers were heavily exposed, certainly more than ample time to detect a disease with a long latent period, such as cancer.

The most extensive occupational studies of long-term exposure to PCBs involved electrical-equipment workers. Many of these employees had daily skin contact with PCBs for many years and may have even inhaled relatively high levels of the chemical, and probably ingested some while eating near their work stations. Aside from occasional skin irritations that disappeared quickly, no significant adverse health effects have been reported among workers in the electrical industry. Four studies are particularly significant.

1. NIOSH (National Institute for Occupational Safety and Health) studied maintenance workers exposed to PCBs at two utility companies.[22] Although their blood PCB levels were much higher than the national background level (12 to 298 ppb compared with 10 to 20 ppb), they did not exhibit any ill health effects, not even chloracne.

2. NIOSH also studied 224 workers exposed to PCBs at an electrical-equipment manufacturing plant and found PCB blood levels ranging from 15 to 3,580 ppb. Despite finding such high levels, again there were no ill effects noted.[23]

3. General Electric has studied the health of 194 workers heavily exposed to PCBs for an average of fifteen years, some for as long as thirty-five years. The first report included studies done on the workers through

1976, and showed no ill effects. A 1979 reevaluation again failed to produce evidence of ill health among these workers.[24]

4. Probably the most comprehensive data concerning the long-term health effects of PCB exposure come from a NIOSH study of 2,500 workers employed by two separate capacitor manufacturing plants.[25] The researchers reported no statistically significant excesses of cancer, with the exception of more liver cancer deaths in one plant. The researchers, however, said this could not be explained by PCB exposure, but by confounding factors. This is particularly noteworthy, since more than 50 percent of these workers were exposed to PCBs on the job for more than twenty years, and some for as long as forty years. NIOSH reported that while the incidence of all cancer deaths expected in a population of a demographic profile similar to that of the 2,500 workers would be 182, only 163 deaths from cancer were actually observed. Also there was no clear relationship between the increasing length of employment in PCB-exposed jobs and the risk of mortality from cancer.

The only factor that correlates with blood PCB level is blood triglyceride level. The interpretation of this correlation is confounded by the fact that PCBs distribute equally among all lipid pools in the body, including those in the blood. This means that for any given PCB body burden the serum PCB level must vary directly with the level of serum lipids. Thus, for any given PCB body burden, increased serum PCB levels are the result, not the cause, of increased serum lipids.[26]

These occupational results should reassure us that general environmental exposures to PCBs are probably not capable of harming health. In point of fact, mean serum levels of heavily exposed but disease-free workers in one study were 500 ppb, with 10 percent over 1,000 ppb. This compares to average PCB levels in the general population of 2–24 ppb.[27]

A. B. Smith, M.D., of the National Institute for Occupational Safety and Health (NIOSH) summarizes the occupational studies of PCBs:

> None of the published occupational or epidemiological studies (including ours) have shown that occupational exposures to PCBs is associated with any adverse health outcome . . . except for the occurrence of chloracne.[28]

But recent research now suggests that the PCB-chloracne association is probably spurious.[29] The most revealing evidence is the fact that in the three largest and most recent studies of capacitor-manufacturing and transformer repair workers, not one case of chloracne was identified.[30]

Finally, two sets of studies have attempted to find a relationship between reproductive or neurodevelopmental effects in humans and low-level PCB exposure.[31] Both sets of studies, however, have many shortcomings and confounders that prohibit one from making any conclusions. Nigel Paneth, M.D., M.P.H., director of epidemiology at Michigan State University comments on what confounded one study set.[32] He notes that the fish-eating mothers had quite different health behaviors. They were, on average, nine pounds lighter than the non–fish eaters. Dr. Paneth comments that a mother's pre-pregnant weight is one of the strongest known determinants of infant birth weight. The fish eaters also had other high-risk health behaviors, including alcohol use, high caffeine intake, and frequent use of over-the-counter medications.

PCBs in Fish

Because of their chemical stability, PCBs discharged into rivers and lakes stay there for long periods. Fish living in these waters acquire the PCBs either through the gills or during feeding. Because fish are unable to metabolize some PCBs, the PCBs accumulate in fatty tissues. In fish-eating fish, levels of accumulation are higher still. Humans consuming fish ingest and accumulate the PCBs as well.

For these reasons, fish are monitored for PCB concentration in contaminated bodies of water. Two studies show that fish eaters have suffered no known ill effects from PCBs.

The Michigan Department of Public Health, under the sponsorship of the U.S. Food and Drug Administration, measured *potential* health effects of higher-than-normal exposure to PCBs because of fish eating. The study involved 182 adults, 105 of whom consumed over twenty-six pounds of Great Lakes fish per year. A significant correlation between blood PCB levels and the quantity of fish consumed was observed. But an evaluation of health histories and current medical problems of the study subjects did not reveal any significant differences between the heavy fish-consuming group and those with lower exposure to PCB-contaminated fish.[33]

Similarly, the Connecticut Department of Health Services conducted an analysis of blood samples and medical histories on persons eating fish from the Housatonic River. Again, although people who ate more fish had higher blood PCB levels, they did not have any associated ill-health effects.[34]

PCBs and Pipelines

PCBs were the coolant of choice for compressors along natural gas pipelines throughout this country until the late 1980s. These natural gas pipelines are studded with compressor stations, at which point there are taps to remove condensate. PCBs were released in this condensate and customarily buried at the compressor stations. Major concern arose beginning in 1986 when soil was found to have PCB levels up to 240 times the EPA-approved levels at some of these sites.[35]

Subsequent investigation by the EPA revealed that almost all ten EPA-designated regions of the United States had PCBs buried along natural gas pipelines. Probably the worst case involved Texas Eastern Gas Company, which had buried PCBs in eighty-nine pits along 10,600 miles of pipeline throughout fourteen states. They have been ordered to clean up the PCBs and replace much of the pipeline, at a total estimated cost of $400 million. In addition, they were fined a record-breaking $15 million by the EPA. Interestingly, the EPA assigned one employee whose sole responsibility was to deal with the Texas Eastern PCB cleanup. Fourteen other pipeline companies were investigated by the EPA for this problem.[36]

While these facts are startling, the bottom line is reassuring. Contrary to some press reports,[37] drinking water wells were not contaminated with PCBs, and at no time was human health threatened by the presence of these PCBs.

Alternatives to PCBs

The alternative materials to PCBs are not without problems. The most important use for PCBs was in electrical equipment, where their flame-resistant characteristics were needed badly. Alternatives to PCBs include other chemicals, like silicone fluids and fluorocarbons, and mineral-oil transformers.

All the substitutes work electrically. However a transformer constructed for use with PCB fluid can't operate at the same power load with a substitute chemical. That transformer becomes less efficient, resulting in a higher operating cost. And that is to say nothing of the safety problem. Many of the alternatives present fire risks, defeating one of the reasons why a fire-resistant alternative was originally sought to mineral-oil. The net effect, then, is the replacement of a hypothetical health risk from PCBs with a product known to lead to an increased fire hazard.

What Are We Doing to Clean Up PCBs?

Many efforts are underway to clean up PCBs in the environment. This, along with the ban and removal of PCBs, ensures that U.S. exposure will decline rapidly. PCB wastes were often discarded in open landfills. Cleaning up the landfills that once served as depositories for PCB waste is an ongoing process that will be expensive in the coming years.

One such landfill is located in Moreau, New York. General Electric paid out $2 million for corrective work at the site. Engineers inserted a hundred-foot-deep impermeable barrier into the ground surrounding the dump and then covered it with a 3.5-foot-thick clay cap.[38]

Cleanup plans for the Hudson River, so heavily contaminated because of industrial discharges, are also under way. From 1947 to 1977 over five hundred thousand pounds of PCBs were discharged into the Hudson River from two General Electric capacitor-manufacturing plants at Fort Edward and Hudson Falls, New York.

The cleanup has been a literal hotbed of debate. In 1984, the EPA issued a "record of decision" recommending no action be taken to clean up the river's sediment. John A. Moore, former assistant EPA administrator for pesticides and toxic substances, issued a statement in 1987 saying that the EPA should not engage in "heroic measures" such as cleaning up the Hudson River. His opinion was that the project, estimated in 1987 to cost $26.7 million, would cause even worse environmental problems (resuspending PCBs from the sediment, thus raising water PCB levels) and is not the wisest investment of our limited environmental-resource dollars. The EPA did recommend that remnant sites containing PCB piles be capped, which is currently being done at General Electric's expense.

New York State's Department of Environmental Conservation (DEC) never agreed with the EPA's no-action approach. They proceeded independently to develop an action plan, which they are still hoping to implement. In December 1989, the EPA agreed to reassess its 1984 decision; as of September 1992, according to DEC, that process is still going on and a final decision is not expected until 1994.[39]

The main goal of the action plan is to dredge the river of a quarter-million pounds of PCBs and bury them in a leakproof landfill. Residents of the proposed site in Washington County continue to oppose such a proposal vigorously. Hudson River–based environmental groups, however, are strongly in favor of such a plan, which they see as necessary to the health of the river and the river-based recreation industry.

The facts clearly speak for themselves, however. All indications are that, as predicted, the Hudson River is cleansing itself of PCBs. PCB levels in the upper Hudson River are declining. A 1977 DEC survey reported 346,000 pounds of PCBs in the upper river. The 1984 survey by DEC found only 151,000 pounds. This decline could be due to transport away from the area or due to biodegradation. If the decline were due to transport, one would expect fish PCB levels in the lower river to be increasing. The good news, though, is that PCB levels in striped bass in the lower Hudson River are actually lower, which is a clear contradiction to the transport theory.

Biodegradation is most likely responsible for the decline. Naturally occurring anerobic bacteria first dechlorinate the PCBs to a certain extent. These lower-chlorinated PCBs are then readily degradable by naturally occurring aerobic bacteria and are also more desirable in that they do not bioaccumulate in humans (either in blood serum or adipose tissue) or in the food chain. It has been found that even the "hot spots"—those areas in the river containing substantial amounts of PCBs—contain basically detoxified PCBs.

The bottom line is that bioremediation is effective and is advantageous for many reasons, including reducing the cost and eliminating the need to find a landfill in which to dispose of the dredged material.[39]

PCBs have also been a big issue in Waukegan Harbor in the state of Illinois, in Lake Michigan's Green Bay, and New Bedford Harbor, Massachusetts. Surveys indicate that these areas are cleaning themselves, as is the Hudson River. The directors of Michigan's Council on Environmental Quality, for example, recently reported that of sixty Lake Huron lake trout sampled in 1989, none exceeded the FDA standard for PCBs of 2.0 ppm. In 1986, 65 percent of sampled trout exceeded that standard.

Research is underway on other new techniques for cleaning up PCBs. Two different researchers have come up with promising chemical-disposal methods and a New Jersey Institute of Technology team has discovered that an aquatic plant can use PCBs as a nutrient.[41] Incineration is probably the best method for PCBs not in rivers and lakes. (As discussed above, PCBs found in rivers and lakes are biodegraded.) A minimum temperature of 1,200° C is required, but incineration turns PCBs back to simple elements with 99.9999 percent efficiency. Some researchers feel that using mirrors to concentrate solar energy not only raises the temperature sufficiently, but also spurs a photochemical reaction that breaks down the chemicals.[42] Public fear of contaminating the air has prevented more widespread PCB incineration. In Canada, for example, discarded PCBs sit in storage, at an annual cost of $150 million. Dr. Philip Jones, founding director of the University of Toronto's Institute for Environmental Studies says, "If all Canada's PCBs went to the nearest cement kiln we could get rid of the problem in six months."[43]

A Perspective

It is only twenty-twenty hindsight that enables us to see that past PCB-disposal practices were wrong. These practices led to the widespread contamination of many of this country's rivers and lakes.

Americans have, over the past few years, been presented with a contradictory array of information about the possible health hazards of PCBs. Certainly we have cause for concern when there is uncontrolled dumping of potentially toxic and possibly cancer-causing agents into our rivers, streams, and lakes. Not only do we run the risk of an adverse effect on human health should the levels become high enough, but we also would be endangering fish and other natural resources.

It is a source of concern when studies indicate that members of the general population—that is, people not working with PCBs—have PCB blood levels ranging from 2 to 24 ppb. (Those who don't eat fish probably have about 5 to 10 ppb.) We still do not know the effect of PCB exposure, and therefore care must be taken in the handling, disposal, and general management of these chemicals.

Although this class of chemicals is indeed persistent, no evidence exists that the normal background levels or even levels among heavily exposed workers are causing damage or posing even a potential threat. PCBs are not new. They have been part of the American industrial environment for over fifty years.

The public should relax its PCB vigilance, just as the EPA has. The EPA deserves a commendation for its late March 1987 announcement of new PCB-cleanup rules. After two years of weighing evidence, the EPA has adopted a comparatively less stringent cleanup policy. This new policy requires cleanups only for spills resulting in a contamination level of more than fifty parts per million. And cleanups needn't be so fastidious, reducing levels to a reasonable level rather than to a squeaky-clean, impossibly expensive result.[44] This will save the government and private industry many precious environmental dollars, as the cost of cleaning up PCBs at ever more stringent levels goes up exponentially. The EPA estimated, for example, the cost of cleaning up all capacitor spills in 1987 to a level of twenty-five parts per million at $54.1 million, but $395 million if cleanup reduced the levels to five parts per million.[45]

Certainly we'd rather not have PCBs or any other contaminant in our bodies. But, though the presence of a chemical warns us of a potential problem, it does not prove a hazard. In the case of PCBs, all studies to date have suggested that heroic, exceedingly expensive corrective measures are unwarranted and that time itself is an important factor in resolving the situation.

NOTES

1. L. Regenstein, *America the Poisoned* (Washington: Acropolis Books, 1982).

2. *Science News* (July 7, 1979): p. 2.

3. C. Glendinning, *When Technology Wounds* (New York: William Morrow and Co., Inc., 1990), p. 128.

4. C. Ricci, "The Breast-Milk Test," *Parents* (August 1988).

5. *Federal Register* 1982, pp. 37342–60.

6. R. Derks, "Weighing the Options of PCB Elimination," *American City and*

County (April 1991): p. 42.

7. H. Urabe, et al., "Present State of Yusho Patients," *New York Academy of Science Annals* 320 (1979): pp. 273–76.

8. T. Kanshimoto, H. Miyata, S. Kunita, et al., "Role of Polychlorinated Dibenzofuran in Yusho (PCB Poisoning)," *Archives Environmental Health* 36 (1981): pp. 321–26.

9. R. D. Kimbrough and R. A. Goyer, *Environmental Health Perspectives* 59 (1985): p. 3.

10. J. Doull and S. Abrahamson, letter to Richard A. Griesemer, Chairman, Environmental Health Committee, Science Advisory Board, U.S. Environmental Protection Agency, reporting the Halogenated Organics Subcommittee review of fifteen draft health advisories for drinking water, SAB-EHC-87-005, 1986, 5–27.

11. E. J. Burger, "Health as a Surrogate for the Environment," *Daedalus: Journal of the American Academy of Arts and Sciences* (Fall 1990): pp. 142–43.

12. R. D. Lyons, "House Votes Ban on Output of PCBs within 3 Years," *New York Times,* August 25, 1976.

13. R. D. Kimbrough, et al., "Induction of Liver Tumors in Sherman Strain Female Rats by Polychlorinated Biphenyl Aroclor 1260," *Journal of the National Cancer Institute* 55 (1975): p. 1453.

14. D. H. Norback and R. H. Weltman, *Environmental Health Perspectives* 60 (1985): pp. 97–105; E. Schaeffer, H. Greim, and W. Goessner, *Toxicology and Applied Pharmacology* 75 (1984): pp. 278–88.

15. J. A. Moore, "Reassessment of Liver Findings in Five PCB Studies for Rats," Institute for Evaluation Health Risks, July 1, 1991.

16. National Cancer Institute, "Bioassay of Aroclor® 1254 for possible carcinogenicity," DHEW Publ. NIH-78-838 (Virginia: Natl. Tech. Inf. Serv., as PB-279 624/IGA, NCI-CG TR-38).

17. Schaeffer, Greim, and Goessner, *Toxicology and Applied Pharmacology.*

18. Moore, "Reassessment of Liver Findings."

19. P. H Abelson, "Excessive Fear of PCBs," *Science* 253 (1991): p. 361.

20. Moore, "Reassessment of Liver Findings."

21. Ibid.

22. A. B. Smith, et al., "Cross Sectional Survey of Two Groups of Workers Occupationally Exposed to Polychlorinated Biphenyls (PCBs) in the Maintenance, Repair and Overhaul of Electrical Tranformers" (National Institute for Occupational Safety and Health, Division of Surveillance, Hazard Evaluations and Field Studies, Cincinnati, Ohio 45226; Lipid Research Center, University of Cincinnati Medical Center, Cincinnati, Ohio 45267, 1981).

23. Ibid.

24. R. W. Lawton, M. R. Ross, and J. Feingold, G.E. draft report on PCBs, 1981.

25. D. P. Brown and M. Jones, "Mortality and Industrial Hygiene Study of Industrial Workers Exposed to Polychlorinated Biphenyls," *Archives of Environmental Health* 36 (1981): p. 120.

26. J. F. Brown, "Polychlorinated Biphenyl (PCB) Partitioning between Adipose

Tissue and Serum," *Bulletin of Environmental Contamination and Toxicology* 33 (1984): pp. 277–80.

27. R. W. Lawton, M. R. Ross, J. Feingold, and J. F. Brown, "Effects of PCB Exposure on Biochemical and Hematological Findings in Capacitor Workers," *Environmental Health Perspectives* 60 (1985): pp. 165–99.

28. A. B. Smith, J. Schloemer, L. K. Lowry, et al., "Metabolic and Health Consequences of Occupational Exposure to Polychlorinated Biphenyls," *British Journal of Industrial Medicine* 39 (1982): pp. 361–69.

29. G. A. Bennett, C. K. Drinker, and M. F. Warren, "Morphological Changes in the Livers of Rats Resulting from Exposure to Certain Chlorinated Hydrocarbons," *Journal of Industrial Hygiene and Toxicology* (1938); C. K. Drinker, "Further Observations on the Possible Systemic Toxicity of Certain Chlorinated Hydrocarbons with Suggestions for Permissible Concentrations in the Air of Workrooms," *Journal of Industrial Hygiene and Toxicology* (1939): pp. 155–59; National Institute for Occupational Safety and Health, "Criteria for a recommended standard—occupational exposure to polychlorinated biphenyls," DHEW Publication No. 77-225; J. W. Jones and H. S. Alden, "An Acneform Dermatergosis," *Archives of Dermatological Syphilology* 33 (1936): p. 1022; J. W. Meigs, J. J. Albom, and B. L. Kartin, "Chloracne from an Unusual Exposure to Aroclor,"*Journal of the American Medical Association* 154 (1954): p. 1417; D. J. Birmingham, "Occupational Dermatology: Current Problems," *Skin* 38 (1964).

30. Birmingham, "Occupational Dermatology"; Smith, et al., "Consequences of Occupational Exposure to Polychlorianted Biphenyls"; Lawton, Ross, Feingold, and Brown, "Effects of PCB Exposure," pp. 165–99.

31. G. G. Fein, J. L. Jacobson, S. W. Jacobson, et al., "Prenatal Exposure to Polychlorinated Biphenyls: Effects on Birth Size and Gestational Age," *Journal of Pediatrics* 105 (1984): pp. 315–20; J. L. Jacobson, S. W. Jacobson, G. G. Fein, et al., "Prenatal Exposure to an Environmental Toxin: A Test of the Multiple Effects Model," *Developmental Psychology* 20 (1984): pp. 523–32. J. L. Jacobson, S. W. Jacobson, and G. G. Fein, "The Effect of Intrauterine PCB Exposure on Visual Recognition Memory," *Child Development* 56 (1985): pp. 853–60; B. C. Gladen, W. J. Rogan, P. Hardy, et al., "Development After Exposure to PCBs and DDE," *Journal of Pediatrics* 113 (1988): pp. 991–95; W. J. Rogan, B. C. Gladen, J. D. McKinney, et al., "Polychlorinated biphenyls (PCBs) and Dichlorodiphenyl Dichloroethene (DDE)," *American Journal of Public Health* 77 (1987): pp. 1294–97.

32. N. Paneth, "Human Reproduction after Eating PCB-contaminated Fish," *Health and Environment Digest* (October 1991).

33. Michigan Department of Public Health, Final Report on FDA Contract 73-2209, "Evaluation of Changes in the Level of Polychlorinated Biphenyls (PCBs) in Human Tissue" (1975); H. E. B. Humphrey, "Evaluation of Humans Exposed to Halogenated Biphenyls," *American Chemical Society Division of Environmental Chemistry Preprints* 30 (1980): p. 272.

34. G. J. Beck, "Housatonic River PCB Study," Statistical Analysis Prepared under Contract from Connecticut State Department of Health Services, 1981.

35. "Clean-up Target: 10,000 Miles of Toxic Soup," *U.S. News and World Report,* November 23, 1986.

36. Ibid.; J. Castro, "Mopping up the PCB Mess," *Time,* November 23, 1987, p. 50.

37. "PCBs High in Wells Near Town," *New York Times,* March 6, 1987, p. 1; *New York Times,* March 17, 1987.

38. *Saratogian,* July 14, 1983.

39. Personal communication with Bill Port, New York State Department of Environmental Conservation, September 30, 1992.

40. Mathematical model of the long-term behavior of PCBs in the Hudson River Estuary, June 1989 (prepared for the Hudson River Foundation); personal communication, Karl Berger, citizen participation specialist at NYDEC, November 11, 1990; J. F. Brown, et al., "Polychlorinated Biphenyl Dechlorination in Aquatic Sediments," *Science* 236 (1987): pp. 709–712; J. F. Quensen, J. M. Tiedje, S. A. Boyd, "Reductive Dechlorination of Polychlorinated Biphenyls by Anaerobic Microorganisms from Sediments," *Science* 242: pp. 752–54.

41. "Bulrushes Decrease PCB Contamination," *Chemistry* 50 (1977): p. 4.

42. S. Siwolop, "Poisons: Now You See 'em, Now You Don't," *Business Week,* June 6, 1988.

43. "PCB Disposal a Big Business," *New York Times,* April 11, 1985; P. Ohlendorf-Moffat, "PCBs—Should You Worry?" *Chatelaine,* April 1990.

44. "EPA Announces National Policy on PCB Clean-ups," *Wall Street Journal,* March 24, 1987.

45. Ibid.

7

PBBs: What Can Go Wrong Will

The Charges

. . . a few hundred pounds of PBB caused a major health disaster in Michigan . . . we continue to produce and market tens of thousands of enormously hazardous chemicals on a massive scale, oblivious to the possible disastrous consequences of our thoughtless action.

—America the Poisoned[1]

When PBB contamination was discovered in 1974 highly contaminated milk and meat were flooding the food chain. . . . As a result, a chemical accident that began with dairy farmers became an environmental disaster that spread, unchecked, into the state's marketplaces. And its frightening legacy remains.

—Who's Poisoning America[2]

The contamination of Michigan was probably the most widespread, and least reported, chemical disaster ever to happen in the Western world.

—The Poisoning of Michigan[3]

Six years ago, Michigan's entire population of nine million discovered it had been endangered by chemical contamination of livestock feed sold to farmers all over the state. The full dimensions of this agricultural disaster are now becoming evident, and at least 40 million people may be affected.

—Atlantic[4]

Investigators have determined that eight million of Michigan's 9.1 million residents are carrying in their bodies toxic chemicals that have caused cattle deaths and caused liver cancer in rats.

—Wall Street Journal[5]

The study confirms scientists' worst fears that PBBs are widely disseminated throughout the state's population and are likely to be retained in their bodies forever.

—*Wall Street Journal*[6]

Reporters [from the *Detroit Free Press*] turned up evidence that testing of meat products now being sold is inadequate and that diseased cattle are still going to market. They reported that one calf dropped dead on the scales in an auction house, and that cows with ulcers on their udder were sold as recently as last summer.

—*Progressive*[7]

The most alarming result is the discovery of serious defects in the immune systems of Michigan, but not Wisconsin, farm residents.

—*Science News*[8]

The Facts

- In a frightening 1973 mishap, PBBs, chemicals with excellent fire-retardant properties, were misidentified as animal feed and delivered to farms in central Michigan, causing devastation to Michigan's agricultural community. Many thousands of cattle, other animals, and contaminated foodstuffs were subsequently destroyed.

- PBB contamination caused serious human stress, disorientation, and financial loss. However, there is no evidence that even heavily exposed humans suffered any serious health damage.

- If given in high enough doses, PBBs can cause liver cancer in rats and mice and have been shown to be injurious to many other animals.

- Although PBBs have been found in human tissues and breast milk, numerous follow-up studies have been conducted on individuals who were heavily exposed to PBBs, and no significant ill effects have been associated with PBB ingestion.

- PBBs were invented and used in the interest of promoting long life and good health by reducing the nation's death and injury toll from fires.

- The PBB contamination of Michigan was a disastrous accident, one attributable to nothing other than human error. There is, in the normal use of PBBs, no environmental contamination problem and no hazard to human health.

A Toxic Accident

Polybrominated biphenyls (PBBs) are a class of chemicals with excellent fire-retardant properties. They were extensively used in plastic consumer products such as telephones, electric typewriters, calculators, hair dryers, television sets, and automobile fixtures, satisfying a demanding need for fire resistance.

The Michigan Chemical Company, the exclusive U.S. manufacturer of PBBs, began marketing them in 1971 under the trade name Firemaster. At this time, there were approximately twelve thousand Americans dying each year, and an additional three hundred thousand seriously burned, in fires. PBBs came on the market in response to new federal regulations for flame-proofing consumer products.

In addition to Firemaster, Michigan Chemical manufactured several distinct products having nothing to do with PBBs, but with similar-sounding names. Many of these trade names ended in *master,* one being Nutrimaster.

Farmers used Nutrimaster, a feed supplement containing magnesium oxide, to increase milk production in their lactating cows. The Nutrimaster was or-dinarily packed in brown bags and the Firemaster in red, each with its own label. Sometime during summer 1973 the plant ran out of the red bags and substituted the brown bags for packaging the PBBs. Although "Firemaster" was stenciled on the bags, a frightening and monumental mix-up occurred: the PBBs were delivered to an animal feed mill in central Michigan.

How this mix-up occurred is uncertain. An attorney for Michigan Chemical explained that the buildings in which Firemaster was manufactured and stored were several hundred yards from the Nutrimaster buildings. Further, it was the practice to load products directly from storage buildings onto trucks for shipments *without* moving them to some common loading area where a mix-up would be more likely.

Nonetheless, the ensuing chain of events was devastating to Michigan's agricultural community. Some five hundred to two thousand pounds of PBB were mixed into feeds that were then widely sold and distributed to Michigan farmers.

A farmer, Frederic Halbert, first suspected a problem in 1973. No ordinary farmer, Halbert held a master's degree in chemical engineering, a factor that would prove to be a great asset in solving the mystery that was about to develop.

Mr. Halbert noticed that over a twenty-day period milk production dropped 40 percent and food consumption dropped 50 percent among his herd.[9]

Suspecting the feed, he stopped using what was indeed contaminated feed after only sixteen days. This change caused consumption to return to normal, but milk production was still off by 40 percent. In addition, weight loss continued. The animals had several other health problems, including abnormal hoof growth, loss of hair, skin anomalies, and reproductive problems. Six months later, twenty-four cows out of Halbert's herd of four hundred were dead. Autopsies revealed liver and kidney changes.

Despite Halbert's persistence in trying to find the cause, PBBs were not linked to the episode until April 1974, nearly nine months after the first contamination occurred. Officials failed to identify all affected farms until the end of 1975. Eventually, all of the eighty-seven feed mills associated with the marketing channel of the involved feed company were identified. All had milk, milk products, or meat with PBB levels at or above the recently set FDA action level. In addition, twenty-four additional feed markets showed PBB contamination.

Thirty thousand cattle were eventually quarantined or destroyed. Other animals became contaminated from two practices: (1) all animal feeds were mixed with the same PBB-contaminated equipment in the feed mills; and (2) dead animals from contaminated farms were sent to a rendering plant for processing and incorporation into feed used for several types of animals. All told, this caused the contamination of about 1.5 million chickens, 6,000 swine and 1,300 sheep.[10] Millions of eggs and large quantities of cheese, butter, and dried milk were also affected.[11]

The losses were staggering. Financially, they were estimated at between $75 million and $100 million or more in the form of destroyed animals and their byproducts, and clean-up costs. In addition, a $270 million lawsuit was brought against the company by the Michigan Farm Bureau; this was settled for around $20 million. Numerous lawsuits were brought by individual farmers. The total cost of the mental stress the farmers and their families had to endure is impossible to quantify.

How Much Contamination?

When the problem was identified, the Michigan Department of Agriculture stepped in and quarantined all contaminated herds and products. The U.S. Food and Drug Administration also became involved in setting tolerances (maximum levels) for PBBs in food. In May 1974 these levels were set at 1.0 ppm for milk and meat, 0.1 ppm for eggs, and 0.3 for feed. However, these were revised downward only a short time later on November 4, as more sensitive analytic techniques became available. The new levels were milk and meat, 0.3 ppm; eggs and feed, 0.05 ppm.[12]

In a report by the Michigan Department of Agriculture dated October 7, 1974, feed levels were reported as high as 13,500 ppm; milk, 595 ppm; poultry-tissue levels, 4,600 ppm; eggs, 59.7 ppm; and cattle tissue, 2,700 ppm.

In a later survey conducted during March 16–21, the Food and Drug Administration found 1–12 ppm in the body fat of dairy cattle and 1–13 ppm in their milk. These levels corresponded to feed levels of 1–14 ppm.

Delay in the detection of the PBB contaminant allowed wide and prolonged distribution of contaminated feed. As a result, experts agree that most of Michigan's nine million people have detectable levels of PBB in their serum and body tissues. Needless to say, concern arose over the potential human health effects of PBB. Not only were the deaths and disease among farm animals alarming, but there was no previous experience of PBB contamination in humans.

Health Effects: Animals

Since the contamination incident in Michigan, numerous studies have been conducted in both laboratory and domestic animals to assess the possible adverse effects of exposure to various levels of PBBs.

Studies conducted on the poisoned cows indicated that adverse effects can occur in cows with as little as 1 ppm of PBB in their tissues.[13] This is significant when one notes that some of the cattle had tissue PBB concentrations exceeding 3,000 ppm.[14] The affected cows exhibited a wide range of abnormalities.

Initially the cows displayed anorexia, decreased milk production, increased urination, and some lameness. About one month after the onset of the decreased milk production, hematomas (severe bruising), which later developed into abscesses, appeared. Weight loss was marked, and this continued even after the PBB-contaminated feed was withdrawn.

Later problems included abnormal hoof growth, loss of hair, thickening skin, and inability to stand longer than momentarily. Cows contaminated during pregnancy often aborted.[15] When the contamination was during the last trimester, offspring were often delivered two to four weeks late. The offspring were unusually large and either were born dead or died soon after birth.

Researchers also found that when cows accumulated 500 grams of PBB in their tissues, which corresponds to blood levels of 1,000 ppm, they lost their ability to fight infections normally.[16] Cows accumulating more than 500 grams of PBB in their tissues died. Pathology reports on these animals show abnormalities in the liver and kidneys. In addition, numerous internal abscesses and ulcers were found.

The effects of PBBs on pigs and their offspring were far less dramatic than in cows. Sows were administered up to 200 ppm of PBB in their feed per day and their offspring did not show signs of toxicity. In addition, the

PBBs did not appear to cause an increase in the number of stillbirths. Autopsies of newborn pigs indicated that PBBs do cross the placenta and enter the fetal tissues, but the newborns received a dose far smaller than did nursing pigs. In fact, as much as 80 percent of the PBB was excreted in the milk.* Increased mortality was noted among piglets nursing from sows that were continued on the feed contaminated with 100–200 ppm of PBBs.

Chickens were also adversely affected in the PBB incident. When chickens were fed a diet containing 80 ppm Firemaster, their egg production plummeted by 95 percent in only three weeks. Although withdrawal of the PBBs from the diet caused production to return to normal, PBBs continued to be excreted in the eggs for some time.

Laboratory studies found PBBs to be carcinogenic in rats and mice, but only at exceptionally high levels. In rats, carcinogenic changes were found in the liver with either a single dose of 1,000 mg, or twelve doses of 100 mg. Some mice displayed changes in their immune systems at relatively low doses, 10 ppm; but such changes were more commonly noticed at doses above 100 ppm. Feeding 390–1,300 ppm PPB in the diet for three- to six-month periods caused minor neurological symptoms in rats and mice; such abnormalities were similar to the neurological problems found in exposed humans.

Some studies indicated that PBBs cause several reproductive problems in rats when high doses (200–1,000 ppm in the diet) are fed early in pregnancy. Researchers have noted increased resorptions and fetal death, and certain birth defects, such as cleft palate, diaphragmatic hernia, and changes in metabolism.[17] The PBB scientific advisory panel appointed by Governor William G. Milliken of Michigan found that "although not a potent teratogen in mice, PBB does produce fetal lethality at levels that have no gross maternal effect."

Health Effects: Humans

Numerous follow-up studies have been conducted both on individuals who were heavily exposed to PBBs and on those who were exposed to trace amounts in their foods. In all of these studies, a control group of unexposed farmers was used as a means of comparison.

Reassuringly, health evaluations of the most heavily exposed failed to prove that significant ill effects resulted from PBB ingestion. For example, a study carried out on a subset of twenty-three farmers experiencing heavy exposure and reporting multiple, disabling health problems failed to link PBB exposure with the problems. Although the farmers complained of such constitutional

---

*Because PBBs are fat soluble and breast milk has relatively more fat than blood, breast milk is the prime route of excretion for lactating mammals.

symptoms as depression, fatigue, weakness, and memory loss, all medical tests were negative. Researchers concluded that the PBBs were not responsible but that reactive depression was.[18]

Neither did PBB-exposed men show abnormalities suggestive of infertility: the number, shape, and movement of sperm were all normal."[19]

Many neurological symptoms were reported, including nervousness, dizziness, depression, and sleep problems. Again, researchers failed to link such symptoms to PBBs, but found stress to be the more likely culprit. Two studies of exposed farmers complaining of memory dysfunction concluded that their memory loss was again induced by stress.[20] Other studies of heavily exposed farmers failed to find physical changes or damage to the brain.[21] Only one study showed a relationship between levels of PBB in the blood and neurological function: higher PBB levels were associated with lower test scores. However, it must be noted that those with the low test scores were those reporting more dizziness, headaches, and blurred vision. Because these symptoms themselves can be a reaction to an event—in this case, PBB exposure—the real causes of the low test scores are in question.

Exposed children were also scrutinized, but did not show any ill health or developmental problems. Even children with significantly high PBB blood levels showed no evidence of impaired developmental abilities when compared with unexposed children.[22] Neither did children who resided on quarantined farms from conception have any medical evidence of ill health. Although parents claimed abnormally high rates of respiratory disease, urinary tract infections, fevers, and increased clumsiness among their children, comparison with nonexposed children revealed no such increase. Even children reported as having loss of appetite and slow weight gain actually measured up equally to controls.

PBBs were linked to some minor abnormalities. One investigation suggested PBBs may have reduced the number of cells produced by the immune system. There were, however, no clinical indications that this caused any ill health. This abnormality was found among heavily exposed farm families and was not related to age or sex.[23]

There were some skin abnormalities among heavily exposed farmers. Three years after exposure stopped some were found to have characteristic acne, hair loss, skin redness, skin peeling and scaling, increased sweating, and abnormal growth of fingernails and toenails.[24]

While there are indeed anecdotal reports of acute symptoms associated with PBB exposure, there is no convincing evidence that human health was threatened. To quote again the PBB Scientific Advisory Panel of the governor of Michigan:

> The panel received no report or data correlating symptoms to body burden of PBB, or abnormal blood chemistry, in a concentration-effect relationship.

The panel received no evidence that significant health effects resulting from PBB ingestion have been documented in man.[25]

As of December 1991, there are still no clinically significant changes among a group of four thousand exposed people who have been studied since the accident. Harold Humphrey, Ph.D., environmental epidemiologist and director of the Michigan Long-term PBB Study for the Michigan Department of Public Health, says that while PBBs are persistent in the bodies of the exposed, there is no indication that they have or are causing cancer, deaths, or other disease. Some new, very sensitive biological markers now indicate that PBBs may have caused some subtle biological changes. Again, however, there has been no measurable or observable significance of such changes.[26]

We must remember that the stress these farmers experienced was severe. Many of them lost farms, had to slaughter hundreds of farm animals and pets, and some were even accused of mistreating their animals. Some farmers complained of feeling guilty for unwittingly contaminating milk and meat products, which resulted in placing most of Michigan at risk.

The anxiety about any effects to children—both unborn and born—was certainly understandable in light of the severe reproductive problems noted in cows. Knowledge of the cows' problems caused fear, which led to anxiety and depression, all of which may have been reflected in how parents perceived their children's behavior and health.

Perspective Or Accidents Will Happen

Murphy's Law states that what can go wrong will. And that's what happened with the mishandling of PBBs in Michigan. This fire-retardant chemical was never intended for any use whereby subsequent food (or for that matter, environmental) contamination could occur through either direct or indirect means; yet, this did happen. The title of one magazine's account of the incident says it so accurately: "Somebody Simply Goofed."

No one gains from such an accident; everyone's best interest is served if we can avoid this kind of catastrophe. In this case, stress and financial burdens were enormous, and they no doubt took their toll. We are fortunate that human health seems to have escaped with just a few minor—and already healed—scratches.

Unfortunately, incidents such as this perpetuate the chemophobic perception that has spread among the American public. Fueled by fear and mistrust, citizen groups call for the banning of "all toxic chemicals." What is the trade off?

Would we rather go back to the days of increased death, disability, and disfigurement caused by fires? Or will we responsibly accept any risks associated with improved technologies?

No one is belittling the public's fears about issues like PBB contamination; the fears are real and justified, but often trace to a lack of understanding. According to Judge David Bazelon, we can achieve better understanding if scientists become more moral.

Scientists must resist the temptation to belittle these concerns, however irrational they may seem. The scientific community must not turn its back on the political processes to which we commit societal decisions. Scientists, like all citizens, must plan an active role in the discussion of competing values. Their special expertise will inevitably and rightly give them a persuasive voice when issues are discussed in our assemblies and on our streets.

It behooves us to understand new technology and accept the uncertainties associated with it when specific problems are to be solved by its application.

NOTES

1. L. Regenstein, *America the Poisoned* (Washington: Acropolis Books, 1982), p. 263.

2. R. Nader, et al., *Who's Poisoning America?* (San Francisco: Sierra Club Books, 1981), p. 64.

3. J. Egginton, *The Poisoning of Michigan* (New York: W. W. Norton & Co., 1980), p. 15.

4. J. Egginton, "The Poisoning of America," *Atlantic Monthly,* October 1979, p. 16.

5. "Study Finds Most Residents of Michigan are Carrying Toxic Chemicals in Bodies," *Wall Street Journal,* October 10, 1977.

6. Ibid.

7. W. Chapman, "Somebody Simply Goofed," *Progressive,* August 1977, p. 30.

8. "PBBs: More Effects and More Exposure," *Science News* (August 13, 1977): p. 100.

9. PBB Scientific Advisory Panel, Report to William G. Milliken, Governor, State of Michigan, on Polybrominated Biphenyls (PBB), May 24, 1976, p. 5.

10. "And Now, Cattlegate," *Time,* May 10, 1976, p. 75.

11. P. R. Werner and S. D. Sleight, "Toxicosis in Sows and Their Pigs Caused by Feeding Rations Containing Polybrominated Biphenyls to Sows During Pregnancy and Lactation," *American Journal Veterinarian Research* 242 (1981): p. 184.

12. Ibid.

13. Michigan Department of Agriculture, PBB Contamination Status Report, Lansing Michigan, October 7, 1974.

14. T. F. Jackson and F. L. Halbert, "A Toxic Syndrome Associated with the Feeding of Polybrominated Biphenyl-Contaminated Protein Concentrate to Dairy Cattle," *American Journal Veterinarian Medical Association* 165 (1974): p. 437.

15. P. D. Moorehead, et al., "Pathology of Experimentally Induced Polybrominated

Biphenyl Toxicosis in Pregnant Heifers," *Journal of the American Veterinarian Medical Association* 170 (1977): p. 307.

16. J. R. Kateley, et al., "Host Defense Systems in Cattle Exposed to Polybrominated Biphenyl," *American Journal Veterinarian Research* 43 (1982): p. 1288.

17. Werner and Sleight, "Toxicosis in Sows."

18. J. K. Stross, et al. "Human Health Effects of Exposure to Polybrominated Biphenyl (PBB)," *Toxicology and Applied Pharmacology* 58 (1981): p. 145.

19. D. Roseman et al., "Spermatogenesis in Men Exposed to Polybrominated Biphenyl (PBB)," *Fertility and Sterility* 32 (1979): p. 209.

20. G. G. Brown and R. Tixon, "Exposure to Polybrominated Biphenyls: Some Effects on Personality and Cognitive Functioning," *Journal of American Medical Association* (1979): p. 523.

21. Stross, "Human Health Effects."

22. M. Barr, "Pediatric Aspects of the Michigan Polybrominated Biphenyl Contamination," *Annals of Research* 21 (1980): p. 255.

23. J. G. Bekes, et al., "Immunologic Dysfunction Among PBB-Exposed Dairy Farmers," *Annals of the New York Academy of Science* 320 (1979): p. 717.

24. J. J. Chanda, et al. "Cutaneous Effects of Exposure to Polybrominated Biphenyls (PBBs): The Michigan PBB Incident," *Environmental Research* 29 (1982): p. 97.

25. PBB Scientific Advisory Panel, 11.

26. Personal communication, Harold Humphrey, Ph.D., Michigan Department of Public Health, December 2, 1991.

8

Can a Single Asbestos Fiber Kill You?

The Charges

A single asbestos fiber can kill you.

—From abatement literature

The Facts

- Asbestos is the name of a group of naturally occurring minerals that separate into strong, microscopic fibers that are heat-resistant, odorless, and very durable.

- Between 1900 and 1980, some 30 million tons of asbestos were used commercially in the United States. It was used for thermal and acoustical insulation, fire-proofing, pipe insulation, cement piping and many other products requiring insulation.

- Asbestos is a proven health hazard. But while several studies have linked asbestos to lung cancer, asbestosis, and a cancer called mesothelioma, these studies examined occupational groups whose exposure levels were several thousand times higher than those presently found inside commercial, residential, and school buildings.

- Risk assessment models have shown that ten years of exposure to an asbestos concentration of 0.001 fibers per ml could cause one case of lung cancer or mesothelioma per 100,000 persons, a relatively insignif-

263

icant environmental risk. But asbestos levels in buildings average only 0.0007 fibers per ml, far below the exposure necessary to produce cancer. And keep in mind that the Occupational Safety and Health Administration (OSHA) allows a time-weighted average of 2 fibers per ml, a level almost three thousand times higher than the average level found in buildings containing asbestos.

- Asbestos removal procedures vary substantially, depending on adherence to worker protection and handling procedures. Requirements state that indoor asbestos levels must not exceed outdoor levels following asbestos removal. But a few studies have indicated that indoor asbestos levels may actually be greater after asbestos removal than they were before.

Asbestos: That Wonder Mineral

Historians suspect that asbestos use dates back to the Stone Age, when it was used to strengthen earthenware pots. Observing that objects made of asbestos didn't burn, the Greeks dubbed this mineral *asbesta,* Greek for unquenchable.[1]

In modern times, the asbestos industry was born of the Industrial Revolution. The great surge in mechanical power demanded an insulation material that would reduce heat loss, resist combustion, and remain intact at high temperatures. Asbestos fit the bill. Indeed, fire-proofing materials made from asbestos are outstanding in their effectiveness. They were also the prime choice for insulating heating sources and electrical wires.

Asbestos was soon used by more than just the power-producing industry. Heavy industry and the construction trade soon demanded large quantities.[2] By the 1890s, asbestos boasted hundreds of applications, and by 1900 cumulative world production reached approximately 200,000 metric tons. By 1980, this volume swelled to over 100 million tons.[3] Asbestos was eventually used in over 3,000 commercial products, from hair dryers to spackling compound.

Not a Single Material

Asbestos, the state rock of California, is naturally abundant. Asbestos is actually not one, but a set of six minerals bearing similar properties. They are fibrous, heat resistant, strong, and conduct electricity. All forms can be milled, spun, and woven like cotton.

Chrysotile is both the most commonly occurring and used form of asbestos; 95 percent of asbestos-containing materials in the United States are composed of chrysotile.[4] The other five varieties of asbestos are crocidolite, amosite, tremolite, actinolite, and anthophyllite, all of which are called amphiboles.[5]

A Difference Greater Than Just the Name

The different types of asbestos have tremendous differences in size and shape, differences that make them significantly distinct health risks.[6] Medical researchers now know that fiber type, shape, and size determine carcinogenic and other disease potential.[7] Asbestos can threaten health when fibers are released into the air. This can occur when asbestos-containing materials deteriorate or are damaged. Once released, the fibers tend to linger for long periods of time. The risk arises when sufficient quantities of certain fiber types are inhaled. Some types of asbestos dissolve in the body, posing no risk at all. Others, however, remain in the body for years and can cause disease; but, to reiterate, only at or above certain critical concentrations.[8]

Because these facts are little publicized, most people think of cancer any time asbestos exposure is mentioned. The critical information that people do not have is that the most common type of asbestos, chrysotile, poses the lowest risk. Amphibole fibers, particularly amosite and crocidolite, pose a far greater health risk.

A Summary of Asbestos-Related Health Risks

The overwhelming majority of asbestos-caused disease occurs from occupational exposure—prolonged exposure at relatively high levels—to amphibole-type asbestos. Such asbestos exposure can cause four diseases: asbestosis, lung cancer, mesothelioma, and pleural disease. All except pleural disease are serious and potentially fatal; pleural disease in itself is benign, but it does place that person at increased risk for asbestosis.[9] All asbestos-related diseases occur after a relatively long latent period, or a lag from time of exposure to onset of symptoms (four to seven years from fibrosis; twenty to forty years for cancers). It is also crucial to remember that critical concentration: nearly all asbestos-related disease occurs in workers who are exposed to asbestos levels several thousand times higher than those found inside commercial, residential, and school buildings. Says Linda J. Fisher of the EPA's office of Pesticides and Toxic Substances:

> The mere presence of a hazardous substance, such as asbestos on an auditorium ceiling, no more implies disease than a potential poison in a medicine cabinet or under a kitchen sink implies poisoning. Asbestos fibers must be

released from the material in which they are contained, and an individual must breathe those fibers in order to incur any chance of disease.[10]

ASBESTOSIS

Although not a form of cancer, asbestosis is generally fatal. In asbestosis, the lung tissue is scarred and the airways become narrowed; this progresses even after a person is no longer exposed to asbestos. The damage to the lung in asbestosis causes breathing difficulties, and, in turn, the heart becomes increasingly deprived of oxygen. Victims of asbestosis eventually die of heart failure. People who smoke and are exposed to asbestos have a much higher prevalence of a more severe form of asbestosis, called interstitial pulmonary fibrosis.[11]

LUNG CANCER

Asbestos generally does not cause cancer by itself, but acts to help, or promote, other substances in causing cancer. The primary carcinogenic agent in most asbestos-related lung cancers is cigarette smoke. In fact, asbestos workers who smoke are over fifty times more likely to get lung cancer than asbestos workers who do not smoke;[12] they are ninety times more likely to get lung cancer than non-exposed nonsmokers.[13] Past occupational exposure to asbestos accounts for about four thousand to six thousand cases of lung cancer per year.[14]

MESOTHELIOMA

This is a relatively rare cancer that is almost exclusively associated with asbestos exposure. A cancer of the membranes lining the lungs and abdominal cavity not associated with cigarette smoking,[15] it initially causes pain and shortness of breath and then death.[16] It can be caused by even short exposures to amphibole type asbestos, particularly crocidolite.[17] This means that even family members of amphibole asbestos workers as well as people who live near mines are also at risk.[18] This type of cancer has a very long latency period, generally of forty to forty-five years.[19] Past exposure to asbestos causes approximately two thousand cases of mesothelioma per year.[20]

OTHER CANCERS

Asbestos workers who smoke have a much higher incidence of laryngeal cancer.[21] There is evidence that asbestos is associated with cancer of the stomach and pancreas,[22] and some weak evidence that it might cause bowel cancer.[23]

Who Is at Risk of Asbestos-Related Disease?

The population at risk of asbestos-related disease has changed over time. In the 1930s and 1940s, asbestos miners and millers were most affected.[24] Pipe fitters, shipyard and insulation workers, and construction crews were most affected from the late 1940s to the 1960s.[25]

Risk over time changes not only because of changing occupational exposures but also because worker safety regulations have been increasingly fortified. Although certain occupational groups in more recent times may have had higher exposures than earlier groups, they may be at less risk because of far superior worker protection laws and practices. Present levels of asbestos in workplaces utilizing current control procedures, in fact, are not expected to produce any measurable impairment.[26]

Contemporary occupational exposure occurs most frequently in fire fighters, building maintenance personnel, repair workers, custodians, and, as discussed in more detail later, asbestos demolition and abatement workers. Nonoccupational exposures can occur when air or water becomes contaminated with asbestos fibers released from asbestos-containing products. It is this concept that has led to the flurry of asbestos removal projects in schools and other buildings.

Asbestos Becomes a Perceived Public Health Concern

Nonoccupational exposure to asbestos first became a public concern in the mid-1970s. Insulation and other asbestos-containing materials—wall plaster, floor and ceiling tiles—began to deteriorate. At a time when asbestos workers of the 1940s through 1950s were coming forward in large numbers with lung cancer, asbestosis, and mesothelioma, which caused the general public to become frightened to think that they—or worse yet, their children—might be at risk from the asbestos being released into schools and other buildings.

The EPA Acts to Limit Asbestos Exposure

The EPA determined in 1971 that asbestos is a hazardous air pollutant as defined by the Clean Air Act of 1970.[27] In 1973 the EPA issued regulations to control asbestos emissions from manufacturing, milling, roadway surfacing, and demolition projects. By far, however, schools have been the central focus of the asbestos issue.

The EPA first required that all schools inspect for friable (easily crumbled) asbestos in May 1982, with the passage of the Asbestos-In-Schools Identification and Notification Rule; this rule also called for parent, teacher, and school worker notification.[28]

In 1984, Congress passed the Asbestos School Hazard Abatement Act (ASHAA) to provide financial assistance to those schools with serious asbestos hazards and concurrent financial need. From 1985 to late 1991, the ASHAA program provided approximately $291 million to more than 1,100 needy school districts and private schools.[29] ASHAA was reauthorized in 1990, calling for revisions to its accreditation plan, which, among other things, would increase training requirements for abatement workers.[30]

On October 22, 1986 President Reagan authorized the Asbestos Hazard Emergency Response Act (AHERA), taking the asbestos issue in schools two steps further. All public and private schools were thus required to inspect for asbestos, develop asbestos management plans and submit them to the state, and then implement appropriate response actions called abatement. Abatement could be in-place management, repair, encapsulation, or removal. AHERA required that all inspection and abatement, mandated to begin by July 1988 in every school judged to be unsafe, be carried out by accredited personnel.[31]

In 1990, the National School Boards Association estimated the cost of abatement work in public schools alone at more than $6 billion,[32] only a portion of which has been or will be paid for by the federal government. The EPA itself estimated the cost of removing asbestos from *all* public and commercial buildings at $51 billion.[33]

In addition to the $291 million EPA distributed to schools under ASHAA, the agency continues to spend a steady stream of cash on other asbestos activities. From 1985 to 1990, the EPA awarded $2.5 million in grants to thirty-nine states for abatement worker certification programs. In 1987 alone, EPA distributed $1 million among seventeen states for the development of inspector and management planner accreditation programs. In 1990, an additional $1.5 million was awarded to various state-level asbestos activities.[34]

It's critical to keep a perspective on the amount of asbestos in schools. At no time were children thought to be exposed to health-threatening amounts of asbestos. As stated above, the average level of asbestos in schools was just 0.0007 fibers per ml, which is nearly three thousand times less than the legal amount allowed by OSHA in workplaces using asbestos (where workers are exposed for eight hours each day, five days per week).

Abatement Doesn't Always Mean Removal

It cannot be emphasized enough that removing asbestos was but one recommendation in the abatement options. As Linda J. Fisher, assistant administrator for Pesticides and Toxic Substances at EPA, told the U.S. House of Representatives,

It bears repeating that, for most situations, EPA under the AHERA program *does not* mandate removal of asbestos. . . . In addition, removal is often *not* a school district's or other building owner's best course of action to reduce asbestos exposure. In fact, an improper removal can create a dangerous situation where none previously existed. Instead of removal, a conscientious in-place management program will usually control fiber releases, particularly when the materials are not significantly damaged and are not likely to be disturbed. *EPA does recommend in-place management whenever asbestos is discovered.*[35]

The American Medical Association agreed with this line of thinking, recommending removal only when damage to the asbestos-containing material is severe and cannot be repaired,[36] or when there might be a significant release of fibers during building renovation or demolition.[37]

Maintaining friable asbestos in place is not only the wisest choice from a health standpoint, but it is also the easiest and most inexpensive way to manage asbestos. *Money* magazine estimated in 1987 that the cost of maintaining asbestos in place in the average home costs approximately $10 to $50, whereas removal can cost up to $5,000.[38]

Effective methods of maintaining asbestos in place, all approved by the EPA, include:

- Enclosure: a material is placed over or around the asbestos-containing material. A dropped ceiling, for example, can be installed below an asbestos tile ceiling.
- Encapsulation: the asbestos-containing material is treated with a sealant that binds the asbestos fibers together or coats them so that they can no longer be released into the air. A special type of duct tape, for example, is used to cover asbestos-containing heating ducts.

The homeowner should exercise discretion when undertaking any home asbestos repair or removal job. If there is uncertainty that the damaged material in question contains asbestos, a reputable testing agency should be called (your public health department can help in choosing such an expert). Be certain that the testing agency doesn't conveniently operate an asbestos removal service as well; testing and abatement services should be totally separate to ensure integrity.

It bears repeating again that just because asbestos is present, there isn't necessarily a health hazard. Concern about the presence of asbestos arises only when the asbestos fibers are released into the air (such as when asbestos-containing materials become damaged) in sufficiently dangerous quantities and are subsequently inhaled.

How Much Asbestos *Is* There in Schools and Other Buildings?

With a few exceptions, the asbestos level in most schools is very low, generally well below 0.001 (mixed) fibers per milliliter.[39] A recent survey of seventy-one school buildings, in fact, found that 80 percent of these schools had asbestos fiber levels *lower* than required by the EPA *after* abatement. Interestingly, all of these schools were scheduled for some abatement work.[40]

Experts have estimated the lifetime risk for schoolchildren exposed to 0.001 fibers per milliliter for a minimum of ten years. (But please keep in mind that many schools and other buildings have levels far below this value; the risk estimates you are about to read are indeed an overstatement of the actual risk.) They estimate that there would be at most one additional death per 100,000 people from asbestos-related lung cancer or mesothelioma, which, if it did occur, would do so much later in life.[41] This theoretical one death per 100,000 is an inconsequential fraction of expected deaths from other causes. Refer to Table 2 for a sampling of other, real risks and how they compare to the asbestos risk. Note, for example, that the known risk of being struck by lightning is far greater than the theoretical, overstated risk of contracting asbestos-related disease from being a student in an asbestos-containing school.

Levels in other buildings also measure at reassuringly low levels. A 1987 EPA study found air levels in a group of federal buildings with asbestos management programs to be so low as to be indistinguishable from levels outside the buildings.[42] Another EPA survey of schools and other buildings found the average airborne asbestos concentration to be just 0.00070 fibers per milliliter.[43] The suggested lifetime cancer risk for thirty years of continuous occupancy of buildings with an asbestos concentration of 0.00070 fibers per milliliter would be 0.4 (theoretical) cases of cancer per million persons.[44]

Why, Then, Is Asbestos Unnecessarily Removed?

Unfortunately, many public and private managers, concerned about liability in an ambitiously litigious society, feel they are taking the simplest and safest course of action by calling for asbestos removal.

Financial motivation is another important reason that the asbestos-removal industry remains strong. An organized asbestos removal industry with a collective self-interest to promote additional removal utilizes effective marketing strategies.[45]

Unfortunately, asbestos removal, even in cases where it is proven necessary, has been synonymous with scam. Many companies go from town to town, ripping out asbestos without conforming to regulatory requirements, essentially leaving a mess worse than any amount of intact asbestos. An EPA study of

Table 1

Published Estimates of Risk from Various Causes

CAUSE	VOLUNTARY OR INVOLUNTARY	LIFETIME RISK OF PREMATURE DEATH (PER 100,000)
Smoking (all causes)	V	21,900
Smoking (cancer only)	V	8,800
Motor vehicle	I	1,600
Frequent airline passenger	V/I	730
Coal mining accidents	I/V	441
Indoor radon	V/I	400
Motor vehicle pedestrian	I	290
Environmental tobacco smoke/ Living with a smoker	I/V	200
Diagnostic X-rays	I	75
Cycling deaths	I/V	75
Consuming Miami or New Orleans drinking water	I	7
Lightning	I	3
Hurricanes	I	3
Asbestos in school buildings	I	1

SOURCE: J. D. Spengler, H. Ozkaynak, J. F. McCarthy, and H. Lee, *Summary of Symposium on Health Aspects of Exposure to Asbestos in Buildings* (held December 14–16, 1988 at Harvard University Energy and Environmental Policy Center), August 1989.

leaving a mess worse than any amount of intact asbestos. An EPA study of asbestos levels after removal found alarmingly high levels of asbestos *after* the removal, increasing ten to one hundred times over the pre-removal levels.[46] The EPA also estimated that at least one half of all asbestos-removal projects are done improperly.[47]

Asbestos-removal workers may claim that containment methods used during removal will adequately protect workers and reduce or eliminate residual asbestos when the job is completed. Most containment methods, however, have been proven inefficient to prevent leakage. Even the most ambitious containment plans produce substantial residues to threaten the health of both removal workers and building occupants alike.[48]

Indeed, removal places the asbestos-removal workers at risk; *Science* magazine stated: "The misguided removal efforts may even have created a new risk group for asbestos-associated disease: asbestos removal workers."[49] In fact, asbestos-removal workers are today the population at greatest risk from asbestos exposure.[50] The Occupational Safety and Health Administration estimates that there will be almost seven casualties per thousand workers, many more deaths than would be expected if the asbestos were left in place.

The American Cancer Society commented about unnecessary asbestos abatement, saying,[51]

> This extensive national remediation effort is presently under question because of its great cost and complexity, uncertainties in non-occupational risk estimates and substantial increases in risk for workers removing asbestos.

Another Reason for Unnecessary Removal

Current federal regulations, which fail to differentiate the types of asbestos and their tremendous difference in risk, are another important reason why unnecessary asbestos abatement work continues. Says Philip H. Abelson, deputy editor of *Science* magazine:

> A puzzling defect in federal legislation and regulations is an arbitrary lumping together of disparate minerals and calling the lot of them asbestos. As a result, chrysotile, a serpentine mineral, is tarred with association with the dangerous amphibole crocidolite. The two minerals differ in composition, color, shape, solubility and persistence in human tissue. Chrysotile is a white mineral. . . . It tends to be soluble and to disappear in tissue. Fibers tend . . . to be excluded from the periphery of the lung. Crocidolite is blue . . . and is relatively insoluble. It persists in tissue. Its fibers . . . penetrate narrow lung passages.

The Harvard Symposium on Health Aspects of Exposure to Asbestos in Buildings, held in December 1988, also concluded:

> This is an important point for public policy, because present U.S. regulations do not consider variations in the biological potency of different fiber categories.

Another puzzling defect in federal performance is failure to give sufficient weight to epidemiological experience relating to chrysotile mines in Quebec. These mines have been operating since before 1900 and have produced about 40 million tons of chrysotile. In keeping with the lax practice of earlier days, mining operations were accompanied by large amounts of chrysotile dust. Wives of miners were heavily exposed; they dwelt in homes near the mines. Despite such heavy exposure, four epidemiological studies of the Quebec chrysotile-mining localities failed to show that lifelong exposure of women to dust from nearby mines caused any statistically significant excess disease.

And Panic Continues

Despite reassuring facts about the lack of an asbestos hazard, the mere presence of asbestos continues to cause panic. *Science* magazine's Abelson says that,

> Panic has not been confined to schools. Building owners broadly have been ripping out asbestos. If anything, the rush to remove asbestos is accelerating. Most people, unfortunately, don't realize that deaths from smoking, drowning, and playing high school football, are orders of magnitude higher than deaths from asbestos exposure.

Dr. B. T. Mossman and colleagues at the University of Vermont wrote in *Science* (January 19, 1991) and echo the fact that the asbestos risk has been overrated:

> The available data and comparative risk assessments indicate that chrysotile asbestos, the type of fiber found predominantly in U.S. schools and buildings, is not a health risk in the nonoccupational environment. Clearly, the asbestos panic in the U.S. must be curtailed, especially because unwarranted and poorly controlled asbestos abatement results in unnecessary risks to young removal workers who may develop asbestos-related cancers in later decades. The extensive removal of asbestos has occurred less frequently in Europe.

The American Medical Association's Council on Scientific Affairs released a position paper on asbestos in early August 1991, echoing the fact that the asbestos risk has been greatly inflated:

> Contrary to what was described as public "misconception," asbestos poses far less risk to the health of the everyday occupants of buildings than that posed by smoking, drug and alcohol abuse, improper diet, and lack of exercise.

The 1988 Harvard Symposium on Health Aspects of Exposure to Asbestos in Buildings concluded:

> In many cases, spending money on asbestos removal will likely decrease funding which might be available to support other public health and educational

measures which could be far more effective in reducing environmental health risks.[52]

An Attempt to Ban Asbestos*

The mass hysteria over asbestos resulted in the EPA banning it in 1987. When the asbestos ban was first proposed in 1987 the EPA estimated it would save 1,500 lives over a fifteen-year period—100 lives per year. The agency was forced to revise the estimated number of lives spared to 200 over thirteen years— 15 per year—after cross-examination hearings brought out the fact that the only category of people at any substantive risk from asbestos were brake maintenance workers.[53] And those workers, approximately 150 of the total 200, are now protected under regulations of the Occupational Safety and Health Administration.

The ban, finalized in 1989, but reversed in the fall of 1991, would have pitted the United States against Nairobi—and the rest of the world. The ban may well have become the basis for a worldwide debate over a double standard in which 200 theoretical American lives spared from cancer are allegedly worth more than millions of lives lost in the Third World. Waterborne diseases, such as malaria, cholera, and dysentery account for 25 percent of all deaths in Asia, Africa, and South America because of a lack of asbestos/cement pipe essential for sanitation.

At the time of the ban, Raymond Savoie, the Canadian minister of mines, said, "This is a political decision, taken in bad faith and without scientific foundation, and it makes me damn angry." He worried the ban would result in a "ripple effect" that would effectively stop the production of asbestos/cement for pipes and construction in the Third World. The U.S. Agency for International Development, in fact, suspended financial support for such asbestos projects at the time.

In the penultimate paragraph of the press release announcing the ban, EPA Administrator William K. Reilly said:

> The rule's ban of asbestos/cement pipe or other products should not be seen as a signal to other nations, especially developing countries, that use of these products should be discontinued. The actions taken in this rule are based on an evaluation of the specific uses of these products in the U.S., the availability of substitutes in the U.S. market and other factors that may be unique to this country. Similar evaluations should be performed in other countries.

---

*Much of this discussion is based on an article by Michael J. Bennett, appearing in *Priorities for Your Good Health* (Fall 1989).

Reilly, however, dropped those comments from his prepared remarks at a carefully stage-managed press conference that drew twenty-one television cameras and almost one hundred reporters. Only under questioning did he concede:

> Asbestos still has great use in developing countries, particularly asbestos/cement pipe for sanitation.

Reilly also noted that there would be little sense in ripping out the more than 200,000 miles of asbestos/cement pipe that carry water to almost everyone in the United States.

But the estimated number of lives saved by the ban and its later revision had to be virtually dragged out of Reilly, as did the fact that almost every other nation, the International Labor Organization, and the World Health Organization have adopted a controlled-use approach to asbestos. The only exceptions, as Reilly noted, are West Germany, Sweden, and Switzerland, and their bans are still under consideration.

Few, if any, of these details were used in press accounts. The most obvious reason is that the media were invited to arrive at the press conference two hours before the commercial interests. The reporters were gone long before most of the commercial interests even showed up. And of course, scientific authorities who have found, almost without exception, absolutely no reason for the ban were not invited at all.

Once again, the media demonstrated that they had been carefully trained, as Edith Efron observed in *The Apocalyptics:*

> As one trains a circus dog, to view apocalyptics in and out of government as fountains of scientific truth . . . [with] consummate credulity in the face of arbitrary edicts brandished by the policy-makers as the voice of science.

Once again, EPA's formidable public relations apparatus proved reporters to be "prisoners of gullibility," as Jim Sibbison, a longtime public affairs officer for the agency, wrote in an article in *The Washington Monthly*, March 1984. Sibbison said:

> Call it hubris, but I came to feel that my fellow EPA press officers were the real reporters, and the reporters were the publicists.

Banning was the central article of faith of the EPA and the environmental lobbyists. "If we can't ban asbestos, we can't ban anything," former EPA Administrator John Moore testified before Congress a few years ago.

Fortunately, the asbestos ban was partially overturned in the fall of 1991, with uses including automobile brake liners, asbestos-cement pipe and construction materials such as asbestos coatings, shingles and paper products allowed once again.

NOTES

1. Robert A. Fowler, *Asbestos Dust Everyone's Problem* (Berkeley: Western Institute for Occupational/Environmental Sciences, n.d.).

2. D. E. Lilienfeld, "The Silence: The Asbestos Industry and Early Occupational Cancer Research—A Case Study," *American Journal of Public Health* 81 (1991): pp. 791-800.

3. Malcolm Ross, "The Geologic Occurrences and Health Hazards of Amphibole and Serpentine Asbestos," reprinted from *Reviews in Minerology* 9A.

4. J. F. Dunn, "Asbestos and Regulatory Philosophy" (unpublished, 1990).

5. M. Ross, "A Survey of Asbestos-Related Diseases in Trades and Mining Occupations and in Factory and Mining Communities as a Means of Predicting Health Risks of Nonoccupational Exposure to Fibrous Minerals," in *Definitions for Asbestos and Other Health-Related Silicates, ASTM STP* 834, ed. Benjamin Levadie (Philadelphia: American Society for Testing and Materials, 1984), pp. 51-104.

6. Ibid.

7. H. Scheier, *Studies in Environmental Science 37: Asbestos in the Natural Environment* (New York: Elsevier Science Publishing Company, 1989).

8. B. T. Mossman, J. Bignon, M. Corn, A. Seaton, and J. B. L. Gee, "Asbestos: Scientific Developments and Implications for Public Policy," *Science* 247 (1990): pp. 249-301; Environmental Protection Agency, "Environmental Backgrounder: Asbestos," March 1989; statement of Linda J. Fisher, assistant administrator for pesticides and toxic substances, EPA, before the Subcommittee on Toxic Substances, Environmental Oversight, Research and Development of the Committee on Environment and Public Works, U.S. Senate, April 26, 1990.

9. I. J. Selikoff, J. Churg, and E. C. Hammond, "Asbestos Exposure and Neoplasia," *Journal of the American Medical Association* 252 (1984): pp. 91-95; H. Skinner, W. Catherine, M. Ross, and F. Clifford, *Asbestos and Other Fibrous Materials: Minerology, Crystal Chemistry and Health Effects* (New York: Oxford University Press, 1988).

10. Linda J. Fisher, April 26, 1990.

11. R. Lilis et al., "Radiographic Abnormalities in Asbestos Insulators: Effects of Duration from Onset of Exposure and Smoking. Relationships of Dyspnea with Parenchymal and Pleural Fibrosis," *American Journal of Industrial Medicine* 20 (1991): pp. 1-15.

12. Skinner et al., *Asbestos and Other Fibrous Materials Minerology.*

13. American Cancer Society, "Cancer Response System #2026," July 12, 1991.

14. American Cancer Society, "Executive Notice on Asbestos," April 20, 1990.

15. Ross, "Survey of Asbestos-Related Diseases"; Fowler, *Asbestos Dust Everyone's Problem.*

16. Skinner et al., *Asbestos and Other Fibrous Materials.*

17. Fowler, *Asbestos Dust Everyone's Problem;* Ross, "Survey of Asbestos-Related Diseases."

18. Mossman et al., "Asbestos," pp. 249–301; Ross, "Survey of Asbestos-Related Diseases"; Skinner et al., *Asbestos and Other Fibrous Materials.*

19. American Cancer Society, "Cancer Response System #2026."

20. American Cancer Society, "Executive Notice on Asbestos."

21. P. J. Landrigan, and Baker, "The Recognition and Control of Occupational Disease," *Journal of the American Medical Association* 266 (1991): pp. 676–80.

22. M. S. Kanarek, in *Non-Occupational Exposure to Mineral Fibers,* ed. J. Bignon, J. Petro, and R. Saracci (Lyon: International Agency for Research on Cancer, 1989), pp. 428–36.

23. B. T. Mossman and J. B. Gee, "Asbestos-Related Diseases," *New England Journal of Medicine* 320 (1990): pp. 1721–30; J. Petro in *Non-Occupational Exposure to Mineral Fibers,* ed. J. Bignon, J. Petro, R. Saracci (Lyon: International Agency for Research on Cancer, 1989), pp. 457–69.

24. E. Whelan, *Preventing Cancer* (New York: W. W. Norton and Co., 1980).

25. Council on Scientific Affairs, American Medical Association, "Asbestos Removal, Health Hazards, and the EPA," *Journal of the American Medical Association* 266 (1991): pp. 696–97.

26. Berry et al. (1980), as quoted in J. D. Spengler, H. Ozkaynak, J. F. McCarthy, and H. Lee, *Summary of Symposium on Health Aspects of Exposure to Asbestos in Buildings,* August 1989, held at Harvard University Energy and Environmental Policy Center, December 14–16, 1988.

27. EPA, Environmental Backgrounder: Asbestos.

28. Statement of Linda J. Fisher, assistant administrator for pesticides and toxic substances, EPA, before the Subcommittee on Environment, Energy, and Natural Resources, Committee on Government Operations, U.S. House of Representatives, September 24, 1991.

29. Linda J. Fisher, September 24, 1991.

30. Linda J. Fisher, April 26, 1990.

31. Ibid.

32. M. Fumento, "Great Asbestos Rip-Off," *Readers Digest,* January 1990, p. 174.

33. EPA, "Study of Asbestos-Containing Materials in Public Buildings: A Report to Congress, United States Environmental Protection Agency," Washington, D.C., February 1988.

34. Linda J. Fisher, April 26, 1990.

35. Linda J. Fisher, September 24, 1991.

36. Linda J. Fisher, September 24, 1991.

37. Linda J. Fisher, April 26, 1990.

38. L. Luciano, "Toxic Hazards in the Home: Sometimes the Best Thing to do is Nothing," *Money,* March 1987, p. 47.

39. Spengler et al., *Symposium on Health Aspects of Exposure to Asbestos.*

40. M. Corn, K. Crump, D. B. Farrar, R. J. Lee, and D. R. McFee, "Airborne Concentrations of Asbestos in 71 School Buildings," *Regulatory Toxicology and Pharmacology* 13 (1991): pp. 99–114.

41. Spengler et al., *Symposium on Health Aspects of Exposure to Asbestos.*
42. Linda J. Fisher, April 26, 1990.
43. Spengler et al., *Symposium on Health Aspects of Exposure to Asbestos.*
44. Corn et al., "Airborne Concentrations of Asbestos."
45. Spengler et al., *Symposium on Health Aspects of Exposure to Asbestos,* p. 27
46. Spengler et al., *Symposium on Health Aspects of Exposure to Asbestos.*
47. *Science,* March 2, 1990.
48. Spengler et al., *Symposium on Health Aspects of Exposure to Asbestos,* p. 25.
49. *Science,* January 19, 1990.
50. Spengler et al., *Symposium on Health Aspects of Exposure to Asbestos.*
51. American Cancer Society, "Executive Notice on Asbestos."
52. Spengler et al., *Symposium on Health Aspects of Exposure to Asbestos,* p. 27.
53. M. J. Bennett, "Beyond Abatement: The Asbestos Ban," *Priorities* (Fall 1989).

9

Deadly Dioxin?

The Charges

. . . 2,4,5-T is a component of Agent Orange, the defoliant used in Vietnam which was later implicated as the cause of birth defects and infant deaths.

—Pills, Pesticides and Profits[1]

Dioxin . . . [is] the most toxic known chemical. . . .

You can't go around spraying deadly chemicals on people's property, where they keep animals and kids. I thought if you could go to the moon you ought to be able to control something like that.

—Hazardous Waste in America[2]

Dioxin can cause severely adverse health effects, and death, at the lowest doses imaginable. . . . millions of pounds of the two ingredients of Agent Orange are still being sprayed, despite the enormous harm they are known to have caused to human health, wildlife and the environment. . . .

The disposal of dioxin wastes is another time bomb ticking across the country. . . .

No one knows the damage that dioxin is causing to public health, but the pervasive presence in the environment and food chain of a variety of toxic chemicals known to cause cancer may play a significant role in the current cancer epidemic. . . .

Nor can anyone say what will be the long-term effects on the American people—the chemical industry's ultimate guinea pigs. By the time the final results are in, it may be too late to take corrective action.

—"Across America, Dioxin," New York Times[3]

The so-called phenoxy herbicides 2,4,5-T, Silvex and 2,4-D, used here to combat aquatic weeds that clog rice fields, are contaminated by dioxins, one of which is the most toxic compound synthesized by man.

—*New York Times*[4]

Humans who have been exposed to it [dioxin] near Love Canal, in Vietnam or in situations such as train wrecks or factory explosions have suffered a variety of severe health problems, including kidney and liver ailments, birth defects and cancer.

—*New York Times*[5]

Dioxin, however, has a short, sexy ring to it, and there is even an x in the middle syllable that brings forth images of the skull and cross-bones on a classic poison bottle.

Suffice it to say, however, that if animal tests are any indication, TCDD can affect about any organ in the body. As a carcinogen, it possesses almost unprecedented potency.

There are also aches in muscles and joints, digestive disorders, nerve changes, and even psychiatric effects—including the hearing of phantom voices.

—*Toxic Cloud*[6]

A 39-year-old man died Wednesday morning after drinking beer and whiskey. Sheriff's Corporal said that the man took four bullets out of a .357-magnum revolver, spun the chamber, said "I'll show you what's real," and fired the gun into his head. The friend told investigators the victim was depressed over an illness related to exposure to Agent Orange during the Vietnam War.

—*When Technology Wounds*[7]

In 1985-86 Sweden and Denmark halted building new incinerators because they produced dioxin in mother's milk.

—*Design for a Living Planet*[8]

The Facts

- Dioxin is highly toxic to some species of animals but less so to others.

- Dioxin is an animal carcinogen only at doses that are toxic to that animal.

- As far as we know, no human has ever died or become chronically ill from environmental exposure to dioxin in the United States. The only human illnesses so far proved to occur from exposure to dioxin are chloracne, a severe acne-like skin disorder and short-term reversible nerve dysfunction. Acute dioxin poisoning can also be toxic to the liver and kidneys.

- There is no conclusive evidence that 2,4,5-T or dioxin causes human cancer, spontaneous abortion, or birth defects.

- Follow-up studies on accidental exposure to high levels of dioxin (for example, Monsanto workers exposed in a 1949 accident) indicate no long-term adverse health effect.

- Some studies, yet to be confirmed, have suggested that exposure to 2,4,5-T and dioxin increases the risk of soft-tissue sarcomas in heavily exposed industrial workers. Even if this link with occupational exposure were confirmed, it would have no bearing on the allegations of the myriad of other complaints, including miscarriage, made by those objecting to traces of dioxin. Further, if the causal link were made for those occupationally exposed to high doses of dioxin-containing herbicides over many years, it would be of little relevance to those of us who might be only occasionally exposed to trace amounts in the general environment.

Hardly a day goes by without an unsettling media report citing yet another contaminated dump with measurable amounts of what is routinely called "the most toxic chemical known to man." Dioxin, many Americans believe, is synonymous with skull and crossbones, signifying illness, cancer, and death. Remarkable it is, and indeed a tribute to the power of the media, that a substance of such infamous reputation has never been shown to cause any deaths or serious harm to humans.

The dioxin saga consists of four separate but related chapters. The first focuses on a fear of dioxin itself; that is, its presence in places like Times Beach, Missouri, the Love Canal neighborhood, and Newark, New Jersey. The question here is: Is the mere presence of dioxin an imminent health hazard and a reason for grave concern?

The second chapter relates to anxiety over a previously widely used agricultural chemical that has traces of dioxin as an unavoidable contaminant. The herbicide 2,4,5-T has been charged with causing a variety of human ills, and, in particular, been cited in some preliminary (but since discredited) studies as causing miscarriage and other reproductive difficulties. As a result of these concerns, 2,4,5-T was first partially and then totally banned as a commercial herbicide. But the question remains: Is there evidence that this herbicide itself, or in conjunction with its contaminant dioxin, causes human reproductive failure?

The third chapter of the dioxin saga involves Agent Orange, that now-infamous defoliant used in Vietnam during the period 1962–70. Veterans claim that a wide spectrum of diseases they now experience and birth defects in their children are the result of their exposure to this chemical (Agent Orange was actually a combination of the herbicides 2,4,5-T and 2,4-D.) And here, too, the question begs an answer: Is there scientific evidence that the wartime use of Agent Orange was responsible for the health problems now alleged by veterans?

And the fourth chapter is about dioxin in the paper and pulp industry. A 1985 EPA survey discovered dioxin in effluent and sludge around some mills where bleached paper is produced. Interestingly, a survey the previous year had found no such association between paper and dioxin. This discovery was puzzling, as dioxin had never been used, or been associated with materials used, by this industry. Around this time, dioxin was also found as a contaminant in various paper and cardboard food-packaging material. Whatever the cause, are the associated levels of dioxin harming human health?

As will be evident from the material in this chapter, the answer to all four questions is no. Obviously there is nothing beneficial about dioxin. And given the chemical's varied toxicity to humans and animals, there is just reason for concern and calm, reasoned, and efficient remedial action to clean up the contaminated areas. Its presence in the environment serves absolutely no useful purpose.* But its mere presence in the environment does not translate into a massive public health disaster. Although dioxin was spread throughout the small town of Times Beach, Missouri, for example, there was no documented case of dioxin-related death or serious illness among the exposed residents.

The charges of health effects related to the pesticides 2,4,5-T and Agent Orange are both confusing and volatile. Only a calloused individual would not respond sympathetically to the veteran who has developed cancer or fathered children with birth defects. Similarly, the passionate appeal of a woman from Oregon recounting the trauma of miscarriage draws an immediate emotional response. But emotional outbursts fail to examine scientific evidence, serving only to cloud the facts. In trying to lay the blame on dioxin, 2,4,5-T, Agent Orange, or any other environmental factor for human illness, we must have data showing that the diverse health effects are appearing at a rate more frequently in the exposed than in the "unexposed" population. The unfortunate reality of life is that people from all walks of life, from all parts of the country, have children with birth defects, suffer premature deaths from cancer, and report the full gamut of human ills. But there is absolutely no convincing evidence that Vietnam War veterans are experiencing more than their share of disease and other health misfortunes, nor is there evidence to indicate

---

*Oddly enough, however, despite being an animal carcinogen, dioxin has also been found to be a potent inhibitor of tumor formation caused by at least two known carcinogens.[9]

correlative miscarriage rates in women living in areas where 2,4,5-T has been sprayed. What has happened instead is that the public has become increasingly anxious—sometimes hysterical—as a result of a media blitz of half-truths, distortions, and nonscientific fantasies about dioxin, 2,4,5-T, and Agent Orange.

The media has led us to believe that environmental dioxin, both present and past, has been proved guilty without a shadow of a doubt. The crime, they say, is death, cancers, birth defects, and numerous other ailments. The jury in this case, they continue, is the scientific community. But, as we shall see, there is a paucity of credible scientists and public health officials stepping forward to say that dioxin and dioxin-containing herbicides are responsible for the alleged crimes.

What we do see on television news programs are interviews with the few same scientists preaching horror stories and doomsday prophecies. How the press successfully hyped the dioxin "danger" throughout the 1980s was summarized succinctly by Joan Beck of the *Chicago Tribune*:

> Newspaper editors and broadcasters, who help set the national agenda by what they choose to report, have hyped the dioxin danger, made it more dramatic by their choice of human interest stories, ignored much of the scientific evidence and used quotes from some scientists whose conclusions weren't justified by their research.[10]

What Is Dioxin?

Seventy-five separate chemical compounds constitute the group labeled dioxins. The most acutely toxic of these is 2,3,7,8-tetrachlorodibenzo-p-dioxin, or TCDD. A stable compound, dioxin breaks down slowly in the environment when unprotected from the ultraviolet rays of the sun. Once it finds its way into the soil, dioxin persists for a long time, remaining tightly bound to soil particles. Since dioxin is highly insoluble in water, it does not migrate very fast through the soil.

Dioxins are not manufactured directly for use in any product. Rather, they are formed as unwanted byproducts in the production of herbicides such as Silvex and 2,4,5-T and in chlorophenol wood preservatives. Dioxins are also formed naturally by the incomplete combustion of wood products and industrial and municipal wastes (although the 2,3,7,8 form is less predominant among the dioxins formed in this way). Dioxin has also been found in the exhaust from diesel- or gasoline-powered vehicles, suggesting that it is formed during the combustion of diesel fuel and leaded gasoline. Dioxin is also a byproduct of bleaching in the paper and pulp industry.

Herbicide 2,4,5-T

2,4,5-T was developed in 1945 and approved for use as an herbicide in 1948. Because this phenoxy-type herbicide was very selective—killing undesirable plants while sparing crops—it was very popular. 2,4,5-T was especially useful in controlling broadleaf weeds and brush along highways and railways, in rangeland and forests, and in wheat, rice, corn, and sugarcane fields. While other phenoxy herbicides, such as 2,4-D are less expensive, they are not as widely useful because some plants are resistant to them.

Although dioxin was discovered as an unavoidable rare contaminant in 2,4,5-T in 1957, it escaped public concern (and appropriately so) until the 1970s, when dioxin became a household word. The EPA restricted the use of 2,4,5-T to rice fields and rangeland in 1979, largely in response to public outcry. With mounting hysteria, all uses were canceled by February of 1985.[11] Experts agree that this banning was without scientific basis, nor did the EPA consider the far-reaching consequences. This highly selective, inexpensive, and efficient herbicide is virtually impossible to replace, and its absence has had a tremendous impact on agriculture.

Michael Newton, Ph.D., professor of forest ecology at Oregon State University, says that there are two herbicides now used in place of 2,4,5-T in forests: triclopir and glyphosap. Both are well-known herbicides with two of the advantages of 2,4,5-T: they are immobile in soil and they have desirable degradation rates. "However, to control all underbrush, a mixture of substitutes, rather than just one product, is required. Further, more applications are required. This, in turn, means more helicopters in the sky. The result: more alarm is generated among the public."[12]

There is no good substitute to kill sagebrush, chaparral oak, and other hardwoods that grow up in rangeland, that when uncontrolled snuff out grass needed for grazing livestock. While substitutes work when combined properly, their expense is prohibitive. Thomas G. Welch, Ph.D., extension rangebush and weed control specialist with the Texas Agricultural Extension Services, describes what is happening in rangelands:

> Fewer acres are being treated and we are therefore seeing an increase in brush infestation. In 5–10 years, we're going to have a major brush problem: there's going to be a loss in grass production [needed for livestock] and there will be soil erosion. Some areas will grow so dense that there will be a loss of habitat for wildlife.

Similarly, Ford Baldwin, Ph.D., extension weed scientist at the University of Arkansas Cooperative Extension Service, says that many products were brought on the market quickly for rice fields after 2,4,5-T was canceled. "There is nothing that will substitute for 2,4,5-T in rice fields. They can get by with other combinations, but remember that nothing has been approved."[13]

WHY 2,4,5-T WAS BANNED: HALF-BAKED SCIENCE

The initial 1979 partial ban on 2,4,5-T was based largely on an epidemiological study in the Alsea, Oregon area linking 2,4,5-T spraying with human miscarriages. The EPA launched this study when eight Alsea area women reported ten miscarriages that they say were associated with 2,4,5-T spraying. Eventually the EPA studied thirteen miscarriages among twelve women. Note that all occurred within the first twenty weeks of pregnancy.

The EPA's preliminary investigation, known as Alsea I, concluded that there was a seasonal variation in the miscarriage rates among the Alsea women compared with a control group from the nearby city of Corvallis. There was, however, insufficient evidence to prove a relationship between the miscarriages and 2,4,5-T spraying. But anxieties intensified and the matter did not end here. The EPA launched Alsea II study, a retrospective evaluation of the earlier investigation. Using hospital records from the years 1972–77, EPA scientists collected information on miscarriages from three study areas: the Alsea region (along the Oregon coast); the city of Corvallis (immediately inland from Alsea); and a sparsely populated rural area near the Idaho border.

Alsea II, released in February 1979, suggested that there *was* a relationship between the use of 2,4,5-T and an increase in miscarriages. It concluded,

> The agency's systematic survey of the occurrence of spontaneous abortions in an area of 2,4,5-T use indicates that there was an unusually high number of spontaneous abortions in the area, and that the incidence of spontaneous abortions may be related to 2,4,5-T in that area.

Based on the findings of this *one* report, the EPA immediately issued an emergency suspension of 2,4,5-T except for use in rangeland and rice fields.

Understandably, when the EPA partial ban on 2,4,5-T was announced, much scientific attention was thrust on the Alsea II study, which had not, at that point, undergone any peer review, which means it was not judged or validated by the scientific community. In the months that followed, however, at least eighteen reviews concluded that the EPA data did *not* support the EPA conclusions.[14]

Scientific experts from Australia, Canada, the United States, and New Zealand delivered extensive, consistent, and unanimous criticism of Alsea II. James A. Witt, a member of the Oregon State University team that published the most extensive critique of the study, said that what the EPA alleged to be a yearly "June peak" of miscarriages was in fact a single year's deviation from the norm. Furthermore, there was no "significant" correlation between the amount of 2,4,5-T used and the number of pregnancy losses, and, except for June 1976, there was not even an "insignificant" correlation.[15]

A study by S. H. Lamm of Tabershaw Associates concluded that both statistically and epidemiologically the EPA report did not support any relationship between herbicide spraying and miscarriages.[16]

A scientific advisory panel set up under the auspices of the Federal Insecticide, Fungicide, and Rodenticide Act found neither immediate nor substantial threat to human health when 2,4,5-T or Silvex was applied to rice, rangeland, orchards, or sugarcane.[17]

While the scientific community was systematically discrediting the results of Alsea II, citing it as just another case of half-baked, non-peer-reviewed government agency attempt at science, the Alsea women quickly became folk heroes in the eyes of the American press. Portrayed by many as helpless victims of corporate neglect and greed, the women became symbols of the natural, environmental struggle to free our country from the onslaught of the giant poisoners.

On October 2, 1979, for instance, WGBH in Boston aired "A Plague on Our Children," a documentary about the "victims" of 2,4,5-T spraying in Oregon, including such excerpts as

> About one hundred miles south of Debby Marano's house is Eve DeRock's valley and farm. . . .She is still sick two years after 2,4,5-T was sprayed there. . . .
>   While the animal studies continue, the spraying continues. And Oregon residents are convinced that their health problems are linked to it.[18]

There was absolutely no mention of the peer-review findings published during the months before the broadcast, findings that showed that the study was statistically flawed and meaningless.

KRON-TV of San Francisco also managed to distort the public's view of the facts in its irresponsible 1979 documentary "The Politics of Poison." Their opening statement said it all:

> What if you and your children were receiving tiny doses of a terrible poison—a synthetic chemical so powerful that an ounce could wipe out a million people? Is that too incredible, too bizarre to believe? And if that were happening, wouldn't the government do something about it? These unbelievable questions face millions of Americans who are exposed to phenoxy herbicides every day. They are in the front line of a symbolic battle—a struggle over what values will prevail in this chemical age. This film is their story.[19]

The message here is, you and your children are receiving tiny doses of a terrible poison, and, no, it is not too incredible and bizarre to believe. These accusations are so easy to make. The incredibility of the accusers is rarely, if ever, questioned—they apparently come from concerned citizens whose aim is the protection of public health and the environment. But we must look beyond their concern, even if the concern appears to be genuine.

Many reasons move people to make outrageous, nonscientific statements about things they don't understand. First, the herbicides and other agricultural chemicals are manufactured by giant corporations; their sales total billions of dollars annually. Perhaps envy causes some to resent another's business successes. Second, and more importantly, it is always easier to blame life's misfortunes on someone else, especially when that someone is as enormous and anonymous as the federal government or the chemical companies. And third, there is a tendency for the general public to accept anecdotal information (especially as it pertains to something as emotional as cancer, birth defects, or other incidents of bad health) as undeniable proof. It is one thing for a Bonnie Hill of Alsea, Oregon, to be curious about why she and some of her neighbors suffered miscarriages; it is something quite different for her observation to be equated with proof of a causal relationship between 2,4,5-T and miscarriages. The facts are, women within and outside areas sprayed with herbicides suffer miscarriages. Spontaneous abortions are common—not rare—among women, with 20 to 60 percent of all pregnancies ending this way. But to reiterate, the scientific community overwhelmingly agreed that the spraying of herbicide 2,4,5-T did not increase the incidence of miscarriage.

Does Dioxin Cause Cancer?

Initially, concern focused on whether or not dioxin causes cancer. But, with the downgrading of dioxin's cancer-causing ability in the early nineties (as you'll read about below), scaremongers, in looking to maintain dioxin's heinous reputation, are now asking if dioxin causes immunotoxic effects. For many years, the scientific world has focused on a single 1978 study, the Kociba study, in which rats were fed high doses of dioxin. The rats appeared to develop a greatly increased incidence of liver cancer. Until 1991, the potential human health effects of dioxin—and resultant public policy about the chemical—traced to that 1978 study. It was on the basis of this study that dioxin came to be called "the most toxic substance known to man." But, as you will read, scientists no longer believe this to be true. Scientists have downgraded dioxin's toxicity, and the general consensus among them is summarized by Vernon N. Houk, M.D., assistant surgeon general and director of the Center for Environmental Health and Injury Control at the Centers for Disease Control, the public health official who ordered the evacuation of a small Missouri town when dioxin was found there: "If it's a carcinogen, it's a very weak carcinogen and federal policy needs to reflect that."

Let's trace the roots of dioxin's heinous reputation, and the current attempts to change that image.[20]

As we already said, the EPA based all of its risk assessments about dioxin on a single 1978 rat study. The primary finding in this study was liver tumors in female rats. Two points about this study, however, are telling and are under intense scrutiny as science has advanced.

First, the liver tumors that developed in the rats were analyzed according to 1975 scientific criteria.[21] Appropriate at the time, but not today, this evaluation suggested that dioxin was highly carcinogenic.

Second, these high-dose experimental results were used to estimate, or extrapolate, the effects of low-dose rat exposure. A second extrapolation, or projection, was then made to predict the health effects of low-dose dioxin exposure in humans. In other words, scientists played two big guessing games, introducing enormous potential for error into their predictions.

It's not just that scientists stretched the limits of a little knowledge to make a lot of predictions. Today, the same scientists seriously question *how* they stretched these facts. Such projections were made according to standard protocol at the time, the linear-dose model. This method assumes one can predict the consequences of low-dose exposure from knowledge of consequences at high doses. The model assumes that some risk must exist at every dose. That's like saying that because excessive calories cause weight gain, anything with calories causes obesity. Many scientists now question whether this *every-dose-has-a-risk philosophy is an accurate assumption.*

Dr. Houk spoke about the inappropriateness of using such a model to judge dioxin's toxicity in humans:

> Many scientists now understand that loading an animal with a chemical for a lifetime, then counting tumors and feeding a mathematical extrapolation model does not necessarily predict the chemical's potential for causing cancer in humans. In the early days of risk assessment this modeling approach was the only game in town. It combined some animal data, statistics and mathematical extrapolation to evaluate what chemicals [have] a potential to produce a specific human health effect. This combination process in its many forms became the basis for science policy. *Scientists now understand that the laboratory rodent is not a small human* [emphasis added].[22]

Further, scientists have found a new, more accurate way to evaluate and classify the information gleaned from animal testing. Specifically, researchers have a more thorough understanding of how tumors develop when animals are fed extremely high levels of a chemical. When the original 1978 liver tumor samples were reevaluated with the new criteria developed from this clearer understanding, scientists were astounded to realize that tumors occurred only when the rats were fed doses large enough to kill cells. This caused surviving cells to divide rapidly, in an effort to replace those cells that had not survived. Such hasty cell division can ultimately result in cancer.[23]

Scientists discovered one additional crucial fact. For dioxin to even become poisonous, it must be given in a dose sufficiently large to activate certain body chemicals, called receptors. Below that critical dose, dioxin cannot possibly exert the toxic effect that leads to rapid cell division. There is absolutely no risk unless that critical dose is reached or exceeded.

Insight magazine confirms that the downgrading of dioxin's toxicity "isn't just one guy's opinion. The body of scientific knowledge on dioxin has exploded in the past 10 years. In the U.S. alone, more than $400 million in federal funds has been spent on research since the Times Beach panic. Among the research have been three major studies of people exposed to the chemical. Each has shown it to be harmless at low and moderate doses. The most recent study, done for the National Institute for Occupational Safety and Health, looked at the health records of 5,172 workers in chemical factories where there were dioxin wastes. Advocates of the dioxin-is-dangerous theory expected that the study would show an inordinate number of stomach, liver and nasal cancers, as well as high rates of Hodgkin's disease and non-Hodgkin's lymphoma. But there was no higher incidence of such diseases."[24]

In an unprecedented action, EPA Administrator William K. Reilly set the regulatory works in action in April 1991. He ordered a re-evaluation of the risks of dioxin exposure. He and other scientists have openly acknowledged the changing situation and have voiced their regrets about how dioxin issues have been handled in the past:

> We're public health officials. When something is worse than we thought, we seem to be able to move very rapidly at gathering the data and making the decision to restrict its use. When something is not as bad as we thought it was, I think it's fair to bring that issue forward too.
> Vernon N. Houk, M.D., Assistant Surgeon General

> In summary, the recent [pathology working group] review of the female rat livers from the Kociba dioxin study indicate a weak tumor response, even following lifetime administration of the compound at toxic levels. The implications of this finding go beyond the mere changes in tumor incidence and the impact of this change on EPA's current risk assessment procedures. The contribution of cell proliferation, which would be expected only at toxic levels, and the comparatively high susceptibility of rats to liver tumor development, also indicate that overly conservative assumptions of human cancer

risk, such as those inherent in EPA's present potency factor, are not war-ranted. *Based upon all of the biological evidence, I do not believe that dioxin poses a cancer risk to humans at any anticipated levels of exposure.*[25]

Robert Squire, D.V.M., Ph.D., Dioxin Pathology Working Group

It's interesting to note how "ABC News" dealt with the news of an updated risk assessment on dioxin in their April 9, 1988 show.[26] They reported that "the new EPA assessment says dioxin is still a dangerous carcinogen, but that it is much safer than once thought." The interviewer then asked Dr. Marvin Schneiderman of the National Academy of Sciences if he had seen the new data. Appropriately, the doctor said he hadn't and added that the new assessment came from a new way of looking at the old data. Dr. Ellen Silbergeld of the Environmental Defense Fund jumped up and said that there simply wasn't any new data, commenting: "Where is the beef in this argument? It doesn't seem to be there." After allowing this tone to be set, the interviewer then explained that risk assessments are based on complex mathematical computer models, saying that "EPA admits its dioxin reassessment was based on a new computer model, not new animal or human data. But critics say dioxin is too dangerous to play number games with." Was the implication that the EPA was trying to hide the fact that they had reanalyzed old data with new, state-of-the-art knowledge?

The downgrading of dioxin's potential toxicity finally hit major news sources accurately in August 1991 when the *New York Times* reported:

In a rare official reassessment, several top Federal health authorities are back-ing away from the position that the chemical compound dioxin is toxic enemy No. 1. Exposure to the chemical, once thought to be much more hazardous than chain smoking, is now considered by some experts to be no more risky than spending a week sunbathing.[27]

EPA Administrator William K. Reilly, in announcing the EPA's review of dioxin's risk said,

I know the stakes and that I'm unraveling something here. There isn't much precedence in the Federal establishment for pulling back from a judgment of toxicity. But we need to be prepared to adjust, to raise or lower standards, as new science becomes available.[28]

The dioxin reappraisal has been fraught with political problems. The Banbury Conference on dioxin, co-sponsored by the Chlorine Institute and the Environ-mental Protection Agency was accused of being a "public relations exercise"[29] for the Chlorine Institute, an industry-backed group. George L. Carlo, Ph.D., chairman of Washington, D.C.'s Health and Environmental Sciences Group, Ltd., addressed the poor reporting and false accusations.[30]

It is neither justifiable nor realistic to assume that the U.S. Environmental Protection Agency, which co-sponsored the conference, is in the habit of paying for the outreach activities of trade associations. Had you seriously considered the published Banbury proceedings, you would have noticed that the chairmen of the conference considered it to be an important and necessary gathering, giving in the preface to the proceedings the rationale that "much of the new biological work and its implications for human health risk [has] yet to make its way into the regulatory arena and, in particular, into quantitative risk assessment." To suggest that the Banbury conference was a manipulation in view of the powerful science considered and the high caliber of the participants is both naive and an insult to all those involved.

Dr. Carlo further commented about the effect of irresponsible reporting of issues:

Irresponsible reporting such as yours is hindering the ability of our government to make important regulatory decisions based on science rather than hysteria. The reevaluation of the EPA dioxin risk assessment is a step in the right direction; reviewing new scientific evidence in rule-making should be termed desirable rather than "unusual." At worst, your article is an irresponsible manipulation of scientists and scientific fact, aimed at perpetuating fear and uncertainty. With an issue as important as dioxin, the American public deserves better. In trying to hang on to dioxin's heinous reputation, some people are focusing on possible immunotoxic effects, looking for evidence that it may increase the incidence and severity of infectious diseases and/ or precipitate or exacerbate the development of allergic and autoimmune diseases. The bottom line is that the jury is still out—and that dioxin's opponents are grasping at straws.

Human Evidence Also Clears Dioxin

Extensive human studies also confirm that dioxin doesn't pose much of a human health threat. High-dose exposure can cause chloracne; however, there is no convincing evidence that dioxin causes any type of disease, adverse pregnancy outcome, or premature mortality. There is a small, increased risk for cancer at very high exposures. Specifically, when blood levels of dioxin exceed six hundred times the recognized background level, there is a very small (approximately one-and-one-half times) increased risk for all forms of cancer combined. Note, however, that such cancers occur only after a minimum of twenty years of exposure. To put this in perspective, consider that smokers are ten times more likely to get lung cancer than are nonsmokers.[30]

Let's review the information available from industrial accidents resulting in dioxin exposure.

SEVESO, ITALY

One of the most publicized chemical accidents in recent years gives us considerable assurance that dioxin is not the health villain the press makes it out to be. On July 10, 1976, in Seveso, Italy, a chemical-reaction chamber exploded at the ICMESA chemical company. A section of the densely populated Seveso community was contaminated by an estimated one to four pounds of dioxin, which was produced during the manufacture of the antibacterial hexachlorophene.

Plants, birds, rabbits, and chickens died soon after the accident. When exposed children and adults complained of nausea, nervous symptoms, and chloracne, local authorities evacuated some five thousand persons from the contaminated area.

An extensive health-surveillance system was activated to study the short- and long-term effects of dioxin exposure. Medical examinations and laboratory tests were performed, pregnant women were closely monitored to record miscarriages and birth defects, and a cancer registry was created to track any new cases of cancer among exposed individuals.

A thorough analysis, conducted by the Instituto Scientifico per lo Studio e la Cura dei Tumori in Genova, Italy, showed that Seveso residents developed chloracne and minor, temporary nerve damage. Some studies uncovered early effects on liver function tests and blood lipids, both of which are insignificant. No other organs or body functions were found to be affected despite the fact that the Seveso population was enveloped by a cloud containing a few pounds of "the most toxic chemical known to man." Having claimed in "The Politics of Poison" that one ounce of dioxin could kill one million people, the staff at KRON-TV might be somewhat interested in this fact. Importantly, there was no increase in the number of miscarriages, birth defects, or infant deaths that could be linked to dioxin, although researchers noted a slight decrease in the overall fertility in the years following the accident. The study period was not long enough to uncover any cases of cancer related to the accident.

Contrast the facts about Seveso with the account rendered by John G. Fuller in his ludicrous book *The Poison That Fell from the Sky*. On the inside cover we read of the residents of the town whose

> children have sickened with a disfiguring and life-threatening disease; old people have died and autopsies have revealed that the chemical fatally attacked them; pregnant women have borne birth-defected babies. . . . At first these symptoms were limited to "Zone A," the area closest to the contamination. Soon there were signs that the residents of "Zone B" were affected; the contamination is apparently still spreading. . . .[32]

On what does Mr. Fuller base these claims? He is not a doctor, public health specialist, epidemiologist, chemist, or any other type of scientist. For if he was, he would certainly be wise enough to consider the work and opinions of his peers. It is clear that this man does not believe in the work of the medical and scientific communities. And if he did take the time to read the literature, he simply ignored it.

Rather than study the incident, Mr. Fuller chose to rush to the scene and churn out a bestseller while the story was still hot. One can only wonder about the hypocrisy involved when someone promotes fear and doom by inaccurate, profit-generating reporting while criticizing the "giant corporate profiteers" who produce the hazardous chemicals as a byproduct of their operations.

At least Thomas Whiteside waited a few years before publishing *The Pendulum and the Toxic Cloud,* also with a strong doomsday theme. The author does acknowledge, however, that the episode at Seveso did not result in the kind of human suffering predicted by Fuller. But Whiteside drops the credibility ball when he says that this lack of suffering is actually an omen that the worst is yet to come.

> In view of the mounting evidence . . . of the potential dangers of dioxin to people, the relatively light scattering of ill-effects so far manifested among the Seveso population tends to illustrate not the lack of dioxin's toxicity to humans, but the mysterious—one might say devilishly capricious—manner in which it can strike and how little is as yet understood about this substance.[33]

In other words, the disaster has not occurred—yet. They want a disaster, and they will wait for it if necessary rather than admit the errors of their prophecies.

MONSANTO PLANT ACCIDENT

In 1949, 288 employees of the Monsanto chemical firm were exposed to dioxin in a plant accident, and 122 of them developed the classic symptom of dioxin exposure, chloracne. Studies over the next thirty-four years on the exposed group of workers did not, however, detect any increased rates of cancer, birth defects, or mortality in general. Nervous disorders were reported in some of the men just after exposure, but, as in Seveso, these subsided without any lasting effect.

The Monsanto accident provided medical researchers with perhaps the only sample on which an assessment can be made of the long-term effects of dioxin among people exposed to a level of the chemical sufficient to cause acute symptoms such as chloracne. The absence of increased rates of chronic diseases such as cancer in the group affected ought to be quite reassuring to residents of areas like Times Beach, Missouri, and the Love Canal in New York, as environmental trace levels of dioxin there were many magnitudes less than the level of exposure in the Monsanto plant.

DIOXIN AND SOFT TISSUE SARCOMA

Studies conducted in Sweden in 1977 on heavily exposed lumberjacks suggested a relationship between phenoxy herbicides and chlorophenols on the one hand and a very rare form of cancer on the other, a cancer called soft-tissue sarcoma (STS). Similarly, in 1983, the United States National Institute of Occupational Safety and Health (NIOSH) published the results of its study of mortality patterns of over four thousand workers who manufactured these products at a number of occupational sites. The individuals involved in the sample population had all been exposed to the dioxin-containing products for ten to twenty years, and some showed evidence of chloracne. NIOSH reported five cases of STS, which statistically amounts to twenty-one times the expected number of cases.

While a twenty-one-fold increase sounds substantial enough to merit the description epidemic, a closer look at the facts leads to a more cautious approach. Although the significance of five cases of STS should not be minimized or disregarded and data do indeed suggest the need for intensive follow-up studies, one must remember that in dealing with such a rare disease as soft-tissue sarcoma, it is statistically easy to achieve a twenty-one-fold increase with just a few cases—in this case, just five.

Other studies have failed, however, to uncover the STS/dioxin link. A 1982 New Zealand investigation focusing on 102 STS patients recorded in their cancer registry between 1976 and 1980 found "no excess for the occupational group involving agriculture and forestry, in spite of the fact that phenoxy herbicides have been used extensively for many years in New Zealand."[34]

Whether or not the dioxin-herbicide-STS cancer link is established, two points are relevant here in evaluating the scaremonger approach to dioxin and the herbicide 2,4,5-T. First, even if the link between STS and occupational exposure were confirmed in later years, the finding would have no bearing on the allegations of myriad other complaints, including miscarriage, being presented by those who maintain that America is being poisoned by dioxin and agricultural chemicals. Second, if the causal link were made for those occupationally exposed to high doses of dioxin-containing herbicides over many years, this circumstance would bear little relevance to those of us who might occasionally be exposed to trace amounts in the general environment.

Times Beach—Health Hazard or Political Panic?

> There are two dangers in toxic wastes. One is the very real threat to health posed by the chemicals themselves. The second is that a hysterical exaggeration of that threat will needlessly frighten people and drive them from their homes.[35]

That quote, taken from the *Wall Street Journal,* was written in the days following the EPA decision to evacuate Times Beach, Missouri. In the mid-1970s, thousands of gallons of waste oil were sprayed on a horse arena and on unpaved roads in the Times Beach, Missouri, area to reduce dust. After horses and other animals in the immediate spraying area died, investigations pointed to dioxin, subsequently found to be a contaminent of the waste oil, as the culprit. The issue, however, lay dormant until December 1982, when flood waters spread the dioxin throughout the small town.

Federal officials were catapulted onto center stage by a critical, environmentally aware public who demanded an expedient remedy to assuage their fears. Soil levels measured a hundred to a thousand times what, at the time, was thought the safe limit of dioxin ingestion. An evacuation was impulsively ordered, at a cost of $33 million. The government's sense of urgency, coupled with research showing dioxin to be very carcinogenic in certain laboratory animals, was the stuff of which headline news is made.

In 1991, the suspicion of exaggerated health risk became a reality. Dr. Vernon Houk, the federal official who ordered the evacuation, said in retrospect:

> Given what we know about this chemical's toxicity and its effects on human health, it looks as though the evacuation was unnecessary.[36]

A closer look at the facts at the time of the evacuation suggests that *despite high soil-dioxin levels, human health was not in jeopardy.* Unequivocally, soil-dioxin levels were high but scientists knew that dioxin binds tightly to soil, a characteristic that made human exposure very unlikely. A *Science* article at the time affirmed this, saying that dioxin "when bound to soil does not pose much of a hazard."[37]

At the time of the evacuation, the Missouri director of health acknowledged that health surveys didn't reveal any problem: "We've seen nothing to alarm us or to make us believe Missourians are feeling acute health effects."[38] In fact, research through 1991 failed to turn up evidence that human health was or has been harmed as a result of high soil-dioxin levels in Times Beach. There weren't even cases of chloracne, a reversible skin condition nearly always associated with significant dioxin exposure.

Again, we stress that the buy-out was based solely on soil analysis. There was not one iota of scientific evidence to raise concern that human health was in jeopardy.[39]

In a related incident, residents of Quail Run Mobile Home Park in Gray Summit, Missouri, were exposed to dioxin after roads were sprayed with dioxin-contaminated waste oil. The exposed residents were compared to residents from three trailer parks without detectable dioxin. The first study was reported in April 1986; it showed no significant differences in the medical conditions between the two groups but did find limited laboratory evidence of immune system depression.[40] Another study conducted two years later failed to produce the same results. Researchers are fairly certain that these results *do not* mean exposed residents recovered; rather, they feel the second study *more accurately reflects the true situation.* The second study was conducted with better controls and consistent testing and reading methods.[41]

While this is good news, it is interesting to note that the results of the first study were highly publicized, first in the widely read *Journal of the American Medical Association,* and subsequently by the *New York Times* and other popular presses. The follow-up study, self-admittedly more accurate, however, was published in the highly regarded, but quite limitedly distributed, *Archives of Environmental Health.* Was the public apprised of the real situation? Quite typically, no.

In June 1983, shortly after the Times Beach buy-out, the American Medical Association (AMA) publicized its concern about the inappropriate media blitz. Believing there was no evidence of health threat, the AMA passed a resolution at its convention, voting to "adopt an active public information campaign . . . to prevent irrational reaction and unjustified public fright and to prevent the dissemination of possible erroneous information about the health hazards of dioxin."[42] But this consensus was never picked up by the press! This carefully researched and prepared statement fell on deaf ears.

Times Beach, like Love Canal, is an environmental problem turned into an environmental fiasco. Decisions and subsequent actions were based on political motivations and not on public health realities. The reality was that (a) dioxin was present, and (b) the public was not being exposed to health-threatening levels of dioxin. We are left with a tremendous sense of frustration and bewilderment over how an agency presumably equipped to deal responsibly with these kinds of problems can be backed into a hasty, panic-stricken approach to solving them.

Retrospectively, Dr. Houk regrets this decision to evacuate, saying,

> Times Beach was an over-reaction. It was based on the best scientific information we had at the time. It turns out we were in error. . . . The only thing I would have done differently, I would have said we may be wrong. If we're going to be wrong, we'll be wrong on the side of protecting human health. I don't think we ever said we may be wrong.[43]

A *Wall Street Journal* editorial from 1983, the time of the buy-out, accurately sums up the feeling of many Americans even today:

> We'd like to be able to read in a newpaper some day that EPA has gone out and cleaned up a toxic hazard problem without its having been turned into a political circus. When that happens we will mark another milestone on the road to political maturity.[44]

The federal government has already spent $138 million at Times Beach, and $400 million simply studying dioxin. Further costs to strip Times Beach of dioxin are estimated at $118 million. Although the last $118 million are not federal dollars, it will ultimately come out of every consumer's pocket as the private industries who foot the bill pass their costs on to consumers. Unfortunately, it may be too late to save this money. Can officials simply take down the signs declaring Times Beach a hazard and say, "life as usual"? The past handling of Times Beach—branding it a toxic waste site—may unfortunately demand present and future remediation.

Agent Orange Is a Red Herring

The ingredients were unique: equal measures of chemical phobia, anecdotal accounts of human tragedy, guilt about the Vietnam War, and the inevitable media hype. Also unprecedented was the yield: $180 million in compensation for thousands of veterans who asserted that the herbicide Agent Orange harmed them and their families. But the background leading to that out-of-court settlement had an underlying taste that was distinctly familiar: the distortion of science to indict and convict an environmental factor as a cause of disease and death, couched in that emerging doctrine "Unless you prove otherwise, my bad luck is your fault."

During the Vietnam War, a number of herbicides were used by Americans to clear the vegetation that provided cover for the enemy. The use of herbicides is widely credited with saving the lives of thousands of American soldiers. The herbicides were also designed to destroy enemy food crops. The herbicides were stored in color-coded drums, from which their names were derived: they included Agent Orange, Orange 2, Purple, Pink, Green, White, and Blue.

Agent Orange was the military code name for a fifty-fifty mixture of the herbicides 2,4,5-T, and 2,4-D, used during the Vietnam War, from 1963 to 1971.[45] These herbicides had been used singly and in combination throughout the world since 1949 with no apparent deleterious human effects. Thus, these were not new chemicals developed specifically for use in Vietnam, although the manner in which they were employed in the war differed from the domestic agricultural use that had primarily been for highway weed control, forest management, and agricultural and residential landscaping.

Although scientists knew that 2,4,5-T was contaminated with dioxin when the spraying began in 1966, all parties concerned accepted the prevailing scientific opinion that trace amounts of dioxin in the herbicide did not represent a health hazard.

In 1969, however, scientists reported a high rate of birth defects in experimental animals exposed to 2,4,5-T and 2,4-D. On that basis alone, in 1972 the U.S. Department of Defense canceled all uses of herbicides in South Vietnam.

The current Agent Orange saga began on the note pad of a claims counselor, Maude de Victor, in the Veterans Administration's Chicago office. As she puts it, "It all started when I picked up the phone and a sobbing woman told me her husband was dying. He had served in Nam and was convinced that his cancer had been caused by chemicals sprayed there." De Victor began keeping track of other vets who called to tell her their woes, ranging from liver disorders to miscarriages suffered by their wives. When she thought her "data collection" was complete, she approached a CBS televison station in Chicago, and in March 1978 the document "Agent Orange: Vietnam's Deadly Fog," a collection of horror stories about "those chemicals," was aired. The program not only won an Emmy, but also generated an enormous amount of fear and anger among veterans. In July of that year, ABC's "20/20" picked up where the Chicago show left off, with another set of segments on devastating terminal illnesses among vets. The crucifixion of Agent Orange had begun—not on the basis of scientific studies, but as a result of anecdotal hearsay.

Not surprisingly, there was an immediate increase in complaints at VA offices around the country. Veterans were now convinced that the defoliants used during the war were responsible for everything that ailed them. In September 1978 Paul Reutershan, a Vietnam vet dying from liver cancer, filed a $10 million federal suit, claiming that his disease was the result of exposure to Agent Orange. Some months later lawyer Victor Yannacone, Jr., filed a new suit as a class action, saying forty thousand veterans and their families may have been involved. Five chemical companies—Dow, Monsanto, Hercules, Diamond Shamrock, and Thompson-Hayward—were the targets of the suit on behalf of "all American servicemen whose health has been damaged because of contact with Agent Orange."

Just after the class-action suit was filed, new headlines about the domestic use of the herbicide 2,4,5-T gave momentum to the veterans' legal push against Agent Orange. Domestically, the Alsea studies claiming increased 2,4,5-T-related miscarriages were released in 1979, lending momentum to the veteran's legal push against Agent Orange. The Alsea women joined ranks with the veterans, both now the media's folk heroes.

A LAWSUIT SETTLED WITHOUT COMPELLING EVIDENCE

The highly publicized Agent Orange trial was scheduled to begin on May 7, 1984. There was little evidence at that point that exposure to Agent Orange in Vietnam was the cause of cancer, birth defects, or liver disorders. Incidence studies simply hadn't been done.

Perhaps the most significant studies completed at that time as a means of testing the legitimacy of claims made by some veterans were the two so-called Ranch Hand investigations, named after the air force spraying team that applied Agent Orange during the war. The twelve hundred or so men who flew the planes and sprayed the herbicide were those most heavily exposed, handling large amounts of it, frequently reporting accumulations of Agent Orange on their clothing. If Agent Orange is indeed the silent killer, then these highly exposed teams would certainly be affected first and most severely.

Neither study could find statistically significant differences in health status between those veterans who worked daily with Agent Orange in Vietnam and those veterans who did not. There was nothing, then, to substantiate claims that cancer, birth defects, and other chronic illnesses were caused by exposure to the defoliant.

As we discussed earlier, neither was there other evidence that high-level dioxin exposure caused human illness. The accidents at Seveso, Italy, and Monsanto's West Virginia plants only resulted in chloracne and temporary nerve disorders.

Bruce E. Herbert, deputy director of the Center for International Security, summed up the state of our knowledge about Agent Orange and health in 1983:

> After nearly five years of almost constant publicity, as of March 1, 1983 only 16,821 veterans have even filed claims with the VA for suspected Agent Orange damage. Of this number less than 8,400 present any certifiable medical condition, whether or not these disabilities can ever scientifically be linked to exposure. Three thousandths of one percent of the 2.4 million men who could have been exposed to Agent Orange in Vietnam is hardly a compelling statistic on which to make assumptions about "unusually large numbers" of veterans suffering latent Agent Orange–induced health impairments.[46]

As the trial began, Judge Jack B. Weinstein bluntly warned both sides about the problems they faced in the impending trial. He told the chemical company and insurance lawyers that they were taking a major risk by entering the courtroom, even though they were scientifically correct in their argument that Agent Orange has never been shown to be a health hazard. Faced with a Brooklyn jury that was certain to be sympathetic to the veterans, the odds were stacked against the chemical companies. On the other hand, the judge warned the veterans' lawyers that their case was a hodgepodge of flaws and inconsistencies, and that ultimately the claims of the veterans would never hold up in an appeals court. Thus the $180 million out-of-court settlement—all of which will ultimately be paid for by the American consumer in higher costs of goods and services, logically passed on by the corporations that settled. As S. Maynard Turk, vice president and general counsel of Hercules, put it,

> Who ultimately pays for this litigation, settlement costs and all? Sad but true— you do. It's the public who pays. . . . All business costs must be passed on in the price of the company's products. A company has two choices: (1) pass on the costs or (2) if it isn't able to pass them on, go out of business. In either case, the public pays the higher cost of lost jobs.

THE EVIDENCE FINALLY COMES IN

Later studies found no evidence that dioxin was responsible for the myriad health complaints reported by Vietnam veterans. The first was the Vietnam Experience Study (VES) ordered by Congress and conducted by the Centers for Disease Control. Approximately nine thousand men who served in Vietnam were compared to an equal number of men who had military service elsewhere. There were four components to the VES study: mortality assessment, telephone interview, medical and psychological examination, and a reproductive outcome assessment. Exposure to dioxin was also assessed.

Results of earlier studies suggested that current blood dioxin levels provide a reasonable reflection of heavy exposures to dioxin fifteen to twenty years past. Using this method, this study found that most U.S. Army ground troops who served in Vietnam were not heavily exposed to dioxin, except perhaps men whose jobs involved handling herbicides. In particular, only 4 percent of the veterans studied had dioxin levels above 8 ppt (parts per trillion).[47]

During the first five years after discharge, the Vietnam group had 45 percent more deaths, largely due to external causes (motor vehicle injuries, homicides, suicides), but thereafter death rates for the two groups were equal.[48]

Although Vietnam veterans reported far more health problems, impaired fertility, and health problems among their children than did other veterans, medical examinations revealed but two minor objective differences in physical health between the two groups. The Vietnam veterans had more hearing loss and had lower sperm concentrations and lower mean proportions of morphologically "normal" sperm cells. Despite these differences in sperm characteristics, however, Vietnam and non-Vietnam veterans have fathered similar numbers of children.[49] The American Cancer Society agrees that birth defects among offspring of Vietnam veterans are probably not caused by exposure to Agent Orange.[50]

Cancer incidence studies revealed no increased risk for five types of cancer: soft tissue and other sarcomas; Hodgkin's disease; nasal, nasopharyngeal, and primary liver cancer. There was an increase in non–Hodgkin's lymphoma for all veterans who had served in Vietnam, but it was highest for navy men who had served far away from areas where Agent Orange was used. In fact, veterans who had served in the region of heaviest Agent Orange use tended to be at lowest risk for non–Hodgkin's lymphoma. There was no evidence, then, that increased risk of non–Hodgkin's lymphoma was related to exposure to Agent Orange in Vietnam.[51]

After researchers at the National Cancer Institute found an increase in testicular tumors in military working dogs who had served in Vietnam, they initiated another study to see if humans were similarly affected. While this 1990 study showed a twofold increased risk of testicular cancer in Vietnam veterans, researchers could not identify specific factors, such as exposure to Agent Orange, as causing this increase. Research continues on this matter.[52]

Although Vietnam veterans reported more adverse reproductive and child health outcomes than did non-Vietnam veterans, medical records revealed equal rates of total, major, minor, and suspected defects among children from both groups of veterans.[53]

THE IMPACT OF THE MISUSE OF SCIENCE

Consider the Vietnam veteran who has been reading about the toxic time bomb that supposedly ticks within him. Many of these men have had a hard time adjusting to American society in the aftermath of our country's most unpopular war. Many others have suffered from the infirmities described—cancer, birth defects, and other health defects, which, as we have stressed, occur in all segments of the human population. A disturbed or sick veteran is going to find it very easy to believe the words of a Barry Commoner or other "expert" who writes of the toxicological time bomb wreaking havoc on the veterans and their families. And they are likely to step forward to detail their misery. These are the kinds of conditions from which big headline controversies are made.

Agent Orange has left its stamp on the lives of many Vietnam veterans, their families, and friends. But the evidence increasingly points to the imprint as being created more by an army of emotional extremists, the professional scaremongers and their media friends, than by the armed forces of the United States. And our society as a whole has been swept up in the wind of the movement, as described by Dr. Archie B. Blackburn: "It may be more acceptable for us, our society, and our leadership to believe that Agent Orange has damaged our youth, rather than to recognize and deal with the logical consequences of warfare."[54]

Dioxin in the Paper and Pulp Industry:
How Much Money Should We Spend to Reduce a Non-Hazard?

A 1985 EPA study discovered dioxin in the discharges and sludge around the 104 paper and pulp mills producing bleached paper (of a total 600 pulp and paper mills in the United States). This finding was perplexing, as dioxin is not used in any processing steps. An investigation revealed that dioxin is a byproduct of bleaching paper; dioxin is not released from those mills that do not bleach with chlorine.

Despite immediate action on the part of the paper industry to reduce dioxin levels, the Environmental Defense Fund (EDF) and the National Wildlife Federation (NWF) sued the EPA in 1988 for not adequately protecting the public from the risks of dioxin. The consent decree reached between the EPA, the EDF, and the NWF specified that the EPA must study the health risks of dioxin and take regulatory action to reduce human exposure.[55]

Although the FDA and the Consumer Product Safety Commission (CPSC) were not parties to the consent decree, they had worked closely with the EPA under their respective jurisdictions conducting risk assessments for paper products. The three agencies have raised the following issues in regards to dioxin in paper products:

1. Pulp and paper mills effluent: Those industries that use bleach release some dioxin in their discharges. Concern was raised that those people living one to two miles downstream from sixty-six of the plants and who ingest significant quantities of fish caught there might be at increased risk from dioxin exposure;[56]

2. Pulp and paper sludge: Some of this sludge is used as compost on cropland. The EPA estimates that less than 5 percent of the 2.5 million metric tons of sludge produced each year by paper and pulp mills is used on farmland, and almost all of it in areas near the mills.

3. Food contact papers: Paper milk cartons and other food-packaging materials can be made from bleached paper products. Trace amounts of dioxin can be measured in such products.[57]

4. Personal paper products under the jurisdiction of CPSC, such as disposable diapers, paper towels, tissues, and dinner napkins, may contain negligible amounts of dioxin.

In response to the effluent issue, the EPA required all mills to obtain permits to release any dioxin in effluent, at any level, by 1993; to obtain the permit, the mill would have to reduce levels to those the government deems safe. By 1995, all mills would have to eliminate dioxin levels in their discharge to zero.[58] Such practices will also reduce the amount of dioxin contained in the sludge.

Dioxin was discovered in milk in 1989, migrating from chlorine-bleached paper milk cartons at levels below one part per trillion (ppt). Although the FDA said that this level did not pose a threat to human health, the American Paper Institute responded by changing their processes to eliminate even this small amount. By the end of 1989, 75 percent of the involved industry had changed over to the new process that reduced dioxin migration to 0.4 ppt, a level indistinguishable from background levels.[59] Nearly all of the remaining mills producing paper milk cartons changed over by the end of 1990. The FDA appropriately assured the American public that milk with even 2 or 3 ppt was safe to drink. The risk, then, is at most negligible at the current 0.4 ppt. Further reductions could cost each company within this industry $20 million to comply.[60]

Greenpeace, however, said that dioxin levels are still not low enough and advocates use of unbleached cartons. They claim that a kindergartner who drinks only one half-pint carton of milk daily (containing 2 ppt dioxin) drinks seventy-eight times the quantity of dioxin estimated to result in a lifetime cancer risk of one in one million. Their estimate, however, assumes a person will ingest that much dioxin in food every day for seventy years, which is highly unlikely.[61]

The Consumer Product Safety Commission concluded that the risk posed by dioxin from the personal paper products under their jurisdiction is negligible and recommended no regulatory action be taken.[62]

Let's put all of this into perspective. To be exact, the amount of dioxin produced by the entire U.S. paper industry is small, less than twenty ounces a year. That contribution represents about 1 percent of the total U.S. releases of dioxin to the environment from all sources.[63] Since the initial 1985 discovery of dioxin in the paper industry, that industry's quick response reduced dioxin in the effluent by 37 percent and in sludge by 38 percent. But at what cost?

Red Cavaney, president of the American Paper Institute, Inc., describes what are most likely unnecessary expenditures:

> Tremendous amounts of public resources, and many hundreds of millions of dollars of private resources, are now being devoted to reducing trace levels of dioxin in paper products and in paper mill effluent and sludge—in many cases down to the parts per quadrillion. In addition, millions of dollars of public and private resources are spent addressing trace levels of dioxin at Superfund sites.[64]

Even the EPA, which has perpetuated this chain of unnecessary action, said at the outset:

Even though dioxin levels in paper products are small enough to be no cause
for alarm, our intention is to reduce these levels even more.[65]

Regulating Dioxin: Interagency Schizophrenia

U.S. regulatory agencies do not agree about the potency of dioxin and suggest
that different safety levels and factors be applied in the various regulatory
processes. The EPA rates dioxin as ten times more potent than does the FDA,
and the Centers for Disease Control (CDC) has yet another analysis of dioxin's
potency. Based on that one lone rat study back in 1978 and the subsequent
mathematical extrapolation, the EPA set the daily intake that produced a cancer
risk of one in a million as 0.006 picogram/kilogram (pg/kg); the CDC at
0.0288 pg/kg; and the FDA at 0.057 pg/kg. Interestingly, other countries used
these same data and set daily acceptable exposures (for a one in a million
risk of cancer) to between twenty and nearly two hundred times higher than
that of the U.S. agencies. Great Britain has set this standard at 10 pg/kg;
Denmark at 5 pg/kg; and Canada at 10 pg/kg.[66]

Distressingly, no one has incorporated, nay even acknowledged, the latest
information from the World Health Organization, which has just completed
an extensive analysis of dioxin's toxicity.[67] In this latest report, WHO identified a no-effect level of 1,000 picograms/kilogram, equivalent to a dose of
100 picograms/kilogram/day. Because of insufficient data on human reproductive effects, they temporarily added a safety factor of ten, yielding a tolerable
daily intake of ten picograms/kilogram/day. They believe, however, that adverse
reproductive outcomes do not occur, and, when such evidence becomes definitive, will recommend a tolerable daily intake of 100 picograms/kilogram/day.

Not only do the agencies not agree, but they haven't yet incorporated
the new criteria for assessing rat-liver tumors. All regulatory action is being
taken based on the outdated risk assessments that regard dioxin as deadly.

Encouragingly, though, a conference on the biological basis for the risk
assessment of dioxin was held in October of 1990. The summary report of
this conference concludes with:

> Overall, the conference achieved its goal of incorporating the most recent
> biological information pertaining to dioxin and related compounds in an effort
> to move closer to a consensus dioxin risk assessment. The conference was
> a milestone in that it has the potential of moving dioxin risk assessment over
> the hurdle of the one-hit theory and the linearized multistage risk assessment
> model. Perhaps most notably, the results of the conference provide a scien-
> tifically sound basis for modifying, at least for dioxin, the U.S. policy position
> that one molecule is sufficient to cause cancer.[68]

One conference participant summarized the problem of moving beyond the old linearized risk model and the interagency disparity:

> A number of participants seemed to be committed to the linearized models, in spite of the apparent scientific consensus to the contrary. This was particularly true for the representatives of EPA and National Institute of Environmental Health & Safety. It is important to note that EPA appears to be isolated from both FDA and CDC with respect to this issue now. . . . [However] the [EPA] administrator might indeed be responsive to the political reality that they are out on a limb, isolated, with a policy which cannot be supported scientifically.[69]

Mr. Cavaney of the American Paper Institute capsulizes the need for a consistent federal government position:

> The need for a consistent federal government position that reflects the most recent science is particularly acute given the current efforts of a number of states to establish water quality standards for dioxin. Under the Clean Water Act, the states have primary responsibility for setting water quality standards, with approval or disapproval from EPA. Many states have concluded that EPA's present recommendation, which is based on EPA's 1985 potency factor for dioxin, is not appropriate. Several states, including Alabama, Maryland, and Virginia, have adopted water quality standards based on the current FDA potency factor (which is ten times less that of the EPA). EPA staff have indicated that the Agency may veto these state standards when they come before the Agency.[70]

Indeed, such was the case when Vernon N. Houk, M.D., assistant surgeon general and director, Center for Environmental Health and Injury Control at CDC, reviewed dioxin studies for the state of Georgia. Subsequent to his review of this information, Georgia adopted a new standard for acceptable levels of dioxin in drinking water, a standard more lenient than that recommended by the EPA. Dr. Houk was reprimanded for "improperly aiding the paper industry's campaign to loosen restriction of dioxin pollution in water" by a House of Representatives subcommittee.[71]

A Perspective: Why the Environmentalists Need Dioxin

Over the past decade, science has progressed at a remarkable pace. The federal government has invested incredible time and finances into trying to understand just how dangerous dioxin is, spending no less than $400 million toward that end.[72] The new findings, as reviewed above, carry enough potential clout to slash multi-million-dollar clean-up budgets across the country. In short: government and private scientists say, unhesitatingly, that they were wrong about dioxin's toxicity.

Why, then, aren't we moving forward to stop unnecessary expenditures related to dioxin?

Very simply, the environmentalists need dioxin. Dioxin isn't the only chemical regulated on the basis of animal studies; in fact, most are. That includes the nearly two hundred chemicals regulated by the outrageously expensive 1990 Clean Air Act. Many have been judged by the same animal-risk model that has been challenged by the recent action on dioxin. If EPA goes forward to regulate dioxin based on human studies—confirming that a mouse is not a little man—they are in effect challenging the basis of the regulation of many chemicals.[73]

It is no use blaming a chemical for the fact that children have been burnt and starved in Vietnam, or that an American community is, rightly, dissatisfied about the way in which commercial and agricultural and civic interest leads to spraying of insecticides and pesticides on citizens. These are more political than toxicological issues. But, it's probably too late to bring back 2,4,5-T, a pesticide incredibly useful for many purposes.

And it may be too late to save further expenditures at Times Beach, as reviewed earlier. We shouldn't, however, waste that $400 million (the figure *before* the EPA's reassessment began in 1991) the federal government has spent carefully studying dioxin. In the words of Dr. Houk: "That research has given us the science base for good scientific judgments. Now let us have the common sense to use it."

NOTES

1. E. Norris, ed., *Pills, Pesticides and Profits: The International Trade in Toxic Substances* (Croton-on-Hudson: North River Press, 1982), pp. 32–33.

2. S. Epstein et al., *Hazardous Waste in America* (San Francisco: Sierra Club Books, 1982), pp. 26, 140.

3. L. Regenstein, "Across America, Dioxin," *New York Times,* March 7, 1983.

4. *New York Times,* April 9, 1983.

5. *New York Times,* January 23, 1983.

6. M. H. Brown, *Toxic Cloud* (New York: Harper and Row, 1987), p. 21.

7. C. Glendinning, *When Technology Wounds* (New York: William Morrow and Co., 1990), p. 59.

8. J. Naar, *Design for a Livable Planet* (New York: Harper and Row, 1990), p. 13.

9. *Cancer Research* (October 1979).

10. J. Beck, "Have the Media Hyped the Danger of Dioxin?" *Chicago Tribune,*

June 30, 1983.

11. EPA press release, March 8, 1985.

12. Personal communication, Michael Newton, Ph.D., October 1990.

13. Personal communication, Ford Baldwin, Ph.D., October 1990.

14. J. M. Witt, "A Discussion of the Suspension of 2,4,5-T and the EPA Alsea II Study," *Northeastern Weed Science Society* (January 8, 1980).

15. Witt, "Suspension of 2,4,5-T Study."

16. American Medical Association, *Agent Orange and Dioxin* (1981), p. 24.

17. Ibid.

18. "A Plague on Our Children" (WGBH Educational Foundation, 1979).

19. "The Politics of Poison," (KRON-TV, 1979).

20. K. Napier, "Re-evaluating Dioxin's Toxicity: Implications for Science Policy," *Priorities* (Winter 1991).

21. R. A. Squire and J. H. Levitt, "Report of a Workshop on Classification of Specific Hepatocellular Lesions in Rats," *Cancer Research* 35 (1975): pp. 3214–24; letter from Robert A. Squire, D.V.M., Ph.D., to EPA Assistant Administrator LaJuana S. Wilcher, May 24, 1990, regarding need for reassessment of potency factor in light of new evidence, submitted in support of Georgia water-quality standard for dioxin.

22. V. N. Houk, "Dioxin Risk Assessment for Human Health: Scientifically Defensible or Fantasy?" Twenty-Fifth Annual Conference on Trace Substances in Environmental Health, University of Missouri, Columbia, Maryland, May 21, 1991.

23. Presentation by Dr. Dawn Goldman to Florida Department of Environmental Regulation, May 1, 1990; letter from Robert Squire to EPA assistant administrator, May 24, 1990.

24. "The Times Beach Fiasco," *Insight* (August 12, 1991).

25. Letter from Robert Squire to EPA assistant administrator, May 24, 1990.

26. ABC News, "The Health Show," number 57 (April 1988).

27. K. Schneider, "U.S. Backing Away from Saying Dioxin Is a Deadly Peril," *New York Times,* August 15, 1991.

28. Ibid.

29. Letter to the editor, *Wall Street Journal,* March 27, 1992.

30. Ibid.

31. Houk, "Dioxin Risk Assessment."

32. J. G. Fuller, *The Poison That Fell from the Sky* (New York: Random House, 1977), front and back flap.

33. T. Whiteside, *The Pendulum and the Toxic Cloud* (New York: Yale University Press, 1979), p. 133.

34. Smith et al., "Do Agricultural Chemicals Cause Soft Tissue Sarcoma? Initial Findings of a Case-Control Study in New Zealand, *Community Health Studies* 6: p. 114.

35. "The Dioxin Scare," *Wall Street Journal,* February 25, 1983.

36. Schneider, "U.S. Backing Away."

37. "Chlorinated Dioxins," *Science* (June 24, 1983).

38. M. Edgar, "Times Beach Residents Pass First Dioxin Tests," *St. Louis Globe-Democrat,* July 1, 1983.

39. Council for Agricultural Sciences and Technology, "The Missouri Dioxin

Controversy: Scientific Overview" (April 1983), p. 3.

40. P. M. Boffey, "Dioxin Link Cited in Abnormalities," *New York Times,* April 18, 1986.

41. R. G. Evans, K. B. Webb, A. P. Knutsen, et al., "A Medical Follow-up of the Health Effects of Long-term Exposure to 2,3,7,8-tetrachlorodibenzo-p-dioxin," *Archives of Environmental Health* 43 (1988): p. 278.

42. P. J. Hilts, "AMA Votes to Fight Dioxin 'Witch Hunt,'" *Washington Post,* June 23, 1983.

43. K. Schneider, "Times Beach Warning: Regrets a Decade Later," *New York Times,* August 15, 1991.

44. *Wall Street Journal,* editorial, February 25, 1983.

45. National Cancer Institute, Office of Cancer Communications, *In Answer to Your Questions about Agent Orange,* October 1991.

46. B. Herbert, "Agent Orange, A Media Myth," *Chicago Tribune,* March 31, 1983.

47. The Centers for Disease Control Veterans Health Studies, "Serum 2,3,7,8-Tetrachlorodibenzo-p-dioxin Levels in U.S. Army Vietnam Era Veterans," *Journal of the American Medical Association* 260 (1988): pp. 1249–54.

48. Centers for Disease Control, *Health Status of Vietnam Veterans,* vol. 1, *Synopsis* (January 1989).

49. Centers for Disease Control Vietnam Experience Study, "Health Status of Vietnam Veterans, Part II. Physical Health," *Journal of the American Medical Association* 259 (1988): pp. 2708–14.

50. American Cancer Society, Executive Notice #EN-52-R, "Dioxins, Furans, TCDD and Agent Orange," August 11, 1989.

51. Centers for Disease Control, "The Association of Selected Cancers with Service in the U.S. Military in Vietnam" (1990).

52. R. E. Tarone, H. M. Hayes, R. N. Hoover, J. F. Rosenthal, et al., "Service in Vietnam and Risk of Testicular Cancer," *Journal of the National Cancer Institute* 83 (1991): pp. 1497–99.

53. Centers for Disease Control Vietnam Experience Study, "Health Status of Vietnam Veterans, Part III, Reproductive Outcomes and Child Health," *Journal of the American Medical Association* 259 (1988): pp. 2715–19.

54. B. B. Blackburn, "Review of the Effects of Agent Orange: A Psychiatric Perspective on the Controversy," *Military Medicine* (April 1983), p. 339.

55. "EPA to Regulate Dioxin in Paper Industry," *EPA Environmental News* (April 30, 1990).

56. "EPA to Regulate Dioxin," *EPA Environmental News* (April 30, 1990).

57. C. B. Mackerron, "Dioxin and Milk Don't Mix," *Chemical Week* (September 20, 1989), p. 15.

58. "Eating Dioxin-tainted Fish May Cause Cancer, EPA Says," *CNI Nutrition Week* (September 27, 1990), p. 6.

59. FDA talkpaper, "Progress in Eliminating Dioxin from Packaging" (April 30, 1990).

60. P. Shabecoff, "Government Says Dioxin from Paper Mills Poses No Major Danger," *New York Times,* May 1, 1990.

61. Mackerron, "Dioxin and Milk Don't Mix."

62. Letter from Sadye E. Dunn, secretary of U.S. Consumer Product Safety Commission, to Charles L. Elkins, director, Office of Toxic Substances, EPA.

63. American Paper Institute news release, "U.S. Paper Industry Pledges Continued Dioxin Reductions," April 30, 1990.

64. Letter from Red Cavaney, president of the American Paper Institute, Inc., to Dr. D. Allen Bromley, director of the Office of Science and Technology Policy; William K. Reilly, administrator, Environmental Protection Agency; and James S. Benson, acting commissioner, Food and Drug Administration, June 14, 1990.

65. "EPA to Regulate Dioxin," *EPA Environmental News.*

66. Testimony of Vernon N. Houk, M.D., assistant surgeon general and director of the Center for Environmental Health and Injury Control, Centers for Disease Control, before the Subcommittee on Human Resources and Intergovernmental Relations, Committee on Governmental Operations, House of Representatives, July 26, 1990.

67. World Health Organization, Summary Report, "Consultation on Tolerable Daily Intake from Food of PCDDs and PCDFs," Bilthoven, Netherlands, December 4–7, 1990.

68. November 1, 1990 letter from the Health and Environmental Science Group to Dr. Robert Smerko of the Chlorine Institute.

69. Ibid.

70. Letter from Red Cavenay to Dr. D. Allen Bromley, William K. Reilly, and James S. Benson.

71. K. Schneider, "Scientist Criticized for Stand on Relaxing of Dioxin Limits," *New York Times,* July 27, 1990.

72. Houk, "Dioxin Risk Assessment."

73. "America's Most Deadly? EPA Takes Another Look," *Politics of the Environment* 2, no. 3 (1991).

10

Air Pollution:
Is It Safe to Breathe in America?

It is still better to be a nonsmoker in Paris than to smoke 40 cigarettes a day in the mountain pastures of Lozere.
>   —Lucien Israel, M.D., *Conquering Cancer*

The Charges

We now know that air pollution is probably killing literally hundreds of thousands of Americans each year. . . .

Air pollution remains a serious problem, a major aspect of [it] being the presence of dozens of chemicals and other pollutants known to cause cancer, disability and death. The presence of just one of these substances—sulfates—is estimated to cause some 200,000 deaths a year among adult whites.
>   —*America the Poisoned*[1]

While Chrysler competes with Buick for the getaway, cancer competes with emphysema for the layaway.
>   —Robert Rienow, *Peter's Quotations: Ideas for Our Times*[2]

Take a deep breath. Hold it in for a moment. The odds are that what you have just inhaled is polluted. In Chicago, Denver, Los Angeles, Washington, D.C., New York, Boston or virtually any urban area you live in, the air you take in every five seconds almost certainly does not meet federal standards. . . . Now you can let it out!
>   —*Design for a Livable Planet*[3]

A first national survey of industrial air pollution, issued by the EPA in 1989 reported that an estimated 2.4 billion pounds of chemicals believed to cause cancer, neurological disease, or birth defects were emitted into the air in 1987.

—Design for a Livable Planet[4]

But now it is time to cast attention onto the less visible, more exotic threat of airborne toxic chemicals, the same kind that were found in the soil at places such as Love Canal. Unnoticed, they are wafting from our factories, our storage tanks, our incinerators and diesel engines—even from the neighborhood dry cleaner. And they are spreading through our global village like a toxic cloud.

—The Toxic Cloud[5]

The Facts

- When the air is heavily polluted, human health suffers. Specific air-pollution episodes have confirmed that pollution can increase respiratory distress and in some cases cause premature death.

- There is no such thing as pure air. Our air always has had, and will always have, some contaminants from both natural and man-made sources. The question then is: How pure do we want our air, and how much are we willing to pay for that?

- There is no evidence whatsoever that air pollution is a major cause of death or disease in the United States today.

- There is ample evidence that the current air standards in this country are more than adequate to protect human health. According to *Science* magazine, with 1987 as a base, emissions were 40 percent lower in the three years including 1990.[6] EPA figures on urban air declined 89 percent, sulphur dioxide by 30 percent, and carbon monoxide by 28 percent.[7]

- Ten million *fewer* Americans were breathing unhealthy air in 1991, as compared to 1989, due to effective reductions in the primary air pollutants, especially carbon monoxide and particulates.[8]

We must breathe to live, and few places today or in the past are free from some contamination by man-made pollutants. Many city dwellers accept pollution as a fact of urban life. Even in suburban areas, it is not unusual to hear the disconcerting report, "The air quality today is unacceptable."

Obviously, the health effects of air pollution are of concern to all of us.

Equally obvious is the reality that air pollution is undesirable. The question is: Is air pollution in the United States as life- and health-threatening as the scaremongers tell us? Is it possible to prevent all exposure to air pollutants? Before going into these questions in detail, a simple five-part answer to these complex questions provides a workable overview.

First, it is clear that in cases where the air is heavily polluted, human health is threatened with increased respiratory symptoms and, in some cases, premature death. In addition, severe air pollution can reduce visibility and harm vegetation, buildings, and other materials.

Second, while 100 percent pure air might seem like the ideal, it is simply not a realistic or affordable goal. The truth is that completely pure air has never existed. Even if it were possible to prevent all human pollution of the air, some contamination (although a relatively small amount) from natural sources—for example, volcanoes*—would be inevitable. This fact is one that the extremists have trouble accepting. When President Reagan was quoted as saying that growing and decaying vegetation in this land is responsible for a majority of nitrogen oxides in the atmosphere, he was properly criticized by the press. It seems that the president had his pollutants mixed up; studies do show that hydrocarbons are discharged in high concentrations from natural processes. But the point he was alluding to is valid despite his factual error—pure air, that is, air with no contaminants, does not exist in nature. But the extremists, as they usually do, made light of the point, as this quote in a *San Jose Mercury News* editorial shows: "Put the president of the Sierra Club in a sealed garage with a tree. Put Reagan in a sealed garage with a running automobile. Wait to see which one of them yells to get out first."

Third, if air pollution is defined as any contaminant capable of causing health effects in large enough concentrations, and if all air pollution is to be eliminated as the scaremongers tell us it should, then we would be forced to live in a much different, but not healthier, environment. An atmosphere void of microscopic particulate material, that is, particulates much smaller than those emitted by man-made activities, is an atmosphere incapable of producing raindrops. As Thomas Burnam explains, "Without at least some air pollution, this planet would be in very poor shape. For raindrops will not form in a completely unpolluted atmosphere; there have to be what meteorologists call hydroscopic nuclei, or small particles in the air around which the drops will take shape. No hydroscopic nuclei, no raindrops, and no rain."[9] What is critical about air pollution is not the presence of pollution, but pollution at a level that causes ill health or mortality.

It is equally as important to recognize that air pollution, even at significant

---

*In one area of Portland, Oregon, half of the respirable particulates in the air on one day in January 1978 came from residential wood burning.

levels, may only affect susceptible people. Susceptibility varies widely, affecting people quite differently. Individuals with preexisting lung disease, such as asthma or bronchitis, are especially susceptible to the effects of pollutants. The very young and the very old also tend to be more sensitive to air pollution. Potential pollutant health effects range from temporary breathing difficulties to long-lasting, irreversible effects and even premature death. When discussing a pollutant, then, it is vital to ask: What levels of a specific pollutant or combination of pollutants cause health problems, and, how does this vary among various segments of the population?

Fourth, the effects of low or even moderate levels of air pollution on human health are not fully understood. Given the impossibility of 100 percent pure air, we know that human beings have always tolerated some degree of air pollution. The question, then, is not whether polluted air is harmful, but at what level does air pollution become a threat to human health?

Fifth, although there is reason for concern about the quality of air, particularly in some American cities, *no evidence exists that air pollution is a major cause of death or disease in this country.* As will be noted below, air pollution in excessive concentrations can exacerbate existing respiratory problems, *but ample evidence exists that the current air standards in this country are more than adequate to protect human health.* Indeed, as the discussion in this chapter will reveal, those who propose even further multi-billion-dollar clean-up programs aimed at achieving purer air are only luring us to squander additional billions for a minuscule or zero return for protecting the public's health. In protesting the environmental alarmists' demands for cleaner air, I. W. Tucker, president of the National Council of Environmental Balance, was on target when he addressed the hysteria over pollution: "Popular views of the media are based no more on facts than the tales told by Pinocchio."

Air-pollution control is controversial in scientific and political circles alike. In part, the controversy is the result of limited scientific knowledge of the relationship between air pollution and health effects. Emotional responses to the perceived health threat of pollution impede unbiased assessment of the real public health risks.

The complexity of the air-pollution problem confounds even air-pollution experts. It's easy to understand, then, why consumers are confused and even manipulated by media reports. Press reports and news commentary are vital to increasing awareness of the problem. But, by failing to apprise the public of background facts and scientific perspective, the media frequently misrepresent critical issues, perpetuating and compounding fear and misunderstanding.

This concept is excellently illustrated by looking at a 1977 news report and the facts behind it. A news article entitled "Premature Deaths Linked to Coal and Oil Burning" stated that as many as twenty-one thousand people east of the Mississippi River would die prematurely each year because of pollution caused by power plants. Going on to cite unpublished data, the news writer speculated that, should the nation turn to coal to replace dwindling oil supplies, as many as thirty-five thousand premature deaths could be expected annually by the year 2010. A close look at the report from which this news report stems is very telling. The original report stated that, because of the uncertainties of statistical calculations, the actual number of premature deaths east of the Mississippi could range from zero to fifty thousand. It also stated that a proposal to burn more coal might, in fact, *reduce* premature deaths by two thousand each year. Finally, and most importantly, it stated that "the uncertainties associated with these calculations are so large that one must question the significance of any specific number."

What you read often isn't all there is to know!

Background

Air pollution is not exclusively a modern-day phenomenon. The Roman philosopher Seneca observed that "as soon as I had gotten out of the heavy air of Rome and from the stink of the smoky chimneys thereof, which being stirred poured forth whatever pestilential vapors and soot they had enclosed in them, I felt an alteration of my disposition."[10]

In 1157, the wife of King Henry II, Eleanor of Aquitaine, could not endure the air pollution caused by wood burning, and she was forced to move.[11]

Early concern about air pollution gave rise to various regulation attempts, as illustrated by an edict issued in Great Britain during the reign of Edward I: "Be it known to all within the sound of my voice, whosoever shall be found guilty of burning coal shall suffer the loss of his head."[12]

Edward II, who concurred in stiff penalties for polluters, had a man hanged outside St. Bartholomew's Hospital for burning coal and filling the air with a "pestilential odor."[13] Fortunately, present-day pollution problems, largely attributable to increasing urbanization and industrialization, are resolved by less-threatening regulations.

The Atmosphere and Air Pollution

Man frequently has little choice about what enters his lungs. Some forms of air pollution, such as cigarette smoke and aerosol sprays, are partially avoidable, but others, such as industrial and motor vehicle emissions, are inhaled involuntarily. Federal regulations were developed to protect the public from involuntary exposures.

The earth's atmosphere is one part of a dynamic ecological system. There is a constant exchange of materials among the atmosphere, the ocean, and the earth. Approximately 500 billion tons of air surround this planet, of which about 21 percent is oxygen, 78 percent nitrogen, and 0.9 percent argon. These gases make up all but 0.04 percent of a clean, dry atmosphere. Carbon dioxide accounts for 75 percent of the remaining volume.

Atmospheric pollution is neither a new phenomenon nor exclusively the creation of man. Natural pollution from volcanic eruptions, grass fires, and gases from swamps and marshes has always existed and will continue to contribute to global air pollution. Wind-blown dust, pollen, and fog are other natural types of airborne pollutants. In general, although natural sources of air pollution contribute 90 percent of emissions, they tend to be diffuse. Man-made pollutants, on the other hand, are often concentrated, and therefore may have more impact on the environment.

There is probably no general agreement on the quantity and type of pollutants present in the atmosphere, nor on what constitutes a pollutant. Some compounds are considered to be pollutants only under certain conditions and at some locations. The concentration of any given pollutant has great variability and depends on the source, topography, and meteorology.

Pollutants are not emitted into the environment in isolation. Contributions from a multitude of polluting sources, both stationary and mobile, result in a complex mixture of chemicals in the atmosphere. This complexity is further compounded by the fact that the atmosphere is an ideal site for a wide variety of chemical reactions and transformations. The movement of the air provides ample opportunity for pollutants from different sources to interact, while the sun supplies energy for these reactions.

Because of the dynamic nature of the atmosphere, many of the pollutants released into the air, known as primary pollutants, are changed through chemical reactions into different, or secondary, pollutants. For example, pollutants such as sulfur dioxide and oxides of nitrogen, emitted as gases, may be converted to sulfate and nitrate particulates, respectively. The amount of a secondary pollutant present in the environment will depend on many factors, including the presence of the various primary pollutants, and catalysts, and the availability of energy for the reaction. Thus it can be seen that both weather and the presence of other sources can strongly influence the pollutant mix.

Meteorologic conditions have profound influence on pollution concentrations. Mixing and transport of emissions are both affected by the relative stability of an air mass in turn, and influence the production of secondary pollutants. The exposure of a population to a given pollutant mixture is also related to atmospheric stability. For example, a stable or slow-moving air mass allows for greater buildup of pollutants while simultaneously resulting in longer exposure times.

In contrast, turbulent air helps to disperse and dilute pollutants. Although during gusty winds a chimney plume may be deflected downward, exposure to a high concentration at ground level in any one place is usually short because wind direction tends to vary. Under calm conditions warm gases rise until they have cooled to the temperature of the surrounding air. The hotter they are to begin with, the higher they will rise. Cool plumes, such as domestic smoke, rise only a little and so are not well dispersed.

Under calm conditions and clear skies, the earth loses heat at night. This results in the formation of a cool, dense layer of air near the earth with warmer air above. As the layer of cooler air thickens, smoke and chimney gases will be trapped beneath the interface of the warm and cool air layers. This is called an inversion. Inversions also occur when a layer of warm air thickens above a layer of cooler air.

Inversions are associated with great atmospheric stability and, therefore, with higher pollution levels. All of the major air pollution disasters, discussed below, have occurred during inversions. Inversions can last from a few hours to several days. The longer the inversion persists, the greater the potential buildup of pollutants. Duration of an inversion is especially important in urban or industrial areas where emissions are high.

Local topography also plays an important role in creating an inversion. Valleys in latitudes where the nights are long provide ideal circumstances for inversions. This is because the air in the valley, simply because it is shaded, frequently remains cool long after the upper air has been warmed by the sun. Unfortunately, these valleys are often precisely the areas in which towns grew up. Rivers there provided transport and it was easier to build roads, railways, and canals in these flat areas. All the major air-pollution episodes have taken place in valleys—the Meuse Valley in Belgium, the valley of the Monongahela River in Pennsylvania, and the Thames Basin in England.

In addition to inversions, other meteorologic conditions influence pollution. Temperature, for example, dictates the amount of fuel being burned for heating or cooling purposes. Humidity and sunlight both influence chemical reactions between pollutants. Precipitation in the form of rain or snow washes the air through which it falls, scavenging pollutants by absorption and adsorption. The downward air currents that often accompany rain can also entrain pollutants, causing them to settle more rapidly than otherwise.

Although the internal stability of an air mass has great importance in relation to air pollution, the larger movements of the air mass itself are also vital. Air masses are mobile, and thus have the potential to transport pollutants long distances. As an air mass moves over an area, it receives emissions from the sources in that area. A given air mass is constantly accumulating pollutants. If the internal stability of the air mass is high, dilution and dispersal will not occur, and this constant enroute collection of emissions will result in the buildup of extremely high pollutant concentrations. It is essential to realize that the pollution levels in a geographical area are not always the direct result of emissions sources in that area. Frequently, an area will inherit pollution emitted from distant sources. This long-range transport of pollutants is of special importance in relation to compliance with federal air-quality standards, as regulation of local sources may ultimately have little effect on the levels of pollution experienced by an area.

In some locations, fugitive emissions may pose a problem. Wind-raised dust is one example of a fugitive emission. Fugitive emissions may greatly increase the apparent pollution in an area. If fugitive sources are not recognized and accounted for in regulatory policy, the burden of such emissions may fall on local man-made sources in the form of lower emissions standards. This stricter regulation of man-made emissions will have little impact on overall pollution levels in locations where fugitive emissions are substantial.

It is also of interest to note that as weather influences pollution, pollution can also affect weather. Certain types of particles, for example, provide a surface on which droplets can condense and thus encourage the formation of fog and clouds. Visibility, though not directly related to weather, is also affected by pollution, especially by particulates.

Sources of Air Pollution

There are several types of sources of man-made pollution, including single (point) sources, multiple (area) sources, and line sources. Electric generating utilities, manufacturing plants, and other industries or facilities with tall stacks are generally regarded as point sources. Residential areas, office buildings, schools, and hospitals are multiple sources. Line sources are highways, expressways, and city streets, where pollutants result from vehicle emissions. All three types contribute to the total pollution in an area.

In general, pollutants may be emitted from these sources: (1) transportation, (2) industrial processes, (3) stationary fuel combustion, and (4) combustion of solid waste.

TRANSPORTATION

Emissions from mobile sources, including both highway vehicles (cars, trucks, buses) and nonhighway vehicles (aircraft, trains), are responsible for the largest mass of pollutants. This stems primarily from the enormous quantity of carbon monoxide emissions contributed by this source category, which constitutes approximately 70 percent of total emissions from transportation. Vehicles are responsible for approximately 40 percent of total nitrogen oxide emissions and 33 percent of total volatile organic compound emissions (e.g., hydrocarbons).

The last two contaminant types are major ingredients in photochemical smog. Overall, emissions from transportation contribute 45 percent of the total air pollution in this country.[14]

INDUSTRIAL PROCESSES

About 15 percent of the total air pollution produced in the United States comes from the industrial processes associated with chemical plants; petroleum refineries; smelters; foundries; fertilizer plants; kraft, pulp, and paper mills; cement plants; and the rubber and plastics industries, to name a few. Industrial processes as a whole contribute approximately 38 percent of all particulate emissions, 46 percent of volatile organics emissions, and about 16 percent of sulfur-oxide emissions.[15]

STATIONARY FUEL COMBUSTION

This category encompasses all fuel combustion in nonmobile combustion equipment, including that by electric utility power plants and industries, and other fuel consumers such as residences, commercial establishments, and institutions. Of all emissions, 29 percent are attributable to this category, mainly in the form of sulfur oxides, nitrogen oxides, and particulates. Of the components of this stationary fuel combustion category, electric utilities generate the most emissions. Two-thirds of all national sulfur oxide emissions are generated by electric utilities, 93 percent of which come from coal-fired power plants.[16]

SOLID WASTE

Included in this category are emissions from combustion of waste, both by open burning and incinerators. Such incineration contributes to the particulate load, and insignificantly to carbon monoxide and volatile organic compound loads. In 1988, only 2 percent of total pollutant emissions came from this source.[17]

Types of Pollution

Pollution is a general term, but pollutants are quite specific. Under the Clean Air Act of 1970 and its amendments,[18] the EPA has established standards for six criteria pollutants. These standards are called the National Ambient Air Quality Standards—NAAQS: carbon monoxide, nitrogen dioxide, ozone, particulates, lead, and sulfur dioxide. The NAAQS include primary and secondary standards. The primary standards are designed with large margins of safety to protect the health of even the most sensitive groups within the population likely to be exposed. Secondary standards protect against adverse welfare effects not directly related to health, such as crop losses, damage to forests and fisheries, and impaired visibility.[19]

PARTICULATES

Particulates can be solid or liquid. The solid variety includes partially burned or unburned fuel particles like smoke and soot, residues from burning, and, among other things, pollens. Particle size is vital to any discussion of the health effects of particulate air pollution, as the size of a particle will ultimately determine its ability to enter and remain in the lung. Particulates are generally divided into three size ranges, each of which has different capacities for entering and affecting pulmonary tissue.

The largest particles fall rapidly because of their size and usually deposit close to their source of formation. When these large particles are inhaled, they tend to become trapped in the nasopharyngeal region and do not reach deep lung tissue. Therefore, particles in the largest size range may be less important in the generation of respiratory health effects, although such substances as sulfuric acid droplets and pollen grains may exert effects in the upper respiratory region. Breathing through the mouth instead of through the nose can alter the deposition of inhaled particles, permitting some of these large particles to reach the lungs. For this reason, particulate effects may vary according to involvement in strenuous activities or exercise.

Particles between approximately 0.1 um and 3.0 um in diameter are abundant and easily suspended in air, remaining there for hours or days. These particles, commonly known as smoke, fumes, or aerosols, are capable of being inhaled deep into the lungs and remaining there. This fact, combined with their wide distribution and long atmospheric residence times, creates the potential for significant impact on health.

The smallest particles, those with diameters of less than 0.1 um, usually exist only briefly before coalescing or attaching to larger particles. Unattached particles of this size behave like gases and, when inhaled, are largely expelled during expiration.

The chemical composition of a particle is also of significance when considering health effects. The toxicity of a particle is directly related to its chemistry.

Of additional importance when considering particulates of respirable size is the ability of such particles to attach and transport other contaminants. In this way, substances such as sulfur dioxide, which would usually not reach deep-lung tissue, may piggyback on the particulates that reach lower-lung regions.

Suspended particulates are emitted into the atmosphere from a multitude of sources, both natural and man-made. Particulates are also formed in the atmosphere from the interaction of various gaseous pollutants. The chemical composition of particulates can be quite complex and varies according to the source of the emission. Carbon and tarlike hydrocarbon particulates and inorganic ash result from the combustion of various fuels. Ammonium sulfate aerosol is formed from the reactions of atmospheric constituents with sulfur dioxide. Locally, industrial activity can produce specific particles of importance only in the immediate environment. Iron oxide from steelworks and dust from cement works are two examples of the latter.

Originally, the NAAQS for particulates was a measure of the total suspended particulate matter (TSP). New data, however, indicate that TSP is not the most appropriate indicator for particulate matter because it includes substantial quantities of larger particles (up to 25 to 45 mm) of less concern to health. A better measure includes only particles less than or equal to 10 um. This new standard, referred to as PM, became effective in 1987.[20]

SULFUR OXIDES

Sulfur oxides are produced when sulfur-containing coal and oil are burned as a fuel source, and when metallic ores are smelted. Oceanic salt spray and certain metabolic processes of bacteria also contribute to the total sulfur load of the global atmosphere. Sulfur oxides enter the atmosphere as sulfur dioxide (SO_2), sulfurous acid (H_2SO_3), sulfuric acid (H_2SO_4), and various particulate sulfates.

Sulfur dioxide is considered one of the world's major air pollutants. It is a nonflammable, colorless gas. The gas, in sufficient quantity, has a pungent, irritating odor. Excessively high concentrations can cause chronic cough.

The largest single source of man-made emissions of sulfur dioxide is the burning of fuels that contain sulfur as an impurity. Coal is the most notable example of this. Once in the atmosphere, sulfur dioxide (a primary pollutant) can be converted to other products such as sulfate through several reactions.

The process by which sulfates are formed in the atmosphere is not yet fully understood. Most atmospheric sulfate is in the form of ammonium sulfate. Recent studies suggest that, typically, 1 percent or less of the sulfur dioxide produced by fossil fuel power plants is directly converted into sulfate. However, sulfuric acid and sulfate aerosol can account for 5 to 20 percent of all suspended particulates in urban air samples. The ability of sulfur dioxide to cause eye irritation is magnified three to four times when humidity is high and conditions are favorable for the formation of sulfuric acid. Thus, measuring sulfur dioxide alone may be insufficient to predict the adverse health effects of a polluted air mass.

CARBON MONOXIDE

Carbon monoxide (CO), a colorless, odorless, and tasteless gas, is a specific form of "urban pollution" caused primarily by incomplete combustion of fuel. The side-stream smoke from cigarettes is also another source, with "secondhand smoke" containing carbon monoxide at levels of 40,000 ppm.

We know that when carbon monoxide is absorbed into the blood stream, it combines with hemoglobin and can thereby cause interference with oxygen transport to such vital tissues as the heart, brain, and muscles. In simple terms, carbon monoxide can displace oxygen in the body. At high levels it can be injurious to health.

Carbon monoxide exposure is a common occupational hazard for garage attendants who frequently work in poorly ventilated enclosures. High concentrations of it have killed people. Carbon monoxide poisoning, in fact, is a frequent killer of teen drivers who leave the engine running and the windows closed while parking.

The introduction of automobile emission controls has significantly reduced the ambient outdoor CO concentration to the point where all the major metropolitan areas are in general compliance with the current air-quality standards—most of the time. But since levels of CO vary significantly from place to place, and from time to time, depending on the volume of traffic, it is impossible to state flatly that there is never any risk to anyone from carbon monoxide in the air. Healthy individuals compensate for the displacement of oxygen when CO exposure is not abnormally high. However, individuals at high risk of cardiovascular disease will be placed under stress in instances where the CO level climbs temporarily higher than the level now considered acceptable.

NITROGEN DIOXIDE

Nitrogen dioxide is actually a secondary pollutant; that is, it is formed spontaneously in the atmosphere from nitric oxide. Nitric oxide is formed when fuel is burned at high temperatures. The two major sources are transportation and stationary fuel combustion. In high enough concentrations, nitrogen oxides can irritate the lungs and cause respiratory infections such as bronchitis and pneumonia.[21]

OZONE

Although ozone in the upper atmosphere is beneficial to life by shielding the earth from the sun's harmful ultraviolet radiation, high concentrations at ground level are a major health and environmental concern. Ozone in outdoor air is recognized as one of the most important air pollutants by NAAQS and has been the most difficult to control within federal standards.[22] Ozone is not emitted directly into the air, but is formed when volatile organic compounds combine with nitrogen oxides in the presence of sunlight. Volatile organic compounds come from many sources: automobiles, chemical manufacturing, dry cleaners, paint shops, and other sources using solvents. At high enough concentrations, ozone can be a respiratory irritant, especially in those with increased susceptibility to its effects,[23] and can interfere with respiratory function in people who are exercising, but not in those at rest. Prolonged elevated ozone concentrations may precipitate asthma attacks.[24]

LEAD

At toxic doses, lead causes severe adverse health effects. Recent reports about lead have been confusing. These reports indicate that there may be more subtle biochemical changes occurring at lower levels of lead in the body than previously thought. The significance of these subtle changes is not known. But this doesn't mean that lead levels are increasing in air, food, or water. In fact, these levels are decreasing. Air lead levels, as noted in more detail below, are not much of a concern because of the stringent requirements for reducing such emissions.[25]

When and Where Air Pollution Has Made People Sick

In a few well-documented episodes, limited periods of polluted air have caused acute illness and contributed to death among certain vulnerable population groups. These "natural experiments" provide convincing evidence that high levels of pollutants are hazardous to our health. They also suggest to us that high-level exposure is necessary before acute adverse effects are seen.

The episodes most frequently cited are those that occurred in the Meuse Valley in Belgium; in Donora, Pennsylvania; and in London. Investigation of these air-pollution episodes revealed that in cases of excessive pollution, the death rate increased over that normally expected. Comparison of this increased mortality rate with the expected mortality for the same period yields the number of excess deaths, or deaths that can be attributed to the pollution.

The Meuse River Valley is an area of concentrated industry containing steel plants, glass factories, lime furnaces, zinc-reduction plants, fertilizer plants, and sulfuric acid plants. During the first week of December 1930, all of Belgium was blanketed by fog. The many industries continuously emitted pollutants into this stagnant atmosphere. Inversion conditions prevailed, and within three days, residents of the Meuse Valley area became ill with respiratory complaints. Sixty deaths were attributed to this episode. For approximately two months the number of deaths continued to exceed the normal expected mortality by more than ten times. For the most part, those who died were the elderly and individuals already suffering from chronic respiratory diseases. The healthy segment of the population was less severely affected, although thousands reported symptoms ranging from throat irritation, persistent cough, shortness of breath, and tightness in the chest, to nausea and vomiting.

The situation in 1948 in Donora, Pennsylvania, was much the same. A temperature inversion with little air movement prevailed over a wide area of the northeastern United States for about five days. Atmospheric contaminants accumulated in abnormal amounts in the industrialized area of Donora, a steel town located in a meandering river valley some thirty miles south of Pittsburgh. During and following this air-pollution episode, extensive medical records were taken, and public reaction questionnaires and surveys were completed. It was found that nearly six thousand persons, more than 40 percent of the area's population, were affected with some symptoms of illness. As in the Meuse Valley, doctors were soon besieged by patients who complained of a variety of ills, including coughing; wheezing; eye, nose, and throat irritation; nausea; vomiting; headaches; weakness; and general muscular aches and pains.

In this episode, as in others, the aged and infirm were most affected. While the incidence of morbidity for the population as a whole was about 40 percent, approximately 60 percent of those over sixty-five years of age reported some degree of illness. Approximately twenty individuals, with a mean age of sixty-five, died as a result of the pollution. Autopsies showed that death was associated with a diversity of ills, all related to respiratory or cardiovascular conditions. Acute irritative changes in the lungs, characterized by capillary dilation, were prominent. Hemorrhage, edema, and purulent bronchitis were also found. Chronic cardiovascular diseases were frequently represented among those most severely affected, indicating that preexisting heart disease had a significant influence on the nature and severity of illness developing during an air-pollution episode.

In the 1952 London incident, as in many past episodes, fog was a factor. Stagnant conditions had prevailed for about four days, during which high levels of pollutants accumulated. Multitudes in greater London became ill with respiratory complaints. Coughing, sore throats, and vomiting were commonly reported. Mortality records for the two-week period during and following the episode showed that four thousand excess deaths had occurred. The victims were predominantly those already suffering from cardiac and respiratory disease, as well as the elderly and very young. Deaths from bronchitis increased nearly tenfold over the number expected. This increase began simultaneously with the increase in pollution and returned to normal levels within two weeks. Excess cardiovascular-related deaths ceased soon after the pollution cleared. The occurrence of an influenza epidemic complicated the interpretation of trends after the episode had passed.

Ten years later, in 1962, similar meteorological conditions in London triggered another pollution episode. Estimates of excess deaths resulting from this inversion ranged from three hundred to seven hundred, as opposed to the four thousand deaths attributed to the earlier episode. The absence of complete data makes it impossible to compare quantitatively the concentration of the two pollutants measured during the episode: smoke (particulate) and sulfur dioxide. The available data do indicate, however, that whereas the sulfur dioxide concentrations were similar in the two episodes, the particulate level (as measured by smoke) was significantly lower in the 1962 episode. However, it is not possible to conclude that the reduced mortality in 1962 traced to this reduction in particulate pollution, as many other changes took place during the intervening decade that could account for the reduction in the number of excess deaths. An example of an important difference between the two episodes was the extensive use of the news media in the later incident to warn individuals of the dangers of the pollution and to caution against unnecessary exposure, especially in cases of susceptible persons.

Limitations of Descriptive Studies of Episodic Pollution

It would be valuable if we could relate the health effects observed in air-pollution episodes to known combinations of pollutant concentrations. Unfortunately, it is not possible to derive this information either from comparisons of morbidity and mortality during and after an air-pollution episode, or from comparisons of data on disease incidence from different geographical areas. In general, descriptive studies can be used to describe associations, but not to test hypotheses or to establish causality.

Two limitations in particular inhibit the usefulness of comparative studies. First, the type of air pollution predominating in various cities differs. In London, New York, Leningrad, and many of the large cities of northerly humid areas, sulfur dioxide, soot, and dust are the major pollutants. Pollution in warmer, less humid cities, such as Los Angeles, Sao Paulo, and Mexico City, consists of photochemical products, carbon monoxide, and hydrocarbons. This difference in pollutant types precludes generalized conclusions on health effects, which may not be identical for all contaminants. Comparative pollution studies frequently fail to make this distinction between the different types of pollutants in an area and cannot pinpoint specific pollutants in a study.

That air pollution can exert a very real adverse effect on health was demonstrated by the acute episodes of Meuse Valley, Donora, and London. These episodes stimulated suspicion regarding the possibility of health effects from less severe pollution exposure, acute and chronic. Many of the analytical epidemiological studies considered in this chapter were conducted with the purpose of determining the existence and degree of adverse health effects resulting from nonepisodic pollution.

The present issue is not whether exposure to extreme concentrations of pollutants can injure health, but whether lower pollution levels similarly threaten health and at what level this increased health risk occurs. It is additionally important to differentiate between health effects that are the result of acute pollution exposure, and those that are attributable to chronic exposure to low-level pollution. Not only is the separation of these effects vital to any scientific consideration of the evidence, but it is also essential to the development of sound regulatory action.

Is Our Air Safe Today?

We have so far in this chapter documented (a) that our air—all air—is polluted at least to some degree, by natural and man-made sources; (b) that the sources of pollution are many and varied; (c) that there are pollutants—and carcinogens—that may be a threat to our health; and (d) that under some specific circumstances involving air inversions and concentrated pollution, an excess of death and illness has been recorded.

The question before us now, however, is, Is the air in America's cities contributing to ill health and mortality today? The doomsayers say positively yes. The mainstream opinion on this is maybe to a small extent. The concerns about air pollution and modern-day health focus on two areas: *acute effects* and potential *long-term effects.*

As was mentioned above, high-level exposure to carbon monoxide can have temporary negative effects on a healthy person. And for those suffering from cardiovascular disease, high levels can be life-threatening. Fortunately, CO levels throughout the country are well within the margin of safety set by EPA.

In general, epidemiological studies of acute health effects support the conclusion that exposure to very high levels of sulfur oxide or particulate matter can have an adverse effect on lung function. In an individual already suffering from respiratory disease, exposure to excessive pollution may result in worsening of that condition. Various studies associate a range of sulfur oxide and particulate levels with decreased lung function in healthy individuals or with the aggravation of preexisting respiratory disease. In general, most studies show adverse health effects only at very high levels of pollutants.

But the most important information to consider is that concentrations of all air pollutants are decreasing. Specifically:

SULFUR DIOXIDE

From 1978 to 1988, there was a 17 percent decrease in sulfur dioxide emissions, responsible for a 30 percent improvement in ambient sulfur dioxide levels. There are continued reductions in sulfur dioxide emissions from fuel combustion.[26] Not only are air sulfur dioxide levels improving, but the attitude of scientists and regulators regarding the possible health effects of sulfur dioxide has relaxed. In 1975 the Environmental Protection Agency called sulfur dioxide "a deadly atmospheric pollutant killing thousands of people each year."[27] Four years later the EPA downgraded its assessment, calling sulfur dioxide "a mild respiratory irritant which must be removed."[28]

The general scientific consensus on the effects of SO_2 on human health can be gleaned through the commentaries of three scientists who specialize in the effects of sulfur dioxide on human health:

> There is no convincing medical evidence that SO_2 below 10 ppm has any adverse health effects, either acute or chronic.
> Dr. Thaddeus J. Murawski, New York Academy of Medicine[29]

> We do not find any association between SO_2 pollution and mortality.
> Dr. Herbert Shimmel, Albert Einstein Medical College[30]

> Man can tolerate exposure to SO_2 up to 25 ppm (that's 1,250 times the current ambient level of 0.02 ppm) with no ill effects. Even at these high concentrations the nasal filters are so effective that very little SO_2 gets into the lungs.
> Dr. Lawrence Hinkle, Cornell University Medical School[31]

CARBON MONOXIDE

There was a 25 percent decrease in carbon monoxide emissions from 1979 to 1988, causing a 28 percent improvement in air quality as measured by carbon monoxide. These improvements occurred despite a 33 percent increase in vehicle miles traveled during the same period. There continues to be a decline in the number of areas in the United States failing to meet carbon monoxide NAAQS.[32]

NITROGEN MONOXIDE

The ten-year span of 1978–88 showed an 8 percent decrease in nitrogen oxide emissions, resulting in a 7 percent improvement in ambient nitrogen dioxide levels. Los Angeles was the only urban area that recorded any violations of the annual nitrogen dioxide level for the period 1979–88.[33]

OZONE

Although there was a 17 percent decrease in volatile organic compounds (VOCs) for the period 1979–88, there was a 2 percent increase in ambient ozone levels. Ozone, primarily a warm weather problem, continues to be the most pervasive ambient air pollution problem in the United States, with 101 areas failing to meet the ozone NAAQS. The warm 1988 summer was conducive to ozone formation, while preliminary data suggest that a cooler, wetter 1989 resulted in lower ozone levels.[34]

New information released in 1992 helps scientists understand why ozone pollution has not been adequately controlled. As we discussed, one of the most important ways to reduce ozone pollution is to control the emissions of VOCs. Unfortunately, regulations over the past twenty years have been based on underestimated levels of VOCs. Scientists now call for a critical reappraisal that will provide more accurate estimates and then more appropriate control measures.[35]

LEAD

By far the greatest improvements in air quality are in the lead category. The years from 1979 to 1988 evidenced a 93 percent decrease in total lead emissions, with a 97 percent decrease in lead emissions from transportation sources. This decrease in emissions resulted in an 89 percent improvement in ambient air lead levels. These improvements are due largely to the increased use of unleaded gasoline and the reduction of the lead content in leaded gasoline. Unleaded gasoline sales accounted for 82 percent of the total gasoline market in 1988. Lead emissions from industrial sources have dropped by more than one-half since the 1970s.[36]

It seems as though proponents of more stringent, expensive regulations have failed to read the facts: 1991 figures confirm that our air is steadily better and justifies a less demanding set of government regulations and controls. The facts speak clearly: three-fourths of the smog problem (outside of California) has disappeared over the past six years, including in major cities such as New York, Philadelphia, Baltimore, and Chicago. A 1992 study by Kay H. Jones, a Seattle pollution consultant and formerly the Carter administration air quality analyst, says it is "ridiculous to treat the rest of America as if it faces Los Angeles–style pollution problems." Jones says three-quarters of the EPA's ozone attainment program is "a total waste of money." Estimates put the total at around $13 billion a year in direct costs, to which should be added major administrative and legal costs.[37]

Jones says the EPA is suppressing the good news in his report, saying the agency "has a powerful vested interest in parlaying bad news, arguing that it needs this to justify its larger budgets and greater regulatory power." Commenting on Jones's report, *Insight* reporter Peter Samuel says: "If the EPA is allowed to suppress the good news discovered by Jones, draconian 'clean air' measures already in place will grind into effect according to the timetable of the Clean Air Act. They are expected to close one-third of the country's oil refineries, shut down tens of thousands of gas stations and heavily impact hundreds of thousands of small businesses such as spray paint shops and dry cleaners. Moreover, motorists will find themselves paying 10 percent to 15 percent more for new 'oxygenated' gasoline and fees for annual emission inspections."[38]

Why Does Los Angeles Continue to Have So Many Air Problems?

Why, despite enacting some of this country's toughest air quality standards, does Los Angeles have more smoggy days than any other U.S. city? In 1991 (the most recent year for which there are data) L.A. had 218 days when the pollution standard index (PSI) was unhealthful (PSI is a combined reading of all five major pollutants—particulate matter, sulfur dioxide, carbon monoxide, ozone, and nitrogen dioxide); the next highest number of days with an unhealthy PSI was 34 and 35 in New York, Philadelphia, and Washington, D.C. What's the scoop?

In addition to the mountains to the north and east that trap lead air and hot sun that worsens emissions, 60 percent of L.A.'s air pollution comes from petroleum-burning vehicles. Cars crawling through traffic jams at 5 m.p.h. let off three times the hydrocarbons as those cruising the speed limit.

Interestingly, oil refineries are not the worst offender: oil refineries emit just one-quarter the hydrocarbons emitted from hair spray used by L.A. residents. It would seem that residents should take the responsibility to drive less rather than ask the government for expensive regulations, the cost of which will ultimately come from their wallets.

Does Air Pollution Contribute to Lung Cancer?

We know that traces of suspected carcinogens, for example, benzo(a)pyrene and other polycyclic aromatic hydrocarbons, can be found in our air. Workers in some industries have been exposed to dangerously high concentrations of carcinogens, but at levels many times higher than the levels in ambient air. We are painfully aware that inhalation of asbestos and various ores in industrial situations increases the odds of those workers developing lung cancer. For example, in Germany during the late-nineteenth century, environmentally induced lung cancer occurred among uranium miners. Workers in coal mines have been afflicted with a number of respiratory ailments, including lung cancer, as a result of exposure to coal tar and volatile substances released from coal tar such as benzo(a)pyrene. Nickel refiners exposed to chromates and chrome ore dust, and iron ore miners exposed to iron oxide, also have an increased risk of developing cancer of the lungs. Thus it is theoretically possible that the cancer-causing agents we breathe each day increase our risk of cancer at the site with which the air is most likely to come in close contact: our lungs.

Unlike cigarette smoking and industrial and occupational exposure, the potential cancer risk from air pollution concerns all of us. Interest in a possible relationship between community air pollution and cancer has come about for two main reasons. First, certain epidemiological studies suggest that smoking habits cannot fully explain the excess cancer mortality in urban residents. Second, as mentioned above, known carcinogenic agents have been identified in urban air.

Lung cancer *does* occur more often in cities than in rural portions of the country. But, in addition to the air being different in these two types of localities, the people and other community characteristics are different. Of minor, though not insignificant, importance is that cities have more facilities for diagnosing lung cancer. Of somewhat more significance is that more city dwellers may have had some type of occupational exposure in the past that predisposed them to developing lung cancer.

One EPA investigation revealed, in fact, that residents in highly industrial areas are at no greater health risk from air pollutants than are people in rural areas. For two days 350 residents of Elizabeth and Bayonne, New Jersey, wore monitors sensitive enough to register the effect of a visit to the dry cleaner. These monitors revealed that the dosage of volatile air toxics from industrial plants was but a fraction of the total inhaled, anywhere from one-half to one-seventieth, depending on the pollutant. The total intake of industrial pollutants was no greater for the urban dwellers than for those in a comparison farm town in North Dakota.[39]

Of specific concern has been the possibility that airborne asbestos, a known human carcinogen, could be posing a general cancer hazard. As discussed in chapter 8, asbestos can be inhaled by persons who install or repair dry walls, roofing, flooring, automobile brakes and clutches, or home heating and plumbing systems, placing them at risk of developing lung disease. But exposure to asbestos in the outdoor environment probably doesn't contribute to lung cancer. As summarized by Drs. Carl M. Shy and Robert J. Struba in *Cancer Epidemiology and Prevention,* it is likely that "low ambient asbestos levels and levels encountered during incidental nonoccupational exposure to asbestos products constitute a very low risk of lung cancer to the general population."[40] Furthermore, the Advisory Committee on Asbestos Cancers to the director of the International Agency for Research on Cancer concluded, after studying the effects of low-level occupational exposure to asbestos, "Excess lung cancer is not detectable when occupational exposures to asbestos have been low, and these exposures have almost certainly been greater than those of the public from general air pollution."[41]

So, then, does air pollution cause cancer? The conclusions of most scientists, offered from the early 1980s through today, are that air pollution probably contributes very little to the cancer burden:

> The assertion that ambient air pollution is a risk factor for cancer, particularly lung cancer is . . . unwarranted.
> —Carl M. Shy and Robert J. Stuba[42]

> . . . air pollution was not found to be a great culprit in causing lung cancer.
> —American Cancer Society[43]

John D. Graham, associate professor of Policy and Decision Sciences at Harvard School of Public Health, told Congress in September 1989 that if air pollution contributes to lung cancer, that contribution is most incidental:

> . . . while there is a logical basis for public health concern, there is no direct evidence that outdoor exposures to toxic air pollutants are responsible for a significant fraction of disease or mortality. The levels of toxics that people breathe in daily life are typically several factors of ten smaller than the levels that have been studied by scientists. Based on a study of 65 toxic air pollutants, the EPA estimates that up to 3,000 additional cancers from [air toxics] may occur each year in the United States. By way of comparison, keep in mind that 900,000 new cases of cancer are detected in the United States each year.[44]

But Graham goes on to qualify these estimates:

> The EPA's widely quoted cancer risk estimates should be treated with caution because they are based on some questionable assumptions—for example, that humans are as sensitive as the most sensitive tested animal species, and that any human exposure to a carcinogen, no matter how small, results in some increase in cancer risk. While these are prudent assumptions to make in the absence of sound data, the EPA has not always been responsive about revising its assumptions in light of scientific advances. For example, the EPA's risk assessment for benzene, formaldehyde, gasoline vapor, and perchloroethylene are scientifically outdated and need to be revised.[45]

The Smokescreen of Environmentalism

The environmental alarmists like to point to carcinogens and poisons in the air of our cities, demanding stricter governmental control of industries, more restrictive air standards, and other measures for constraining technology "in the interest of health." Interestingly, they pay only minimal attention to the problems of indoor pollution, despite the fact that we spend more than sixteen hours a day inside, not outside, breathing the indoor air. Air quality experts now rate indoor air pollution far ahead of outdoor air pollution in significance. Wood-burning stoves, popularized during the 1970s energy crisis, for example, emit three thousand times the level of particulates that natural gas does. Byproducts formed and often not ventilated can cause cancer, heart disease, and central nervous system disorders.[46]

The average person breathes indoor air 65 percent or more of the day. Yet the existing regulations being put in place by environmentalists, and those that they have on the drawing board, relate almost exclusively to outdoor concentrations.

Sealing up one's home with insulation, caulking, and weather-stripping certainly helps keep the cold air out, but it also traps undesirable indoor pollutants. The World Health Organization cites the cigarette as the number one source of indoor pollution. Cigarette smoking indoors contributes significant amounts of nicotine, polycyclic aromatic hydrocarbons, carbon monoxide acrolein, formaldehyde, and many other substances.[47] Many substances in cigarette smoke are irritants and cause nasal discomfort, cough, sore throat, and sneezing. The nonsmokers inhaling secondhand smoke have been shown to undergo changes in the heart rate and the systolic blood pressure, and to suffer from small-airway dysfunction.

In addressing this number one source of indoor pollution, the cigarette, the National Academy of Science has stated,

> The constituents of tobacco smoke are well documented as hazardous, the prevalence of population exposure is very high, and there is an increased incidence of respiratory tract symptoms and functional decrements in children residing in homes with smokers, compared with those homes without smokers. These considerations and recent evidence of increased lung cancer among nonsmoking women living with smoking husbands, have led us to conclude that indoor exposure to tobacco smoke has adverse effects. Public policy should clearly articulate that involuntary exposure to tobacco smoke ought to be minimized or avoided where possible.

Cigarette-induced air pollution, however, doesn't interest the environmentalist.

Clean Air, Efficiently, in America

There is now substantial evidence that the current ambient air standards in this country are more than adequate to protect our health. But has our health improved since 1970 as a result of the new, stringent air-quality standards? No study has ever been done that answers that question. A study in New York City, however, noted that although the levels of SO_2 dropped 90 percent between 1969 and 1976, there was no change in the daily mortality rates.[48]

It is not surprising that everyone is in favor of clean air. But at what cost? The Clean Air Act was a hot item in Washington in the 1980s. Although sweeping changes that were sought by some and feared by others were expected in the summer of 1982, they did not come along until 1990. Despite the fact that air quality has improved dramatically over the past ten years, the Clean Air Act as amended in 1990 calls for exceedingly expensive further improvements, estimated to cost industry and consumers an additional $19 billion to $21 billion by the mid 1990s; industries already spend an estimated $32 billion each year on clean air.[49] In addition, some of the improvements demanded by the amendments are not yet achievable with current technology. Proponents of the changes argue that the best way to encourage the invention of new technologies is to set standards that cannot be met with current technology.[50] However, as *The Economist*[51] pointed out before passage of the amendments:

> If [standards] add sharply to the cost of new cars and factories, people and businesses may keep their old, much dirtier, ones for longer. And there is an international dimension. This is not just a question of investment and jobs moving abroad (so slowing economic growth) if clean-air standards are too high. It is also that the air crosses boundaries; if the steel industry moves its coke ovens to Mexico, which has much laxer clean-air standards than the United States, air quality over the continent could get worse, not better.

And, many improvements have already been made to the limits of technology. Car exhausts have already had 96 percent of their pollutants taken out.[52] The 1990 bill sought to raise that to 98 percent; some members of Congress wanted to push for 98.7 percent clean air.[53] The new bill calls for tougher tailpipe standards to be phased in with 1994 car models, with possibly tougher standards by 2003.[54]

Over the next decade, electric power plants must make sharp reductions in sulfur dioxide emissions—ten million tons per year, to be exact, as measured from their 1980 level.[55] The cost to New York City electric customers will be approximately $3.6 billion in new scrubbers alone.[56] That cost, of course, will have to be passed on to consumers, in rate increases from 15 to 30 percent.

Seven leading U.S. economists, including Nobel laureates James Buchanan,

George Stigler, and Milton Friedman, sent President Bush a letter in response to the Clean Air Act amendments. They warned the president that the "unduly stringent and extremely costly provision" of the Clean Air Act alone "could seriously threaten this nation's economic expansion." Not only are the astronomical costs cause for concern, but tens to hundreds of thousands of jobs may be lost as businesses move across the border to Mexico.[57]

Many experts, in fact, have estimated the cost of the 1990 amendments. The Office of Technology Assessment, for example, has estimated the cost of bringing levels of volatile organic compounds down to the new standards; the staggering figure: $8.8 billion to $12.8 billion per year.[58] The Department of Energy (DOE) estimated in 1992 that a 20 percent reduction in carbon dioxide emissions from 1990 levels by the year 2000 is technically feasible but would require a carbon tax of about $500 per metric ton to discourage use of fossil fuels; the ultimate cost to consumers would be an additional $1.30 per gallon of gasoline. This would also reduce the size of the U.S. economy by 1.4 percent, according to DOE.[59] The same experts estimated that the health benefits of such a reduction to be at most $1 billion, and as little as $250 million.[60] Finally, these experts say that $10 billion invested in smoking-cessation programs, radon control, and better prenatal and neonatal health care, for example, would contribute far more to improving public health and well being.[61]

Breathing Easy

No one is in favor of pollution. There is no question that the public health and the environment should be protected from harm. It is equally indisputable that it is necessary and reasonable to pay for this benefit to health and environment. However, we should know what we are paying for with our regulatory dollars and what health benefits we are getting in return.

By tightening air-quality standards, would we be paying for prevention of a real or only a hypothetical risk? Is it desirable to pay a great deal of money for very strict regulations based on the most cautious interpretations of ambiguous or flawed data?

There are no easy answers to these questions. Some will feel that it is worthwhile to protect against any possible health effects, regardless of the cost. Others will decide that costs must be justified by solid scientific evidence of benefits in preventing ill health. Either way, it is important to realize that air-pollution regulatory decisions cannot be made in a vacuum. The economic consequences of these regulations are real. We must be sure that the benefits of regulations for protecting human health are equally real.

The results of studies from a variety of sources using different methodologies indicate that whatever the health effects of air pollution in general, sulfur dioxide pollution is unlikely to be responsible for any significant impact on the rate of respiratory symptoms or disease. There is more evidence suggesting that particulate matter may adversely affect health, but the effect of low levels of particulates has not been well documented.

Perhaps it is time for air-quality regulations to reflect both the economic and health needs of individuals. This is not to advocate the protection of the public pocketbook at the expense of the public health. It is reasonable, however, to question the wisdom of those who focus only on a single aspect of a complex environmental issue.

NOTES

1. L. Regenstein, *America the Poisoned* (Washington: Acropolis Books, 1982), pp. 189–90.

2. L. J. Peter, *Peter's Quotations: Ideas for Our Times* (New York: William Morrow, 1977), p. 392.

3. J. Naar, *Design for a Livable Planet* (New York: Harper and Row, 1990), p. 77.

4. Ibid., p. 78.

5. M. H. Brown, *The Toxic Cloud* (New York: Harper and Row, 1987), p. 104.

6. P. H. Abelson, "Major Change in Chemical Industry," *Science* 255 (1992): p. 1489.

7. *Media Watch* (July 1992).

8. *Los Angeles Times,* November 21, 1991.

9. T. Burnam, *The Dictionary of Misinformation* (New York: Crowell, 1975), p. 3.

10. A. C. Stern et al., *Fundamentals of Air Pollution* (New York: Academic Press, 1973).

11. Ibid.

12. Ibid.

13. L. Chamber, "Classification and Extent of Air Pollution Problems," in *Air Pollution,* ed. A. C. Stern, 3rd ed. (New York: Academic Press, 1976).

14. USEPA, *National Air Quality and Emissions Trends Report, 1988,* EPA document 450/4-90-002 (Research Triangle Park: Office of Air Quality Planning and Standards, March 1990).

15. Ibid.

16. Ibid.

17. Ibid.

18. L. D. Grant and B. D. Jordan, *Basis for Primary Air Quality Criteria and Standards,* EPA document 60010-88-045 (Research Triangle Park, USEPA, 1988).

19. American Lung Association, *Health Effects of Ambient Air Pollution* (New York: American Lung Association, 1989).

20. Grant and Jordan, *Primary Air Quality Criteria;* USEPA, *Air Quality and*

Emissions.

21. USEPA, *Air Quality and Emissions;* Grant and Jordan, *Primary Air Quality Criteria;* American Lung Association, *Ambient Air Pollution.*

22. W. S. Beckett, *Yale Journal of Biology and Medicine* (1991).

23. Ibid.

24. Grant and Jordan, *Primary Air Quality Criteria;* USEPA, *Air Quality and Emissions.*

25. USEPA, *Air Quality and Emissions;* Grant and Jordan, *Primary Air Quality Criteria.*

26. USEPA, *Air Quality and Emissions.*

27. J. J. McKetta, "The U.S. Energy Picture—We're Still in Trouble," p. 19.

28. Ibid.

29. Ibid.

30. Ibid.

31. Ibid.

32. USEPA, *National Air Quality and Emissions.*

33. Ibid.

34. Ibid.

35. R. Stone, "NRC Faults Science Behind Ozone Regs," *Science* 255 (1992): p. 26.

36. USEPA, *National Air Quality and Emissions.*

37. P. Samuel, "A Breath of Fresh Air," *Insight* (April 6, 1992): pp. 20–21.

38. Ibid., p. 21.

39. E. Faltermayer, "Air: How Clean is Clean Enough?" *Fortune,* July 17, 1989, pp. 54–60.

40. D. Schottenfeld and J. F. Fraumeni, *Cancer Epidemiology and Prevention* (Philadelphia: W. B. Saunders Co., 1982), p. 342.

41. Ibid.

42. Ibid.

43. American Cancer Society, *Cancer Prevention Study,* 1959–1979, no. 8605 (1979): p. 2.

44. "Air Toxics: How Serious a Threat," *Consumer's Research* (March 1990).

45. Ibid., 21.

46. "Now They Tell Us," *Time,* April 1, 1991, p. 31.

47. J. D. Spengler and K. Sexton, *Science* (July 1, 1983): p. 9.

48. M. Eisenbud, "Levels of Exposure to Sulfur Oxides and Particulates in New York City and Their Sources," *Bulletin of the New York Academy of Medicine* 54 (1978): pp. 9911–11011.

49. Faltermayer, "Air"; "Air Toxics"; "Clean Air Bill Passed by House," *Chemical Marketing Reporter* (May 28, 1990); "Cleaning the Air Can Foul Up the Economy," *The Economist* (February 10, 1990).

50. "Cleaning the Air."

51. Ibid.

52. D. Brock, "Everybody's Smog," *Insight* (February 10, 1992).

53. "Cleaning the Air."

54. "On the Horizon: Cleaner Air," *Consumer Reports* (January 1991), p. 6.

55. A. J. Krupnick and P. R. Portney, "Controlling Urban Air Pollution: A Benefit-Cost Assessment," *Science* 252 (1991): p. 522.

56. S. Kindel, "Profiting From Pollution," *FW* (November 27, 1990): pp. 49–50.

57. C. Lochhead, "Economists Say Federal Rules May Choke U.S. Productivity," *Insight* (November 19, 1990).

58. Krupnick and Portney, "Controlling Urban Air Pollution," p. 523.

59. "Carbon Dioxide Cuts Are Costly, DOE Says," *Chemical Engineering News* (December 16, 1992): p. 12.

60. Krupnik and Portney, "Controlling Urban Air Pollution," p. 524.

61. Ibid., p. 525.

11

Water Pollution: Does It Threaten
Your Life and Health?

There are virtues which become crimes by exaggeration.

—Alexander Dumas, 1841

The Charges

Yet nearly two decades after Congress passed the Safe Drinking Water Act, the water flowing from the nation's taps is anything but pristine. . . . In the early summer, half the rivers and streams in America's Corn Belt are laced with unhealthy levels of pesticides. . . . In enacting the Safe Drinking Water Act in 1974, Congress envisioned a major overhaul of the nation's drinking water supply system. It called on the Environmental Protection Agency to determine what substances were contaminating the nation's drinking water and to assess the potential health effects, establish legal health limits and intervene where the states failed to enforce them. By all accounts, that vision has failed.

—*U.S. News and World Report*[1]

Drinking water in New Orleans, derived from the Mississippi River, contains over 200 synthetic organic pollutants, including a wide range of known chemical carcinogens and many yet unidentified and untested chemicals.

—*The Politics of Cancer*[2]

What looks, tastes, and smells clean enough to drink, but isn't? Boston's water, and the water of thousands of communities across the United States, including New York City, San Francisco, Seattle, Scranton, Pa., and Portland, Maine, according to federal standards.

—The Christian Science Monitor[3]

[There is] little or no effort . . . to prevent, monitor or even note the discharge of toxic chemicals; so the poisons were free to disrupt aquatic food webs, accumulate in fish, birds, and wildlife, or end up as a chemical alphabet soup in a glass of drinking water or the morning cup of coffee of citizens who mistakenly believe their drinking water has been purified.

—Malignant Neglect[4]

Repeated warnings by environmentalists for over a decade have recently been confirmed by various government studies and reports, documenting the contamination of American water supplies and systems with cancer-causing health-destroying chemicals. . . . When the thousands of synthetic chemicals are produced each year for killing insects and other purposes, we end up drinking large amounts of them, since most chemicals introduced into the environment eventually end up in our water supplies. The drinking water of every major American city contains dozens of cancer-causing chemicals and other toxins.

—America the Poisoned[5]

Nearly one in five Americans drink tap water containing excess levels of highly toxic lead.

—U.S. News and World Report[6]

But common sense would lead us to believe that chemicals in our water are dangerous and cause cancer. The incidence of cancer has risen steadily since 1900. . . . More frightening than this present-day rise in cancer is the fact that the disease will probably become much more prevalent in the future; by its very nature cancer takes a long time to develop after exposure to carcinogens. . . .

—Organic Gardening[7]

The Facts

- Water contaminated by bacteria and other infectious organisms, a significant cause of disease and death throughout history, today remains the most important concern as regards water quality around the world.

- The potential for acute chemical poisoning through drinking contaminated water is real. There has been some contamination of groundwater in parts of the United States, and there is just reason to do something to correct this, but no evidence whatsoever exists of any epidemic of health damage caused by contaminated water.

- Traces of cancer-causing chemicals are in our water supply, but the levels at which they are present pose no significant risk of cancer to the human population. To use as an old adage, "It's the dose that makes the poison."

- Although our water does not pose an imminent hazard of causing cancer and other diseases, there is just reason to ensure cleaner, more fishable and swimmable waters. This, however, should be motivated not by the belief that we are faced with a major public health problem, but by the desire to ensure quality, as well as quantity, of water.

The messages we get about the quality of the water we drink are unsettling. We read of "midnight dumping" of toxic wastes into rivers and streams, and of a series of unpronounceable poisons and cancer-causing substances such as asbestos getting into some water supplies. What is the truth about the quality and safety of the water supply of the United States?

Essential for Life

In many ways, the problems and potential problems of water pollution are far more complex than those of air pollution. The physiological necessity of water and the sheer universality of exposure to it, since it is the "sink" or final receptacle for most all of our environmental agents, makes it perhaps our most important health issue.

The pesticides on the farm, the fertilizer on the front lawn, the oil from the old car, and the sewage in the overflowing septic tank all manage to find their way into our vast network of water bodies. The complex process of environmental transport results in the deposition of countless materials in surface water and groundwater supplies.

Although environmental alarmists focus on the quality of water, fearing death and disease from chemical contamination, it is the quantity of water that poses the larger concern. We tend to take water for granted, but indeed it is a precious commodity. As Fred Powledge writes in his book *Water,* "Americans . . . are accustomed to having unlimited supplies of inexpensive clean water at their immediate disposal. It is almost always there whenever we turn on the tap. . . . We have acted as if water were like air—free, so omnipresent as to exist beyond our conscious thought."[8] But water is not free, and not unlimited. Curiously, though, most environmental groups give little or no attention to this aspect of our country's potential water problems.

Water: Above and Below Ground

The water we draw from our taps each day comes from one or two sources. About half of the public water supply comes from surface water: rivers, streams, reservoirs and lakes. The remainder comes from groundwater, mainly from underground geological formations, called aquifers, that can store significant quantities of water. The soils and geological formations contribute dissolved and suspended particles to the water and also serve as a filter to remove contaminants. Sometimes groundwater is clean enough to drink without further treatment, sometimes not.

Ground and surface water have different vulnerabilities to pollutants.

Water and Disease

Contemporary concern about drinking water focuses almost exclusively on developing cancer and other chronic disease from long-term exposure to chemicals in water. In reality, however, the most significant risk today differs little from the risks a century ago: this real, age-old risk is from bacteria and other pathogens that carry waterborne diseases.

Indeed, scientists at least 150 years ago knew that water could cause serious infections. In 1854 John Snow used epidemiological principles to contain a cholera outbreak in London. By looking at the residences of the victims, Snow noticed that the majority clustered around the Broad Street pump, which was the common source of drinking water for people in the neighborhood. Further investigation revealed that untreated sewage was being dumped into the Thames River (the source for the pump) at a location upstream from where the drinking water was drawn.

The principles of water treatment were developed during the latter part of the nineteenth century and the early part of the twentieth. The advent of filtration in the late 1880s brought a dramatic decrease in the incidence of typhoid fever. When chlorine was introduced as a disinfectant in 1908, the incidence of cholera and typhoid diminished even more dramatically.

Water pollution was a very real problem in turn-of-the-century America, but not as we think of it today. Natural pollution, such as that caused by improper sewage disposal and nuisance algae blooms, were typical issues of the day. But by 1924 there was growing concern that our nation's streams should also be kept safe from industrial waste discharge. In the July 1924 issue of *American City and County,* J. Frederick Jackson of the Connecticut Department of Health outlined the dangers facing the quality of freshwater streams because of continual dumping of industrial wastes. Fishermen were upset as fish began disappearing from many favorite fishing sites. Industrialists, on the other hand, argued that the waterways provided the best sink to dispose of all types of wastes. The public generally favored working out a compromise but it was demanding concessions from the dischargers. Jackson cited investigations showing the benefits of waste treatment for bringing effluents within acceptable limits for discharge.[9]

Interestingly, the concerns of people like Fred Jackson parallel some of our present water-pollution concerns. There was a need for give and take between the parties arguing the extremes. He addressed the importance of educating the public about the seriousness of the issue. Today the public is aware of the urgency of this matter, but is it aware for the right reasons?

Warnings about our waning water supply began much before the environmental movement of the 1970s. In 1959 futurist author Alvin B. Toffler wrote of the necessity to conserve and protect our water:

> Experts warn that unless we stop the reckless practice of pouring filth into our rivers and streams, we simply won't have enough clean water for our needs. . . . The time has come to mount an all-out effort to protect our water supply. Every citizen can play a vital part.[10]

Toffler was not alone in his assessment of the problem posed by water pollution. Bernard B. Berger, chief of the Water Supply and Water Pollution Research Branch at the Sanitary Engineering Center in Cincinnati, was quoted in *U.S. News & World Report* as saying, "The burden on water is increasing. . . . It's going to take a lot of effort just to stay even with the problem. . . ."[11] Citizens like Toffler and Berger were expressing a legitimate cause for both public and scientific interest. A few of the contamination episodes at the time included:

- Passaic, Clifton, Nutley, and Harrison, New Jersey, had to switch to alternative sources of water after Passaic River pollution killed thousands of fish.

- Baker, Colorado, residents complained about the poor-tasting water they were getting. It was then discovered that the creek from which the water was drawn was fed raw sewage from six upstream communities.

- The U.S. Department of Health, Education, and Welfare reported that "approximately 30,000 persons in southwestern Colorado and northwestern New Mexico were using Animas River water that ranged 40 to 160 percent above maximum permissible levels of radioactive content."[12]

Although waterborne diseases affect a relatively small percentage of America's water systems, the problem of waterborne disease in this country far surpasses that of chemical contamination. When there are sporadic outbreaks (see below), they are largely as a result of an accident in treatment, an error by a water plant operator, an equipment malfunction, or the use of water that has not been disinfected. But in the developing world, waterborne agents, which contaminate water largely via fecal waste, represent a major public health problem. Typhoid fever, bacillary dysentery, and cholera are just a few of the agents that cause illness and early death.

A cholera epidemic, in fact, hit parts of South America in the early 1990s, affecting 158,000 people per three-month period and killing 1,140 people in the first months of the epidemic. Experts estimated that three million Brazilians would also be affected in 1991. The epidemic is linked to improper water disinfection, which is said to be forty years behind the times in these South American countries.[13]

In the United States, there were 261 outbreaks of waterborne disease between 1978 and 1984, involving 72,000 illnesses.[14] Unfortunately, there has been a steady increase in the number of waterborne disease outbreaks since the 1960s.[15]

Many infections occur in water supplies the public thinks are the safest. Pristine mountain streams are perceived as "pure" and "natural," but they are easily polluted by microscopic organisms from animal excrement. Water from mountain streams should be disinfected as stringently as water from any other source intended for human consumption. The EPA stresses that infections caused by contaminated water occur exclusively in water systems in violation of current microbiological standards.

The type of pathogen causing this disease has changed dramatically since the turn of the century. Early in the 1900s diseases associated with drinking water were largely due to bacteria. Today, viruses and protozoa dominate the picture. The largest contributor is the protozoa *Giardia lamblia;* other contributors include the Norwalk Virus and the hepatitis A virus. Some data indicate that these pathogens are less susceptible to inactivation by chlorine than are bacteria.[16] New laws have been enacted to deal with these nonbacterial water pathogens.

Specifically, the 1986 amendments to the Safe Drinking Water Act addressed this increase in waterborne diseases due to viruses and protozoa.[17] All public water systems using surface water or groundwater under the direct influence of surface water must filter and then disinfect water (unless certain water-quality source requirements and site-specific conditions are met).

The associated cost savings of filtering to prevent a community outbreak are much larger than can be measured. "You have to look beyond the cost of simply preventing the disease in the people who would be affected. The costs are larger than their medical costs. You have to consider the whole community's costs of boiling water, buying bottled water and remediating what caused the outbreak," says Stig Regli of the EPA's Office of Drinking Water.

The EPA says that certain systems already do filter water, and they are known to have one-tenth the chance of having an outbreak than are nonfiltering systems.

Chemicals and Water Treatment

Many people are very concerned that the conventional water-treatment chemicals fluoride and chlorine are causing cancer and other diseases. To be sure, there have been accidental poisonings—for example, the acute fluoride poisoning that occurred in New Mexico in 1978. A malfunction in the fluoridation system resulted in approximately thirty-four illnesses.[18] Events like this are exceedingly rare, and scientific, medical, and dental communities overwhelmingly support the addition of fluorides (up to approximately 1 ppm) to reduce the incidence of dental caries, particularly among children.

Despite the unquestionable efficacy of fluoridation in strengthening teeth and preventing cavities, nearly 40 percent of tap water in the United States remains unfluoridated. Misguided antifluoridation activists have persuaded some local governments and voters to reject fluoridation. They claim fluoride causes cancer, sickle cell anemia, Down's syndrome, and even AIDS. To date, however, there is no scientific evidence that properly fluoridated water has ever caused an adverse health effect.[19]

One of the major public health accomplishments of this century is the addition of chlorine to our water. Chlorination drastically reduced the U.S. typhoid mortality rate[20] and is credited for reducing all types of waterborne diseases. Treatment with chlorine is effective primarily because as a disinfectant it successfully kills sufficient numbers of bacteria and other pathogenic organisms to prevent human infection. A further advantage of chlorine disinfection is the presence of a residual. That means that a small amount of chlorine remains in the water after the treatment is completed to provide disinfection throughout the system, ensuring high efficiency in removing pathogens.

The amount of chlorine added to water is dependent on several factors, most importantly the level of bacterial contamination. Filtration reduces bacteria levels, thereby reducing chlorine demand. The water source is also important. Since groundwater has relatively fewer bacteria and suspended solids than does surface water, it generally requires significantly less (or no) chlorination than does surface water.

Concern about chlorination arose in the early 1970s, when scientists discovered that byproducts such as chloroform and other trihalomethanes (THMs) are formed in the process.[21] Chlorine reacts with some natural organic material, such as humic acids (from decaying leaves and grass in the sediment), to form THMs, of which there are ten varieties.[22] Subsequent studies revealed the presence of chloroform in almost every chlorinated water supply. Concern mounted after high-dose animal studies at the National Cancer Institute (NCI) demonstrated a carcinogenic effect of chloroform.[23] In 1992, the NCI released the results of extensive studies confirming an association between drinking chlorinated water and the risk of developing bladder and rectal cancer.[24] According to their June 30, 1992, report, 18 percent of approximately 8,100 cases of rectal cancer each year can be attributed to drinking chlorinated water, as can 9 percent, or 4,644 cases, of bladder cancer. In contrast, say experts at NCI, the more significant causes of bladder cancer are cigarette smoking and occupational exposures, responsible for 70 percent of such cancers in men and 40 percent in women.

But the most critical perspective lies in considering the consequences of not chlorinating water. The World Health Organization estimates that twenty-five thousand people die each day from diseases carried by inadequately sanitized water; in a year, that amounts to 9.1 million deaths. This risk of death from not chlorinating water, then, is of gargantuan proportions when compared with the chances of contracting cancer from drinking chlorinated water. One must also bear in mind that although contracting cancer may be devastating, many cancers—including rectal and bladder cancers—are treatable or even curable.

Several drinking water experts reiterate the thought that not chlorinating water has far worse consequences than chlorinating. Stig Regli, an engineer in the EPA's Office of Drinking Water, says,

> There are indeed risks to chlorinating water, but we have to consider the risks of not chlorinating. When we set the standards for the amounts of chlorination by-products in water, we do so very conservatively. That is, we project for cancer to the point that at most one person in 100,000 may have a lifetime risk of getting cancer. Again this is an extremely conservative estimate, and we know with certainty that there would be far greater morbidity and mortality from not chlorinating water.[25]

Jack Sullivan, deputy executive director for government affairs at the American Waterworks Association agrees that this issue must be considered from a risk-management perspective:

> We most certainly have to balance the possible chronic health risks of chlorinating with the known acute risks of not chlorinating. The risk of microbiological contamination is far too great to make a snap decision about changing the maximum contaminant level of trihalomethanes in water. It will be some time before a new ruling is made. We are confident that the existing rule is adequate at this point in time.[26]

The American Cancer Society issued a statement on water chlorination in August 1981, saying:

> [There] may be an indication of human carcinogenicity from water chlorination. The evidence is indirect and the level of increased risk is not great. Further observations are needed to be more certain that other cancer risk factors in the population (cigarette smoking, other chemical exposures) have been adequately accounted for in such studies.[27]

There are engineering methods that effectively reduce the amount of chlorination byproducts formed. The most effective way of reducing chlorination is to reduce the organic matter in water before chlorinating. This is done by filtering water through activated charcoal. A limited number of water treatment plants already use this technology and have effectively lowered the amount of THMs and other chlorination byproducts.

It seems prudent to continue the research into the potential health effects of chlorination byproducts, but also to remember that not chlorinating water would be far more threatening to health.

Groundwater Pollution

Groundwater was once thought to be virtually immune from contamination. In the late 1960s, however, synthetic organic chemicals were discovered in groundwater sources of drinking water in several states, with increasing discoveries of such contamination made in the 1970s.

There are a number of ways through which groundwater becomes contaminated, including the infiltration of polluted surface water, improper disposal of hazardous wastes (that is, from unlined lagoons), septic and on-site wastewater systems overflow, through malfunctions allowing entrance of bacteria, accidental spills and leaks, improper animal waste disposal, and mining wastes. Contaminants found in groundwater include a wide spectrum of pollutants. Inorganic ions (chloride, nitrate, heavy metals), synthetic organic chemicals (pesticides), and pathogens (bacteria, viruses, parasites) have all been found in American groundwater. Once contaminated, groundwater by its very nature is difficult to clean up. Sometimes polluted groundwater can be filtered through an activated charcoal filter. Many times, however, an entire aquifer or series of aquifers must be temporarily or permanently closed in response to contamination.

Water: Above and Below Ground

GROUNDWATER

Most of the media and magazine coverage of groundwater pollution has centered around the episodes where industrial chemicals, pesticides, and gasoline have been the invaders of once pristine drinking-water wells. Examples of such incidents include:

- A state of Michigan report released in 1979 listed 268 contaminated sites (83 percent by hazardous substance, oil, or gas) and suspected contamination in 381 sites; potentially polluting activity has or is taking place at over 50,000 sites. Determining the extent of the pollution will cost from $2.9 million to $46.1 million.[28]

- Organic chemical contamination forced the closing of nearly one hundred drinking-water wells in Jackson Township, New Jersey, in 1972. Chemicals found included benzene and trichloroethylene (TCE).[29]

- Bedford, Massachusetts, lost four wells supplying 80 percent of its drinking water when they were found to be contaminated with up to 500 ppb TCE and 2,000 ppb dioxane.[30]

- A shallow aquifer outside of Denver was contaminated when chemical wastes infiltrated into the groundwater from unlined holding ponds.[31]

- Gray, Maine, was the site of sixteen well closings in 1977 because of contamination from a number of chemicals. They were located near a facility that processed waste oil from a tanker spill. Municipal water lines were extended at a cost of $500,000.[32]

- Groundwater in the San Joaquin Valley was contaminated with the pesticide DBCP. According to state health department employee John Gaston, approximately 35 percent of the wells in the valley have been affected.[33]

- In Battle Creek, Michigan, fourteen city wells and eighty private wells were closed due to the presence of vinyl chloride, TCE, and benzene.[34]

- In Perham, Minnesota, eleven of thirteen people who drank from a well became ill from arsenic poisoning. During the 1930s, an arsenic-treated pesticide was buried in the area. When the well was tapped in 1972, the arsenic became a health hazard.[35]

• During the summer of 1978, Elkhart County, Indiana, residents were alarmed to find their water coated with an oily substance. The EPA was called to investigate. Several volatile organic compounds were found. The source is believed to be a leak in an ARCO pipe some dozen years earlier. The groundwater flow presumably brought the chemicals to the water supply of the affected neighborhood.[36]

While acknowledging, however, that chemical contamination of our water supply can cause acute health problems (that is, can cause people to become ill shortly after drinking it), we must keep some perspective here. Between 1978 and 1984, there were a total of 261 waterborne disease outbreaks involving approximately 72,000 people. Only a minute fraction was traced to chemical contamination. In 1984, for example just 1 percent of cases was due to chemical contamination. The overwhelmingly vast majority were from naturally occurring pathogens like those that cause gastroenteritis.[37] There is no evidence whatsoever of any epidemic of health damage from contaminated water in the United States.

A classic and reassuring example is the contamination of wells serving Woburn, Massachusetts. Unfortunately, some wells did have to be closed permanently because of contamination by industrial discharge. This is disconcerting, and we certainly would like to prevent further episodes of groundwater contamination. However, several independent studies failed to prove that exposure to the water was responsible for childhood leukemia, the main allegation, or any other illness.[38]

The important point to remember in all instances of accidental water contamination is that there is a thorough inspection system in every municipal water system to detect contaminants. So, while contamination can occur because of an accident or because of carelessness, a complex water treatment and testing process ensures that contamination will be detected. The polluted aquifer or stream can then be treated or actually diverted from the water supply, protecting all consumers.

To prevent further loss of aquifers or surface water sources because of chemical contamination, and to prevent future waterborne disease outbreaks, it is imperative to protect groundwater via compulsive regulation. Currently, groundwater in this country is protected by eight separate pieces of legislation: the Safe Drinking Water Act;"[39] the Clean Water Act;[40] the Resource Conservation and Recovery Act;[41] the Federal Insecticide, Fungicide, and Rodenticide Act;[42] the Toxic Substances Control Act;[43] the Surface Mining Control and Reclamation Act;[44] the Comprehensive Environmental Response, Compensation and Liability Act ("Superfund");[45] the Food Security Act; and the Uranium Mill Trailings Radiation Control Act of 1978.[46] In 1992, the EPA issued final regulations for twenty-three additional chemicals, bringing the total number of drinking water standards to eighty-four. These regulations will be enforced beginning in 1993.[47]

The total annual cost of complying with this regulation, including costs for treatment, testing, and monitoring, is expected to be about $46 million.[48] In addition, EPA estimates that another $150 billion will be required to make the necessary infrastructure repairs to bring U.S. systems up to the new standards.[49] The Office of Management and Budget (OMB) says that EPA's risk assessments used to determine these new drinking water standards are too conservative. OMB says that the new regulations go beyond health protection and result in excessive costs for treatment. Using antimony as an example, the agency says EPA has set a contaminant level 150,000 times more stringent than the level at which laboratory rats experience toxic effects. As a result, says OMB, annual household water bills could increase from $534 to $3,651, with higher costs incurred by smaller systems that have more work to do to come into compliance with these new regulations. The EPA responded to these allegations, saying that it does not have to consider cost effectiveness.[50]

Historically, the laws did provide a framework for protecting groundwater, but the overall approach was ambiguous and confusing. In 1984, the EPA administrator convened a task force to develop a groundwater strategy to identify the issues clearly and to deliver a more integrated approach. The Groundwater Protection Strategy adopted in 1984 made great strides in ensuring the quality of groundwater. Further efforts in this regard were strengthened in 1989 with the formation of the Groundwater Task Force.[51] In addition to this greatly improved coordination at the national level, many states have made great individual strides towards protecting their drinking water.

As mentioned earlier in the chapter, our concern about our water supply must include the availability of water. The quantity of groundwater is diminishing at an alarming rate in some parts of the country. Along the Gulf Coast, in the Southwest, and in California, water mining has caused a vast reduction in the supply of available groundwater. Water mining is a process by which water is pumped out of the ground at a rate faster than it is replenished. Aquifers such as the Ogalala under the Western plains are dropping rapidly. Computer projections have estimated that the groundwater table in Houston[52] will drop fourteen feet over the next forty years. In Phoenix, fissures as deep as four hundred feet split the earth. Craters have also occurred in parts of Florida where the earth has "dried up." The resource known as groundwater is simply not infinite. It must be preserved and used wisely in the future.

SURFACE WATER

Surface water, as its name indicates, refers to water above ground. Surface water is more vulnerable to contamination than groundwater, and there have been more cases of accidental spills, with resultant human disease and death. As mentioned earlier, industrial dumping of mercury into Japan's Minimata Bay and Agano River in the 1950s and 1960s led to the poisoning of large populations of fish, a local food staple. Many residents ingested the fish for some time before the contamination was discovered. As a result, there was widespread mercury poisoning, with symptoms ranging from memory loss and nervous disorders to blindness and death.

In this country, industrial polluting with PCBs (see chapter 5) and kepone (see chapter 4) has led to fishing bans because of pollutant levels found in fish tissue.

Surface waters are regulated by the Clean Water Act. Industrial dischargers must be granted a permit before they can legally discharge effluents into a body of water.

In general, great strides have been made in cleaning up our nation's streams, rivers, and lakes. However, many bodies of water are still suffering serious pollution episodes. Some examples are:

- Triana, Alabama, where the Centers for Disease Control tested blood from local residents in 1979 and found that 25 percent had five times the national average level of PCB and ten times the average level of DDT. Indian Creek, a tributary of the Tennessee River, was contaminated with the same pollutants. The source was a nearby U.S. Army missile base where four thousand tons of chemicals were left in a swamp.[53]

- In 1974 the EPA discovered that New Orleans water contained measurable amounts of sixty-six chemical compounds. The Mississippi River is the source of New Orleans drinking water.[54]

- The General Accounting Office listed twenty miles of Colorado streams as being void of all aquatic life in 1978. The cause—drainage from area mining.[55]

- For approximately twenty-five years the Reserve Mining Company in Northern Minnesota dumped tailings (leftover debris) into Lake Superior. Many pollutants were in the discharge, including asbestos, which is a proven carcinogen when inhaled. The company agreed to foot the bill to filter drinking water for Duluth, Minnesota, and three other towns at a cost close to $1.9 million during the early 1980s.[56]

Dumping of toxic chemicals—even at approved levels—into our water supply does not sound very appetizing, to say the least. The problem with toxic wastes in surface water is largely one of unsightly appearance, cost to consumers for cleanup, and impact on recreation. The Clean Water Act was enacted in 1972 with a goal of rendering all waters "fishable and swimmable" by 1983. When it was reauthorized in 1986, that goal had not been realized by a majority of the states.

During the first fifteen years of the national program to clean up and control water pollution under the Clean Water Act, attention was focused on "point sources." These include municipal and industrial discharges into rivers and lakes. The widespread and costly improvements in sewage treatment and in controlling industrial wastes, however, failed to effect large improvements in water quality. Clearly identified as the main obstacle in further improvements is nonpoint source pollution.[57]

Nonpoint sources include runoff from agricultural practices, such as excess fertilizer, pesticides, and animal waste; urban stormwater runoff, including road salt, soil, lawn, and garden chemicals; acid mine drainage; bacteria and nutrients from livestock, pet wastes, and faulty septic systems; and sediment and byproducts from timber, construction, and excavation activity. In 1987, the Clean Water Act was amended by the Water Quality Act specifically to address nonpoint source pollution. In 1989, the first federal money—$40 million—was appropriated for nonpoint source pollution.

Considerable controversy arose when the Clean Water Act came up for reauthorization in 1992, and some experts predicted it would not be funded. Competing for limited resources is the Resource Conservation and Recovery ACT. Opponents point to the fact that the U.S. has spent nearly $590 billion (in 1990 dollars) on water pollution control under this law since 1972, without reaching the goal of zero discharge of pollutants into U.S. waters. Revisions expected in the 1992 rewrite include a water conservation section but no wetlands protection provision.

It strengthens water quality standards by requiring EPA to publish criteria for conventional, nonconventional, and toxic pollutants needed to protect human health and ecosystems, including sediments. It also establishes several new grants programs, including $3 billion for a program to help states control nonpoint source pollution, and $2.5 billion for a program addressing the problem of combined sewer overflows. Finally, it requires EPA to develop a plan for using Superfund's Toxic Release Inventory data to develop effluent guidelines, verify discharge permits, and target enforcement.[58]

Is Our Water Polluted With Lead?

At toxic doses, lead causes severe adverse health effects. Recent reports about lead, however, have been confusing. These reports indicate that there may be subtle biochemical changes occurring at lower levels of lead in the body than previously thought. The significance of these subtle changes is not known. But this doesn't mean that lead levels are increasing in air, food, or water. In fact, these levels are decreasing.

In November 1986 it was announced that one in five Americans was consuming water with lead at toxic levels.[59] However, the EPA report[60] from which these news accounts originated was based on outdated figures from an unidentified number of tap water samples. These figures were then used to project the possible number of people exposed to lead in drinking water— yielding an unreliable conclusion.

Some homeowners do have a problem with excessive lead in their drinking water. However, the problem is due to contamination within the home, not from water supplies or the water company. Many older homes have lead pipes, and many new homes, built prior to June 1986, have copper pipes soldered with lead. Soft and acidic water tends to leach metals, including lead, into water.[61] Water coolers, with their lead soldered pipes, have also been identified as a lead source. To be sure, it is not the water supply but rather materials inside individual homes that cause the problem. Unfortunately, consumers today still read alarming accounts of how drinking water is contaminated with lead, without these qualifying remarks.[62]

In 1992, in fact, critics claimed that the EPA was not doing its job in protecting the quality of drinking water, saying that 42 million Americans— among them 250,000 children—were drinking harmful levels of lead in their drinking water. This stems from EPA's tightening up of standards for allowable levels of lead in drinking water, decreasing the standard from 50 ppb (parts per billion) to 15 ppb.[63] But administrators of state and local water companies say they cannot afford to keep pace with EPA's evolving standards—which, we might add, may be more than necessary to protect human health.

Does Polluted Water Cause Cancer?

A review of recent popular books, articles, and newspaper stories clearly reveals that the primary consumer concern about water is whether or not drinking water causes cancer.

Theoretically, it is possible that a water supply could contain enough cancer-causing agents to increase cancer risk in a population exposed to it for a lifetime. For example, our experience with the radium dial workers indicates that human beings ingesting large quantities of radioactive material (in this case, swallowing the paint used to create luminescent watch dials) had a significantly higher rate of bone cancer. Thus, for example, if our water supply was contaminated with sufficiently higher quantities of radium, it seems likely that this would elevate cancer mortality. The questions, then, are, Are there carcinogens in our water supply? If so, are they there at high enough levels to cause cancer?

Given the fact that we now have analytical techniques that permit us to detect chemicals at concentrations well below one part per billion (that is the equivalent of one square foot in thirty-six square miles, one bad apple in two million barrels, or one pinch of salt in ten tons of potato chips), the answer to the question of whether we can detect carcinogens in our water supply is yes. The carcinogens we speak of here are those that cause cancer in laboratory experiments—and, in at least one case, a substance that has been shown to cause cancer when inhaled by humans, namely, asbestos. The more important question for practical effect is, At what level do these carcinogens occur and what is the evidence linking them to cancer?

The level of carcinogens in the American water supply is extremely low and, according to most public health experts, poses no significant risk of cancer to the human population. Doll and Peto, in their classic work *The Causes of Cancer,* looked at the question of water pollution and cancer and concluded, "It is not plausible that any material percentage of the total number of cancers in the whole United States derives from this source."[64]

One concern that they did have was the presence of asbestos in some local water supplies; for example, those of New Orleans. Asbestos, as reviewed in chapter 8, has been clearly shown to increase risk of lung cancer, mesothelioma, and other diseases when inhaled, and there is the suggestion that some asbestos workers were at greater risk of gastrointestinal cancer because of ingestion of dust through the respiratory passages. Furthermore, asbestos fibers are present in varying concentrations in surface waters (and subsequently drinking waters) around the country. They enter water supplies mainly from construction products such as cement and from mining activities, as noted in the previously mentioned case of Duluth, Minnesota.

Schottenfeld and Fraumeni, in what is considered the essential textbook on cancer epidemiology, *Cancer Epidemiology and Prevention,* reviewed the literature available on asbestos exposure from water and concluded that "most epidemiologic studies of populations served by water containing high concentrations of asbestos have failed to yield . . . conclusive results [of an association between asbestos in water and cancer]."[65] Stating that some evidence suggests a positive correlation between asbestos and cancer, the authors recommend continued research in this area.

There is some evidence that drinking water with high levels of the metal arsenic may cause skin cancer. It is based mainly on studies conducted in Taiwan, where waters contain arsenic in much higher concentrations than do those in the United States. Schottenfeld and Fraumeni state, "On the basis of existing evidence, it is not possible to conclude that arsenic, or any other metal present in drinking water, causes cancer in humans by ingestion of ambient trace amounts. However, the broad distribution of these metals in drinking water indicates a need for further study in this area."[66]

Experts on a committee at the National Cancer Institute led by Herman Kraybill, Ph.D., are compulsively studying the water/cancer connection. The committee said there are too many uncontrolled variants to draw any conclusions. They concluded:

> While the experimental and epidemiologic studies provide some presumptive evidence, one cannot establish, with any degree of assurance as yet, any causality relevant to cancer from these micropollutants. There is serious concern, however, about those contaminants with the realization that [they] may contribute to the total cancer burden. Thus, control and reduction technologies in water treatment are recommended.[67]

The water/cancer question challenges science for two main reasons. First, it is difficult to detect and measure trace contaminants. Second, science doesn't understand how such contaminants work together, or cancel each other, in the process of causing cancer. Future study can and will supply answers to many of the unknowns that cloud the picture today. But the evidence that has been collected to date clearly refutes the claim that we as a society are subject to a dangerous risk of cancer from drinking water.

Should I Switch to Bottled Water?

Americans drank three times as much bottled water in 1986 as they did in 1976. This consumption continues to increase. There is, however, no scientific evidence that bottled water is healthier than water direct from your tap, except when your tap is known to be contaminated at unhealthy levels. All water comes from the same places: wells, rivers, streams, or springs. Some bottled water comes from springs, but most comes from the same public water supply as tap water.

Whether bottled or from the tap, all water must meet strict bacteriological standards. This is where the similarity often ends. Public water supplies are usually disinfected with chlorine gas or chloramines, which may impart an objectionable taste to the water. Most bottled water companies, on the other hand, use ozone (a form of oxygen) for disinfecting. Ozone is more expensive, but is often more desirable to consumers because it leaves no aftertaste. Ozone, however, is less stable than chlorine and less potent as a long-term disinfectant. Bottled water held for long periods may, therefore, be at risk for contamination. In 1985, tests conducted on bottled water at the Santa Clara Water District's Rinconada Water Treatment Plant found that the bacteria levels in randomly sampled bottled water were between 5 to 2,300 times greater than in the public water supply.

A 1992 analysis of thirty-seven bottled waters found that twenty-four were out of line with one or more requirements of the U.S. drinking water standards. The study's authors, of the University of Delaware, Drexel University, and Mobay Corporation, said of the results, "It is unlikely that a survey of community water supplies would find as high a degree of noncompliance. Maybe we'd all be better off drinking tap water!"[68]

Bottled water suppliers sometimes use misleading promotional literature. Remember that despite claims to the contrary, the chemicals added to filter and disinfect public drinking water make it safer, not less healthful. Don't be misled by overly ambitious marketing strategies. Since there is no evidence that bottled water is healthier than tap water, the decision to use bottled water should be based solely on taste, mineral composition, cost, and personal convenience.

Conclusion

Fortunately, we in America are acutely aware that we must protect both the quantity and quality of our drinking water supplies. Luckily, too, water pollution has abated during the past decade. But there are still many projects to carry out and dollars to spend before we attain the Clean Water Act's goal of "fishable and swimmable" waters throughout the country. It is imperative that we attack these issues with clarity of mind and our purpose well established, not in a state of hysterical confusion over a public health risk that does not in fact exist.

NOTES

1. B. Carpenter, "Is Your Water Safe?" *U.S. News and World Report,* July 29, 1991, p. 48.

2. S. Epstein, *The Politics of Cancer* (San Francisco: Sierra Club Books, 1987), p. 34.

3. E. A. Brown, "New U.S. Standards Squeeze Cities, States," *The Christian Science Monitor,* February 5, 1991.

4. Environmental Defense Fund and Robert H. Boyle, *Malignant Neglect* (New York: Alfred A. Knopf, 1979), p. 84.

5. L. Regenstein, *America the Poisoned* (Washington: Acropolis Books, 1982), p. 169.

6. *U.S. News and World Report,* November 24, 1986.

7. C. Keough, "The Slow Poisoning of Our Water," *Organic Gardening* (March 1990): p. 139.

8. F. Powledge, *Water: The Nature, Uses and Future of Our Most Precious and Abused Resource* (New York: Farrar, Straus and Giroux, 1982), p. 3.

9. J. F. Jackson, "Stream Pollution by Industrial Wastes and Its Control," *American City and Country* (July 1924): pp. 23–26.

10. A. B. Toffler, "Danger in Your Drinking Water," *Reader's Digest,* March 1960, pp. 82–83.

11. "How Pure is Your City Water?" *U.S. News and World Report,* February 29, 1960, pp. 52–54.

12. Toffler, "Danger in Your Drinking Water," pp. 81–82.

13. J. Brooke, "Feeding on 19th Century Conditions, Cholera Spreads in Latin America," *New York Times,* April 24, 1991.

14. National Research Council, *Drinking Water and Health,* vol. 7 (Washington, D.C.: 1987).

15. L. Harter et al., "A Three-State Study of Waterborne Disease Surveillance Techniques," *American Journal of Epidemiology* 109 (1979): p. 364.

16. National Research Council, *Drinking Water and Health,* pp. 14–24.

17. 54 *Federal Register* 27486.

18. G. F. Craun, "Disease Outbreak, Caused by Drinking Water," *Journal of Water Pollution Control Federation* 53 (1981): p. 1134.

19. National Research Council, *Drinking Water and Health,* vol. 1, 1977; vol. 2, 1980; vol. 3, 1980; vol. 4, 1982; vol. 5, 1983; WHO, *Guidelines for Drinking Water,* vol. 2, *Health Criteria and Other Supporting Information* (Geneva: WHO, 1984); M. C. Mahoney, P. C. Masca, W. S. Burnett, and J. M. Melius, "Bone Cancer Incidence Rates in New York State: Time Trends and Flouridated Drinking Water," *American Journal of Public Health* 81 (1991): pp. 475–79.

20. K. P. Cantor, "Epidemiological Evidence of Carcinogenicity of Chlorinated Organics in Drinking Water," *Environmental Health Prospectives* 46 (1982): p. 187.

21. T. A. Bellar et al., "Asbestos Bodies in Lung Parenchyma in Relation to Ingestion and Inhalation of Mineral Fibers," *Environmental Research* 14 (1977): p. 286; J. J. Rook, "Formation of Haloforms During Chlorination of Natural Waters," *Journal of Society Water Treatment and Examination* 23 (1974): p. 234.

22. 52 *Federal Register* 25726, July 8, 1987.

23. Cantor, "Epidemiological Evidence of Carcinogenicity."

24. "Chlorinated Drinking Water and Cancer Risk," National Cancer Institute press release, June 30, 1992.

25. Personal communication, Jack Sullivan, deputy executive director for government affairs, American Waterworks Association, November 1, 1990.

26. Personal communication, Stig Regli, Environmental Protection Agency, October 30, 1990.

27. American Cancer Society, *Cancer Response System, #2678,* August 8, 1991.

28. D. E. Burmaster and R. H. Harris, "Groundwater Contamination: An Emerging Threat," *Technology Review* (July 1982): p. 56.

29. Ibid.

30. Ibid.

31. Ibid.

32. Ibid.

33. "How Safe Is Your Water?" *Newsweek,* November 1, 1982, pp. 89–90.

34. Ibid.

35. National Water Well Association, *Ground Water Pollution Control* (undated pamphlet).

36. Northern Indiana Health Systems Agency, *A Search for Safe Drinking Water,* August 1981.

37. National Research Council, *Drinking Water and Health,* vol. 7.

38. J. W. Grisham, *Health Aspects of Disposable Waste Chemicals* (New York: Pergamon Press, 1986), pp. 300–302.

39. 42 U.S.C. section 300f–300 j–10.

40. 33 U.S.C. sections 1251–1387.

41. 42 U.S.C. sections 690i–699k.

42. 7 U.S.C. sections 136–136y.

43. 15 U.S.C. sections 2601–2629.

44. 30 U.S.C. sections 12010–1328.

45. 42 U.S.C. sections 9601–9675.

46. 42 U.S.C. sections 7901–7925.

47. D. Hanson, "Drinking Water Limits Set for 23 More Compounds," *Chemical and Engineering News* (June 1, 1992).

48. Ibid., p. 19.

49. J. Dimeo, "Drinking Water Regs Draw Comment," *American City and Country,* August 1991.

50. Hanson, 1992, p. 19.

51. USEPA, "Progress in Groundwater Protection and Restoration" (Washington, D.C. 1990).

52. *National Wildlife,* February/March 1983, p. 36.

53. *National Wildlife,* August/September 1980, p. 33.

54. Powledge, *Water,* p. 216.

55. K. Barton., "The Other Water Pollution," *Environment,* June 1987, p. 15.

56. Powledge, *Water,* p. 216.

57. 55 *Federal Register* 35248.

58. L. R. Ember, "Clean Water Act Is Sailing a Choppy Course to Renewal," *Chemical and Engineering News* (February 17, 1992): pp. 18–21.

59. M. Weisskopf, "Dangerous Amounts of Lead in Much Drinking Water, EPA Says," *Washington Post,* November 6, 1986; S. Wellborn, "Pouring Lead From the Tap," *U.S. News and World Report,* November 24, 1986.

60. USEPA, "Reducing Lead in Drinking Water: A Benefit Analysis," draft final report EPA 230-09-86-019, December 1986.

61. P. D. Elwood et al., "Hardness of Domestic Water and Blood Lead Levels," *Human Toxicology* 2 (1983): p. 645; T. D. B. Lyon et al., "Corrosion in Solder Jointing Copper Tubes Resulting in Lead Contamination of Drinking Water," *British Corrosion Journal* 12 (1977): p. 41; M. R. Moore, "Influence of Acid Rain Upon Water Plumbo-solvency," *Environmental Health Prospectives* 63 (1985): p. 121; W. N. Richards et al., "Lead Hazard Controlled in Scottish Water Systems," *Journal of the American*

Water Works Association 76 (1984): p. 60; J. C. Sherlock et al., "Reduction in Exposure to Lead from Drinking Water and Its Effect on Blood Lead Concentrations," *Human Toxicology* 3 (1984): p. 383; H. F. Thomas, "Domestic Water Usage and Blood Lead Levels," *Public Health* (London) 94 (1980): p. 294.

62. B. Carpenter, "Is Your Water Safe?" *U.S. News and World Report,* July 29, 1991, pp. 48–55; *Consumer Reports,* January 1990, pp. 30–31.

63. Dimeo, "Drinking Water Regs Draw Comment."

64. R. Doll and R. Peto, *The Causes of Cancer* (New York: Oxford Press, 1981), p. 1249.

65. D. Schottenfeld and J. F. Fraumeni, *Cancer Epidemiology and Prevention,* (Philadelphia: W. B. Saunders, 1982), p. 350.

66. Schottenfeld and Fraumeni, *Cancer Epidemiology.*

67. H. F. Kraybill, "Evaluation of Public Health Aspects of Carcinogenic/Mutagenic Biorefractories in Drinking Water," *Preventive Medicine* 9 (1980): p. 212.

68. Newscripts, "Bottled Water Analysis Makes Interesting Reading," *Chemical and Engineering News* (December 16, 1991).

12

Does "No Nukes" Mean Better Health?

How extraordinary! The richest, longest-lived, best protected, most resource-
ful civilization . . is on its way to becoming the most frightened. Chicken
Little is alive and well in America. Is it our environment or ourselves that
have changed? . . . There are risks from numerous small dams far exceeding those from nuclear reactors. Why is the one feared and not the others?
Is it just that we are used to the old or are some of us looking differently
at essentially the same sorts of experience?

—Aaron Wildavsky, 1979

Nothing in life is to be feared; it is to be understood.

—Madame Marie Curie

The Charges

Any dose of radiation is an overdose.

—Dr. George Wald[1]

The truth is that we are courting catastrophe. The permissive policy supported by the American government in effect turns us into guinea pigs in
an experiment to determine how much radioactive material can be released
into the environment before major epidemics of cancer, leukemia and genetic
abnormalities take their toll.

—*What You Can Do! Nuclear Madness*[2]

Good evening. The world has never known a day quite like today. It faced
the considerable uncertainties and dangers of the worst nuclear power plant

361

accident of the atomic age. And the horror tonight is that it could get much worse.

—Walter Cronkite
"CBS Evening News," 30 March 1979[3]

During the accident at Three Mile Island, a hundred thousand people were almost exposed to excessive doses of radiation, because men in power within both the private and public sectors, through fear, greed or incompetence, put politics, economics or pride before the public health and safety.

—Mark Stephens
Three Mile Island[4]

The nuclear industry has been killing people every day for years in the form of cancer leukemia deaths for the workers, and because we haven't declared the workers to be lepers, we let them procreate and thus they spread their radiation damage into the population at large.

—Dr. John W. Gofman[5]

Among the most rapidly growing diseases today are AIDS, Chronic Epstein Barr Virus, Lyme disease, *Candida Albicans,* herpes, septicemia and several other immune-deficiency ailments mentioned. . . . The rise of these maladies in recent years, particularly among people born in the nuclear age, may be related to the huge amounts of low-level radiation released since 1945.

—*Deadly Deceit*[6]

But most of us have not really comprehended how pervasive the nuclear threat has become. Worldwide there are about 340 nuclear power plants, and that could grow by century's end to 600, each holding a deadly threat. . . . Even while the awesome force of the atom spreads, we still do not fully comprehend its dangers, except that it poses the possibility of our extinction and the death of the earth.

—ABC News special: "The Fire Unleashed"[7]

The Facts

- Nearly all of our yearly exposure to radiation comes from natural background radiation (79 percent) or ionizing radiation used in medical tests (18 percent). The remaining 3 percent comes from consumer products.

- Careless use of radiation and radioactive materials (or simple ignorance of its potential hazards) generally early in the twentieth century caused human illness and death, including a number of types of human cancer.

- The scientific consensus is that low-level exposure to radioactivity, of the type to which we might be exposed if we lived near a nuclear power plant, is not hazardous to human health.

- Since 1942, when the first nuclear reactor began operating in this country, not one nuclear power plant has experienced an accident in which health-threatening amounts of radioactivity have been released to the environment in the United States.

- Follow-up investigations on the much-publicized Three Mile Island incident found no health effects on humans or animals, except for the mental stress induced by the misinformation that was widely spread, primarily by the media.

- The "problem" of nuclear wastes is manageable.

- The human health risks of nuclear power are minimal when compared with the everyday risks of cigarette smoking, alcohol consumption, driving, and even flying in a commercial aircraft.

- The need for nuclear power in the United States is real.

- The Chernobyl reactor accident in the Soviet Union could not occur here for several reasons. Most notably, the type of reactor involved was of an obsolete design unique to the Soviet Union.

Introduction

As more and more intricate technologies have found their way to the market during the twentieth century, Americans have become increasingly concerned with the concept of health risks. Many now believe that modern man has created a world that is inherently more risky than ever before.[8] For example, the radiation associated with nuclear power operations is widely viewed as one of the greatest risks to human life and the environment.

Why are nuclear power and radiation of such great concern to so many Americans? There is no simple answer. An enormous amount of information about nuclear technology is available to the public, but deciding on whom or what to believe may be quite confusing when one is confronted with conflicting accounts of the same issue.

Background

Atoms are the basic building blocks of matter: they are the smallest unit of an element that can combine with other elements. Smaller particles, such as protons, neutrons, and electrons, make up atoms.

For any specific element, such as oxygen, iron, chlorine, or carbon, all the atoms contain the same number of protons in the central core (the nucleus). In addition, the nucleus contains neutrons. These uncharged particles may be present in different quantities in individual atoms of the same element. When two atoms of the same element contain different numbers of neutrons they are called isotopes and are named by the sum of the number of protons (constant) plus neutrons (variable) in the nucleus. Thus U-235, U-238, and U-239 represent isotopes of the element uranium containing (in the nucleus) 92 protons plus 143 (U-235), 146 (U-238), or 147 (U-239) neutrons. In addition, all atoms contain negatively charged particles (electrons) in shells (clouds) surrounding the nucleus. In the resting state the number of electrons in any atom is equal to the number of protons, thus providing electrical neutrality.

Isotopes may be stable or radioactive; the latter have unstable nuclei and emit three types of radiation: alpha, beta, or gamma. Each of these possesses different properties and varying ability to cause harm.

Alpha particles contain two protons and two neutrons, so they have a mass four times that of a proton and a charge twice that of a proton. They are stopped by a few inches of air or a thin layer of a denser substance, such as a sheet of paper. Their ability to cause harm from outside the body is minimal because they are absorbed by the body's layer of dead skin cells and do not reach living tissue. However, they are potentially hazardous when emitted within the body.

Beta particles are identical to electrons. They will penetrate paper, but can be stopped by a sixteenth- to a half-inch of heavier material. High levels of external beta radiation may cause skin burns, but the radiation generally will not damage major organs.

Gamma rays can best be described as packets of energy with neither mass nor charge. They are similar to X-rays. In terms of radiation coming from outside the body, gamma rays are the greatest concern. They can be highly penetrating, capable of going through several inches of lead, several feet of concrete, or several yards of packed earth.

Radiation can cause damage when it is emitted from outside the body, as with gamma rays, or when it comes from inside the body. When radioactive materials are taken into the body either through ingestion or inhalation, all three types of radiation can reach major organs and cause damage. Alpha particles are considered the most hazardous inside the body because they have a much greater mass and electrical charge than electrons.

Natural Radiation

Radiation exists naturally in the environment. The amount present in a specific place is primarily determined by the geography and topography of the region. Cosmic rays that originate from the sun are one of the two major sources of natural radiation. Solar cosmic rays are protons accelerated by electric and magnetic fields around the sun. The atmosphere serves as an absorber for most of the sun's cosmic rays. Therefore, the amount of radiation exposure from the sun increases in proportion to altitude.

Radioactive material within the earth's crust is the other major source of natural radiation. A number of elements including potassium, radium, uranium, and thorium contain isotopes that are naturally radioactive. The average layer of soil measuring one foot deep and one mile square (1.7 million tons of soil) contains four to five tons of uranium, six tons of thorium, and one gram of radium. Some of the decay products of these elements are gases that continually escape from the soil. Most radiation comes directly from the ground from building materials and from radioactive materials inside our bodies, such as radioactive potassium in muscles.[9]

Because of these factors, the overall background radiation doses in cities or regions differ greatly. For example, Denver has almost twice the natural background radiation found in most spots in Florida.

Some inhabited areas of Brazil have measured levels of background radiation six times the average for the United States. In fact, plants growing on a hill in the state of Minas Gerais absorb so much radioactive material from the soil that they can be X-rayed simply by placing their leaves in contact with X-ray film.

Measuring Human Radiation Exposure: Terminology

Radiation terminology is difficult to understand, but essential in any discussion of radiation exposure. Here are the basics:[10]

Rad: amount of radiation absorbed per gram of body tissue.

Gray: 100 rad (an international term for rad, gradually replacing the rad).

Rem: a term that expresses the damage potential of any particular type of radiation dose; the rad is multiplied by a quality factor to determine the rem.

Sievert: international unit expressing damage potential of any particular type of radiation dose.

How Much Radiation Are We Exposed To?

On the average, Americans are annually exposed to approximately one-third rem, or 360 millirems of radiation from all sources, including naturally occurring radiation, medical uses, radiation from consumer products, radiation from occupational activities, nuclear power production, and miscellaneous environmental sources (including nuclear weapons testing fallout).

By far the largest contributor to this dose is natural background radiation, contributing 79 percent. It has recently been estimated that as much as two-thirds of this natural background dose is caused by radon and its decay products. The other third is equally divided among cosmic radiation, terrestrial radiation, and internally deposited radionuclides.[11]

Medical procedures contribute approximately 18 percent of the annual dose (smaller than previously estimated) and consumer products about 3 percent.[12] Radiation from occupational activities, the entire nuclear power process and other miscellaneous sources, including nuclear weapons testing fallout, together contribute less than 1 percent of our annual exposure, or less than a thousandth of a rem.[13]

Radiation and Adverse Health Effects

As with all toxic substances, the degree of radiation hazard is dependent upon the dose or exposure. Radiation is dangerous in high doses. At very high doses, about four thousand times the annual background radiation dose, radiation can cause acute sickness and death. At doses that are lower, but above one hundred times the annual background dose, an increased risk of cancer has been observed.

Information about the types of disease caused by excessive radiation exposure and the doses of radiation necessary to induce acute illness and cancer has been gathered by studying a number of occupationally exposed groups, patients subject to inappropriate therapeutic use, and survivors of the atomic bombs dropped on Japan during World War II.

For example, during the early 1900s young women employed in watch-manufacturing factories painted luminous dials on watch faces using a material containing radium. In the course of their work these women commonly "tipped" the end of their brushes using their tongue and lips. This resulted in ingestion of significant amounts of radiation. Of some seventeen hundred workers employed in this trade, forty-eight died from bone cancer. Normally, less than one person would be expected to die from bone cancer in a population more than twice that size.

Unfortunately, watch-dial painters were not the only unsuspecting victims of excessive radiation in the days before its hazard was known. About fifteen thousand British patients treated with high levels of radiation in hopes of alleviating the great discomfort of ankylosing spondylitis (a painful disease that causes the spine to stiffen) were administered doses of X-rays averaging 370,000 millirads. This procedure resulted in ten times more leukemia deaths than would normally be expected.[14]

The atomic bomb attack on Japan that ended World War II not only killed many people, but also, sadly, presented the medical community with unique long-term health problems. Thousands of survivors had been exposed to doses of radiation much greater than normal background levels. Medical and epidemiologic follow up has enabled us to learn a great deal about radiation's effects on human health and on the levels of radiation necessary to cause those effects.

By comparing the intensity of radiation exposure in a given area with the resulting numbers of fatalities, researchers found that a single exposure to 1 million millirads will be lethal to every one and a 450,000-millirad exposure will cause about half of the exposed population to die within a month.[15]

Cancer and reproduction patterns among a hundred thousand survivors of the atomic attack on Nagasaki were studied by the Radiation Effects Research Foundation (RERF).[16] Average exposure had been 20,000 millirads per person, or the equivalent of four hundred chest X-rays. RERF found that the increase in cancer incidence caused by the radiation exposure at this level was minimal, finding that radiation accounted for just one of every five hundred cases of cancer in the exposed group.

Human reproduction was also affected by the radiation shower in Japan. Women pregnant at the time of exposure gave birth to a higher than expected percentage of children with birth defects. An increased incidence of genetic defects has been seen in offspring of animals exposed to radiation in laboratory studies. However, such genetic effects have not been shown for the Japanese A-bomb survivors. According to a *National Geographic* in-depth review:

> Surprisingly no genetic evidence suggests generations to come are doomed. Tests on mice and fruit flies show harmful results. So why not humans? Spontaneous abortions, perhaps, or some remedial effect of the lengthy human gestation period. Said Dr. [Jacob] Thiessen [of RERF], "We would like to find some directly measurable effect. Right now we don't see anything."[17]

Radiation Levels That Will Cause Cancer and Birth Defects

As a result of epidemiologic studies done on human populations after the above-mentioned episodes, we know that radiation at relatively high doses can cause cancer, birth defects, and other adverse health effects. The key issue, then, is whether people in the general environment are exposed to hazardous levels. Fortunately, those exposed to environmental background radiation have experienced few health problems from this background radiation.[18] For example, residents of Denver receive twice the U.S. average (because of their high altitude) yet they have one of the lowest overall cancer rates in the United States.

A cause-and-effect relationship between radiation and cancer has been shown only at levels above 20,000 millirads, with the most solid evidence from exposure of 100,000 millirads or more.[19] As the level of radiation exposure decreases, the evidence of a carcinogenic effect becomes less detectable. Most studies on the human health effects of lower levels of radiation reach the same conclusion—there is no convincing evidence that a single exposure to 20,000 millirads or less will cause cancer. There have been some studies, in fact, which show a beneficial effect of low-level radiation.[20] However, to be on the safe side, regulations regarding radiation doses are based on the assumption that the effects of radiation are proportional to the dose even at levels below which no effects have been observed.

If nuclear power plant operations substantially increased overall radiation exposure to people, the possible adverse effects of the radiation would be an important health concern. But the average dose to a U.S. resident from the 110 reactors currently in commercial operation is estimated at less than one millirem per year,[21] substantially less than the 20,000 millirads that studies have found to be hazardous. People living close to a nuclear plant are exposed to a radiation dose ranging from a few millirads in the plant's immediate vicinity to 0.05 millirads at locations fifty miles from a plant.[22] Nuclear energy produces little real impact on human health or the environment compared to the burning of fossil fuels. The health risk imposed on those living near a fossil fuel plant are significant and well documented, as opposed to the imagined risks of living in the vicinity of a nuclear power plant.[23]

Indeed, epidemiological studies of people living in these areas confirms that there is no health risk associated with living near a nuclear plant. Cancer incidence and mortality studies in the vicinity of nuclear installations in England and Wales during the period 1959-80 concluded that there had been no general increase in cancer mortality. The only exceptions were leukemia in young people and a small increase in multiple myeloma and Hodgkin's disease in people twenty-five to seventy-four years of age.[24] A companion study compared mortality due to leukemia and Hodgkin's disease in people who lived near potential sites to that of people who lived near existing sites and found no difference in mortality between the two groups. They hypothesized that existing and potential sites might share unrecognized risk factors other than the radiation.[25]

The National Cancer Institute (NCI) also investigated cancer mortality among populations living near nuclear facilities, with a special focus on childhood leukemias in light of the British findings. Their study, released September 19, 1990, showed no general increased risk of death from cancer for people living in 107 U.S. counties closely adjacent to sixty-two nuclear facilities, including fifty-two commercial nuclear power plants, nine Department of Energy research and weapons plants, and one commercial fuel-reprocessing plant. The rate of deaths from sixteen types of cancer, including leukemia, were compared to cancer rates in 292 similar counties without nuclear facilities. According to John Boice, Sc.D., chief of NCI's Radiation Epidemiology Branch,

> From the data at hand, there was no convincing evidence of any increased risk of death from any of the cancers we surveyed due to living near nuclear facilities.[26]

Nuclear industry workers receive an average exposure of 400 millirem per year, which, over a forty-seven-year working life, may reduce their life expectancy by ten days. By comparison, occupational accidents reduce life expectancy for the *average* U.S. worker by seventy-four days, and for miners and construction workers by three hundred days. Occupational diseases, stress, and other factors reduce life expectancy in many occupations by eight hundred to fourteen hundred days.[27] Spending one's entire life as a radiation worker increases one's risk of dying of cancer by about 4.94 percent.[28]

Experts, however, caution that this 4.94 percent excess may be falsely elevated. Says Geoffrey R. Howe, Ph.D., of the National Cancer Institute of Canada:

> This interpretation requires considerable caution. The observed excess incidence of cancer is limited to a relatively short period of time at the end of the follow-up interval, to an excess incidence of leukemia primarily in one dose group, and to an excess incidence of lung cancer, which is difficult to interpret in the absence of smoking data.[29]

Dr. Howe concludes with:

> It is somewhat ironic that public concern over the potential hazards of normally operating nuclear facilities receives much greater attention than the far greater risks imposed by such voluntary life-style factors as smoking, drinking and diet.[30]

People living near the highly publicized Three Mile Island nuclear power plant accident received an average dose of one millirad. This amounts to one chance in seven million of getting a fatal cancer from that exposure; or, putting it another way, their increased risk of death is the same as they would face in four extra street crossings or four puffs on a cigarette.[31] In fact, the risks of evacuation from the Harrisburg area were greater than the risk from radiation exposure for the residents who remained.[32]

Other Health Effects of Ionizing Radiation

There is currently no evidence that exposure to low-level radiation of the amounts indicated for the general U.S. population is responsible for AIDS, Chronic Epstein-Barr Virus, Lyme Disease, *Candida albicans,* herpes, septicemia, and several other immune-deficiency ailments often mentioned by antinuclear activists.[33]

Atoms Into Electricity

Fission (the splitting of an atom) is the source of nuclear energy. In the reactor core, a neutron strikes the nucleus of a uranium atom causing the nucleus to split apart. The fragments of the nucleus travel at high speed (they have a high amount of kinetic energy). The energy is transformed into heat. As the fragments collide with other uranium nuclei, these subsequently split apart, perpetuating a controlled chain reaction. The heat of the reaction is captured and used to generate steam, much as one generates steam by placing a kettle on a hot plate. The steam, in turn, is used to drive turbines that spin generators, producing the desired product, electricity.

The reaction process results in the conversion of some of the uranium fuel to fission products like strontium 90 and elements like plutonium. Periodically, spent fuel—fuel that has been "used up"—must be replaced. Removed from the reactor as fuel rods, the spent fuel is commonly referred to as high-level radioactive waste.

SAFEGUARDS

Elaborate safeguards are built into all nuclear plants to reduce the chance of an accident and to minimize the damage to the public, environment, and plant in the event of an accident. Multiple barriers are constructed between the fuel and the public. These include the fuel casing, reactor vessel, and the steel-lined, reinforced containment structure. Of utmost concern is the possible loss of the water that cools the nuclear reactor. (This is separate from the water that is converted to steam to run the turbines.) In the absence of coolant water, the nuclear core may be damaged and radioactive materials released inside the reaction chamber. Therefore, if a coolant pipe bursts, a backup core-cooling system injects cooling water into the reactor core.

In the unlikely event of a breakdown of all coolant systems, the released radioactivity is contained in an airtight building. An additional safeguard is provided by nozzles within the structure. They are designed to spray water to condense the steam and wash the radioactive materials from the atmosphere into a collection tank in the sealed building.[34]

WATER DISPOSAL

Contrary to popular belief, the disposal of high-level radioactive waste is a technologically manageable problem. Public protest, however, prevents the nuclear power industry from going ahead with establishing nuclear waste sites. Such protest, in fact, is the single largest impediment to building new reactors.[35] The major problem with high-level waste is not its longevity, but its very high level of radioactivity when it first leaves the reactor. For this reason, spent fuel rods are placed in water for temporary storage. Natural decay reduces much of the radioactivity. After a few hundred years, the radioactivity in the waste ceases to be especially dangerous. But because the wastes do remain radioactive for up to five hundred years, they must be carefully stored to ensure isolation from human contact.

Good news for the nuclear waste issue came in 1992, when scientists at Sandia National Laboratory in Albuquerque, New Mexico, and at Texas A&M University announced a new class of materials that can selectively extract cesium from solution. These materials, called silico-titanates, have up to sixty times the efficiency of a model zeolite compound for removing cesium from radioactive wastewater solutions. They could, for example, be used to treat radioactive wastes such as those stored at the Hanford nuclear research facility near Richland, Washington.[36]

Currently, fuel rods are stored in storage ponds at reactor sites. However, the Nuclear Waste Policy Act of 1982 mandates construction of a permanent underground disposal facility in a stable geological formation. Liquid waste will be concentrated into a solid material by mixing with inert material (glass or ceramic) and encasing the resulting inert solid in an appropriate container. A number of suitable sites have been located, but a final selection has yet to be made. Some scientists now feel that such wastes would best be stored in above ground concrete blockhouses. These "monitored retrievable storage" facilities would be advantageous if uses are found for the wastes as future technologies are developed. For example, enrichment processes may someday be capable of turning today's waste into tomorrow's reactor fuel, thus changing a long-term storage need into a short-term one.

The total volume of high-level waste is surprisingly small. Of all the waste generated at a nuclear power plant, 99 percent of the radioactivity is contained in just 1 percent of the volume of wastes. A thousand-megawatt plant will annually produce only two cubic meters of high-level waste, or a volume of waste capable of fitting under the average dining-room table.

Most nuclear plant radioactive wastes are considered low-level wastes—such items as discarded workers' gloves, paper, plastic, test tubes, glass—and are similar to radioactive wastes produced at medical facilities and research laboratories. These materials can be safely buried at low-level waste facilities in such a manner as to exclude groundwater and rain penetration with a layer of soil added for shielding. Low-level wastes are much less of a problem than many other of the ordinary chemical wastes encountered in a number of industries.

The nuclear power process results in neither the production of exhaust and combustion gases nor the generation of any chemical wastes. Nuclear power does produce fission products that remain locked in the fuel until removed, reprocessed, and stored, and some radioactivity that is circulated within the closed cooling system.

OPERATING SAFETY RECORD OF THE NUCLEAR POWER INDUSTRY

The first controlled nuclear reaction began in Chicago in 1942. As of September 1992, 110 nuclear power plants were supplying 22 percent of the nation's electricity[37] with no air pollution. All told, there have been over 400 plants in operation worldwide.

Throughout the fifty-year history of nuclear power generation in Western countries an excellent safety record has been achieved—not one commercial nuclear power plant has suffered an accident in which health-threatening amounts of radioactive material have been released into the environment.*

The USCEA has concluded that today's nuclear plants, which have accumulated more than 1,350 reactor years of operation, are more efficient than at the start of the decade.[38] The nuclear power industry has vigorously pursued new-technology research and development, new technologies that incorporate automatically activated safety systems.[39] The nuclear industry has established the National Academy for Nuclear Testing to improve training standards and consistency of all nuclear plant operators. All operators must be regularly trained and recertified. The nuclear industry continues to be a leader in safety. In fact, the comprehensive emergency plans required of all commercial nuclear power plants have been used to evacuate people for non-nuclear emergencies.[40]

Kenneth Carr, ex-chairman of the Nuclear Regulatory Commission (NRC), agrees that nuclear power is safe:

> There is little question that the safety of nuclear power plants today is much better than it was a decade ago. . . . I attribute this enhanced safety to the

---

*The Chernobyl reactor accident in the Soviet Union is discussed below.

vigorous NRC regulatory and inspection program, to the improvements made and being made and to the desire of the nuclear industry to achieve excellence. The bottom line is that the public is being better served today than ever before.[41]

In 1992, Westinghouse Electric Corporation submitted to the Department of Energy a 7,300-page, 18-volume safety analysis of a new type of reactor it is developing. This new generation of reactor adds yet another safety feature, in that it is intended to be "passively safe," immune to operator error and constructed with far fewer parts than conventional nuclear power plants.[42] This new design offers an economic advantage as well: Westinghouse estimates it can build this reactor for $900 million (1990 dollars), compared to a price tag of $4 billion on current units. At this price, nuclear plants are competitive with natural gas plants, because their fuel costs much less.[43]

Another safeguard was introduced in 1992, when the NRC approved a regulation for renewing nuclear power plant licenses. According to NRC chairman Ivan Selin, the rule is tough and requires considerable effort by utilities to perform technical analyses to demonstrate that their plants are safe and that their licenses should be renewed.[44]

What Happened at Three Mile Island?

During the early morning hours of March 29, 1979, a pump responsible for transporting water to the steam generator malfunctioned in the Three Mile Island (TMI) nuclear facility in eastern Pennsylvania. This incident was the first in a series of human and mechanical errors that make up what is widely considered to be the worst U.S. nuclear power accident in history. Antinuclear groups point to the TMI experience as the ultimate proof of the danger of nuclear power, but a close look at what actually happened reveals that the safety apparatus built into a nuclear power plant does in fact ensure that the public health and environment will be protected in the event of a mishap.

Three Mile Island was a serious accident—in fact, a disaster—an economic one, causing more than a billion dollars' worth of damage. Fortunately, it was not the health disaster the public thought it was. Although the consequences of such economic disasters are enormous and not to be ignored, the most important consequences of this or any other accident are the effects on human health. How close did we come to a catastrophic release of high amounts of radioactive materials?

Some have said that if a reactor core is heated uncontrollably and reaches approximately five thousand degrees Fahrenheit, it might melt through the bottom of the containment vessel, resulting in an enormous, health-threatening release of radiation. Before TMI, some believed that if the core of a reactor was uncovered for even a short period of time (more than a few minutes), a "meltdown" could not be avoided. At TMI the core was uncovered, except for steam, for a number of hours, yet a meltdown did not occur. The emergency water-cooling system was mistakenly turned off, yet the steam in the vessel served as a sufficient coolant to keep the core from melting.

The official body established by President Carter to study TMI, the Kemeny Commission, concluded that damage was contained despite many human errors and a few mechanical failures. Its report concluded:

- If a meltdown would have occurred (and it wasn't even imminent), radiological releases would not have been increased significantly.

- The airtight building did not fail. More importantly, it would *not* have failed if there had been a meltdown.

- Neither the reactor vessel nor the containment building would have been ruptured by a steam or hydrogen explosion.

- If the complete core had melted down, it probably would not have melted through the concrete base mat of the containment building.

The Kemeny Commission also reassured us that there is absolutely no evidence suggesting that human or animal life was threatened by the accident. Neighbors of the plant received a maximum exposure to 70 millirads and *an average of only 1 millirad due to the TMI malfunction.*[45] To put this into perspective, a person receiving the maximum might have been exposed to more radiation from two medical chest X-rays.

At TMI, despite everything that went wrong, we learned that the back-up systems and safeguards built into U.S. designs really work. Before TMI it was generally thought that if temperatures within a reactor core got high enough to melt the fuel, the fuel would melt through the bottom of the containment vessel and result in an enormous, catastrophic release of radiation. At TMI, when the emergency water-cooling system was mistakenly turned off, the core was uncovered and a portion of the fuel did actually melt. But the other safeguards built into the plant kept even this serious accident from threatening the health and safety of the public. The water in the TMI containment building retained virtually 100 percent of the radioactivity, and the building maintained its integrity.

Ten years after TMI, we understand more clearly than ever that the safety features in nuclear plants are both essential and effective. But, just as important, we are also beginning to understand just how badly America needs nuclear power. It is nonpolluting. It doesn't depend on the political stability of other nations thousands of miles away. And, as TMI showed us, it is safe.

And What Happened at Chernobyl?

On April 26, 1986, a serious accident occurred at the Chernobyl Atomic Power Station in the Soviet Union. Serious damage to the core and a fire were followed by the release of a large amount of radioactivity into the environment. Many people were hospitalized for radiation exposure and there were thirty-one deaths among the firefighters and emergency personnel working directly at the scene. In the aftermath, over 100,000 people had to be evacuated from the area.

Several important factors assure us that this type of accident could not occur in the United States. First of all, the Chernobyl reactor design is unique to power plants used inside the Soviet Union. This design is not at all comparable to commercial reactors in the United States and in other Western countries. Most significantly, the Chernobyl reactor's design makes it unstable during low-power operation; at the time of the accident, the reactor was indeed being operated at low power. Secondly, multiple operator errors significantly contributed to the escalation of the accident. Operators were performing experiments at the time and made a series of crucial mistakes that resulted in an uncontrollable reaction that destroyed the reactor core and released large amounts of radioactivity.[46] Reassuringly, key Soviet scientists acknowledge the superiority of U.S. designs. And top U.S. nuclear power experts are certain that this type of accident could not happen in a U.S.-style power plant.[47]

What Is the Likelihood of a Serious Nuclear Power Plant Accident?

The possibility of a health-threatening accident is remote. In 1972 the Nuclear Regulatory Commission contracted a study of the risks of an accident associated with nuclear power plants. Researchers estimated that the probability of a nuclear accident killing more than one hundred people in any one year is one in a hundred thousand.[48]

Can Materials Used for Power Plants Be Used for Illicit Weapons?

Plutonium *is* produced during the generation of electricity in a nuclear power plant. This type of plutonium, called Pu-240, is not, however, suitable for the manufacture of weapons.[49]

Plutonium for weapons is more simply and cheaply produced in simple low-pressure, low-temperature research reactors. Indeed, the nuclear-weapons capability of all nations possessing nuclear bombs preceded their nuclear power programs. Proscribing nuclear electric power plants achieves nothing if the goal is to prevent illicit nuclear-weapons proliferation.

Conclusion

Low-level radiation from natural background sources and nuclear power plants is not a significant health threat in the United States. The 360-millirad average total annual exposure (from all sources, including natural radiation) is far less than the level necessary to induce either immediate or delayed health effects. Less than 0.1 percent of this exposure comes from nuclear power sources. Epidemiologic data on large populations in areas where the natural background radiation dose is twice the national average show no increase in either cancer incidence or birth defects, the two major concerns regarding low-level radiation exposure.

The nuclear power industry has been beset by numerous economic and regulatory problems and by the opposition of a frightened public. In the words of Secretary of Energy Admiral James D. Watkins:

> A litigious, overly complicated licensing process, paranoia about the technology, and political barriers to handling nuclear waste, have virtually foreclosed the nuclear option in this country. Despite congressional direction to explore the possibility of creating a permanent waste repository in Nevada, the State of Nevada has used the courts and the press to block us from doing what the law requires us to do. A recent ninth circuit decision may clear the way, at last, but it appears that Nevada is not through litigating yet.
>
> As if all this weren't bad enough, those living on Long Island have the privilege of witnessing and paying for the dismantling of a completed, licensed nuclear power plant. If operating, the Shoreham plant alone could displace 21,000 barrels of oil per day.[50]

Similarly, Massachusetts' Yankee Atomic Electric Company nuclear plant closed permanently in early 1992.[51] Overall, Americans daily consume 17 million barrels of oil, and half of that is imported.[52] Turning to nuclear power can significantly reduce that oil consumption, making us independent of foreign oil sources.

The future of nuclear power hinges on how we can change an unfairly tarnished image. Although three-quarters of the American public agrees that nuclear power plays an important role in our nation's future energy need, just one-quarter favor nuclear energy.[53] Unfortunately, we not only have to overcome a lack of understanding of the facts, but also Hollywood slamming the nuclear power industry, as it did in the 1991 "Simpsons" series. *Media Watch* summarized their slam on nuclear power:

> Homer Simpson, the bumbling father in the series, works at a nuclear power plant because, as his high school guidance counselor told him, "It's one of the few outfits around that won't require a college education." The plant is a disaster waiting to happen, thanks to employees like Homer who sleep on the job and ignore danger signs. As a result, the facility wreaks havoc on the environment, as Homer's son learns when he catches a mutated fish at a nearby lake. After hundreds of health and safety violations are found, the plant is shut down and its owner runs for governor.

Matt Groening, the show's creator, told *Mother Jones* that the anti-nuclear bias is deliberate: "We flirt with disaster in every show. . . . One of the things that makes me happiest is how unfair this is to the nuclear power industry."[54]

But it is crucial to recognize that now, and even in the future should the industry undergo sizable growth, the impact of nuclear power on the total levels of radiation in the general environment will be negligible. The levels contributed by natural background and medically related uses of radiation are simply far greater.

There is no scientific basis supporting the restriction or elimination of nuclear power because of alleged health effects caused by the release of radiation from nuclear power plants.

NOTES

1. Dr. George Wald, in Jon Naar, *Design for a Livable Planet* (New York: Harper and Row, 1990), p. 158.

2. H. Caldicott, *What You Can Do! Nuclear Madness* (Brookline: Autumn Press, 1978), p. 36.

3. M. Stephens, *Three Mile Island* (New York: Random House, 1980), p. 4.

4. Ibid., p. 6.

5. J. W. Gofman, testimony before California Assembly, April 1979, as quoted by Bernard L. Cohen in "Radiation Fantasies," *Reason* (March 1980): p. 24.

6. J. M. Gould and B. A. Goldman, *Deadly Deceit* (New York: Four Walls Eight Windows, 1990), p. 135.

7. ABC News, "The Fire Unleashed," June 6, 1985.

8. C. B. Popescu, "Risk and Reason," *ACSH News and Views* 4 (1983): p. 8.

9. C. E. Cobb, "Living with Radiation," *National Geographic,* April 1989, pp. 403–437.

10. Ibid., p. 415.

11. National Academy of Sciences Committee on Biological Effects of Ionizing Radiation (BEIR V), *Health Effects of Exposure to Low Levels of Ionizing Radiation* (Washington, D.C., 1990).

12. Ibid.

13. Ibid.

14. E. M. Whelan, *Preventing Cancer* (New York: W. W. Norton, 1978), p. 116.

15. M. Eisenbud, *Environment Technology and Health* (New York: University Press, 1978), p. 313.

16. L. A. Sagan, "Medicine on the Midway," *Bulletin of the Medical Alumni Association* (University of Chicago Division of the Biological Sciences, Pritzker School of Medicine) 34 (1979).

17. Cobb, "Living with Radiation," p. 420.

18. B. L. Cohen, *Before It's Too Late: A Scientist's Case for Nuclear Energy* (New York: Plenum Press, 1983), p. 69; International Symposium on Areas of High Natural Radioactivity, Academy of Science of Brazil, June 1975; High Background Radiation Research Group (Ministry of Health, Beijing), "Health Survey in High Background Radiation Areas in China," *Science* (August 22, 1980).

19. R. E. Linnemann, "Medical Aspects of Power Generation, Present and Future," *Medical Research Engineering* 13 (1972): p. 9.

20. T. D. Luckey, "Physiological Benefits of Ionizing Radiation," *Health Physics* 4e (1982): p. 771.

21. BEIR V, *Health Effects of Exposure*, p. 18.

22. E. Kahn, R. Brunchard, et al., *Radiological Surveillance Study at a Boiling Water Nuclear Power Reactor,* BHR/DER 70-1 (Rockville, Md.: U.S. Department of Health, Education and Welfare, Environmental Health Service, Bureau of Radiological Health, March 1970); L. Rogers and C. Gammerstfelder, "U.S. Regulations for the Control of Releases of Radioactivity to the Environment in Effluents from Nuclear Facilities," International Atomic Energy Agency Symposium, U.S. Headquarters, New York, August 10–14, 1970; Linnemann, "Medical Aspects," p. 8.

23. J. W. Naylor, regional director of an environmental engineering consulting firm and a member of the Long Island Architects and Engineers Committee on Environmental Resources, in *Newsday,* September 28, 1989, p. 79.

24. D. Forman, P. Cook-Mozaffari, S. Darby, et al., "Cancer Near Nuclear Installations," *Nature* 329 (1987): pp. 449–505.

25. P. Cook-Mozaffari, S. Darby, and R. Doll, "Cancer Near Potential Sites of Nuclear Installations," *The Lancet* (November 11, 1989), pp. 1145–47.

26. S. Jablon, Z. Hrubec, J. D. Boice, and B. J. Stone, *Cancer in Populations Living Near Nuclear Facilities,* vols. 1–3 (Bethesda, Md.: National Cancer Institute, Division of Cancer Etiology, Epidemiology and Biostatistics Program, July 1990)—later published in the *Journal of the American Medical Association* 265 (1991): pp. 1403–08.

27. American Council on Science and Health, *Health Effects of Low-Level Radiation* (New York: American Council on Science and Health, 1988).

28. S. Wing, C. M. Shy, J. L. Wood, et al., "Mortality Among Workers at Oak Ridge National Laboratory—Evidence of Radiation Effects in Following Through 1984,"

Journal of the American Medical Association 265 (1991): pp. 1397–1402.

29. G. R. Howe, "Risk of Cancer Mortality in Populations Living Near Nuclear Facilities," *Journal of the American Medical Association* 265 (1991): pp. 1438–39.

30. Ibid.

31. B. L. Cohen, "How Dangerous Is Radiation?" *Ascent* (1981): p. 11.

32. American Council on Science and Health, *Health Effects of Low-Level Radiation.*

33. Gould and Goldman, *Deadly Deceit,* p. 135.

34. Eisenbud, *Environment,* pp. 319–20.

35. *New York Times,* June 23, 1992.

36. R. Baum, "Cesium Cut from Radioactive Waste," *Chemical and Engineering News* (July 13, 1992): p. 26.

37. *Christian Science Monitor,* May 9, 1992.

38. J. Graham, *Nuclear News,* February 1, 1990, p. 29.

39. EIA Annual Energy Outlook, 1990, p. 30.

40. USCEA, Key data on nuclear energy.

41. K. Carr, chairman of the Nuclear Regulatory Commission, in *Washington Post,* letter to the editor, April 6, 1990.

42. T. W. Lippman, "New Reactor Designs Cheer Nuclear Power Proponents," *Washington Post,* July 4, 1992.

43. Ibid.

44. *Chemical and Engineering News* (December 9, 1991).

45. G. W. Casarett, W. J. Abrahamson, M. A. Bair, A. D. Bender, et al., President's Commission on Three Mile Island, *Technical Staff Analysis Report of the Radiation Effects Task Group* (Washington, D.C.: October 1979).

46. U.S. Department of Energy, *Nuclear Energy: Answers to Questions* (Washington, D.C.: U.S. Department of Energy, 1988).

47. E. G. Remmers, "Putting the Risks into Perspective: Nuclear Power," *Priorities* (Spring 1989): p. 9.

48. Eisenbud, *Environment,* p. 320.

49. S. McCracken, *The War Against the Atom* (New York: Basic Books, 1982), p. 36; Brookhiser, interview, p. 150.

50. Admiral James D. Watkins, U.S. Secretary of Energy, in a speech on October 11, 1990 before the Heritage Associates.

51. *Wall Street Journal,* April 14, 1992.

52. *Washington Post,* May 28, 1992.

53. *Christian Science Monitor,* May 8, 1992.

54. L. A. Reznowski, "Cartoons Promote Liberal Message," *Media Watch* (March/April 1991).

13

Should We Cut the Power?

The Charges

For a century electric lines have made our lives easier. Now some biologists argue that they're also making our lives shorter.

—Discover[1]

We have evidence that man-made electromagnetic fields from power lines are far more productive of serious health effects than cigarette smoking.

—New Yorker[2]

These high-voltage lines generate electric and magnetic fields, which may be linked with cancer and other harmful effects.

—Design for a Livable Planet[3]

A judge rules that students at a Florida elementary school cannot play in a major portion of their schoolyard because of nearby power cables.

—Journal of the National Cancer Institute[4]

The U.S. Environmental Protection Agency has concluded that there is a significant link between exposure to extremely low-frequency (ELF) electromagnetic radiation and the occurrence of human cancer.

—Nature[5]

Chronic exposure to the electromagnetic fields spawned by high-voltage power lines may result in disturbances in human biological cycles and diminished immune response—and a lessening of resistance against infectious diseases, leukemia, and cancers. Exposure to electroradiation can also cause birth defects and genetic diseases like Down's syndrome.

—When Technology Wounds[6]

The Facts

- A small number of laboratory studies on cells in culture medium have shown that electromagnetic fields (EMFs) may cause biological effects in living tissues. However, these biological effects have not been proven hazardous.[7]

- There is still no evidence that EMF causes or promotes oncogenic, or cancer-causing, changes in normal cells.[8]

- The studies showing leukemia, lymphoma, and cancer of the nervous system in children exposed to magnetic fields from residential 60 Hz electrical power-distribution systems suggest, but *do not prove,* a *causal* link.[9]

- Studies in Colorado and Sweden suggested a small increase of cancer in children and adults living near high-voltage transmission lines, but these findings were not confirmed in similar studies conducted in Rhode Island, Washington state, and England.[10]

- A study of leukemia in adults conducted by the University of Southern California did not find any connection between the occurrence of leukemia and the use of electric blankets.[11]

What Are Electromagnetic Fields?

Electric and magnetic fields are found throughout nature and in all living things. Recall that a compass works because the earth has a magnetic field, created by flowing charges in the earth's molten interior.[12]

There are electric and magnetic fields wherever there is electric power. The electric fields result simply from the strength of the charge. The higher the voltage, the stronger the electric field. It is the motion of the charge that creates magnetic fields. As with electrical fields, the stronger currents produce stronger fields. Any electrical device, such as a hair dryer, that is plugged into a wall socket and turned on generates both electric and magnetic fields. Turned off but left plugged in, that hair dryer will still have an electric field but will no longer have a magnetic field because the charges are not moving. Unlike the electric field, the strength of the magnetic field will change with the setting chosen. When the dryer is operated on high heat setting and draws more current, the magnetic field is greater than when the dryer is on a lower heat setting and drawing less current.

People have become worried about high-voltage transmission lines because they have heard that the magnitude of the electric field is determined by voltage, and that electric fields are most intense nearest high-voltage transmission lines.[13]

The electromagnetic force from any type of electrical power source or power-using item is actually a type of radiation. And that's where the fear comes in. But what most people don't understand is that this type of radiation is at the very low end of the electromagnetic spectrum, very distinct from high energy and high frequency forms of radiation such as X-rays and cosmic radiation, which carry a significant cancer risk in sufficient doses. Electromagnetic forces are referred to as extremely low frequency radiation, or simply as ELF.[14] They carry too little energy to break chemical bonds or to deposit significant heat in tissue.[15]

The strength of the electric and magnetic fields associated with power lines, wiring, and appliances depends on several factors in addition to the voltage. Trees and houses serve as effective barriers, as does furniture inside the home. In addition, the strength of the field diminishes very quickly with increasing distance.

The Beginning of the Controversy

Two independent researchers, Nancy Wertheimer, Ph.D., and Edward Leeper, Ph.D., began the ELF controversy in 1979 when they released their analysis of deaths from childhood cancers in the Denver area during the years 1950 to 1973. Alarmingly, their results suggested that many of the homes occupied by cancer victims were close to electrical transformers, distribution lines and outside wiring classified by these researchers as having a "high-current configuration."[16] Their results indicated that leukemias, lymphomas, and cancers of the central nervous system were two to three times more likely in "high-current" homes. Publication of these alarming results began this charged controversy. It also brought much criticism from the scientific community.

The public was not apprised of one crucial caveat: this study, as judged by epidemiological experts, was wrought with methodological errors. Wertheimer and Leeper never actually measured the electromagnetic forces in the homes. Instead, they simply estimated the field strength. This is problematical because estimation is only accurate in simple situations, like a transmission line crossing an open field. It is just not possible to accurately estimate more complex situations, such as inside a home, where the home itself and its furnishings serve as barriers to electromagnetic fields.[17] They also failed to control for any confounding factors, such as exposure to chemicals and other substances that may have been significant in the development of the cancers.

The Controversy Continues—A Report Blown Out of Proportion

The EPA draft report "Evaluation of the Potential Carcinogenicity of Electromagnetic Fields" was released for very limited peer review in June 1990 with a very clear cover letter stating, "[The report] has not yet been formally released by EPA and should not be construed to represent Agency policy"; in addition, it was marked, "Draft: do not cite or quote."

Nonetheless, *Nature,* under the headline "Cancer risks seen in electromagnetic fields," presented alarming and incomplete excerpts from the EPA draft. The *Nature* article begins as follows:

> After two years surveying the existing evidence, the U.S. Environmental Protection Agency has concluded that there is a significant link between exposure to extremely low-frequency (ELF) electromagnetic radiation and the occurrence of human cancer.

It also selectively quotes:

> The several studies of leukemia, lymphoma and brain cancer in children exposed to magnetic fields from residential 60 Hz electrical power distribution systems, supported by similar findings in adults in several occupational studies also involving electrical power frequency exposures, show a consistent pattern of response.

What the draft report said at the end of the sentence, and what the *Nature* article conveniently omitted from its pivotal statement is *"which suggests, but does not prove, a causal link."*

The same paragraph contributes valuable, qualifying information:

> Evidence from a large number of biological test systems shows that these fields induce biological effects that are consistent with several possible mechanisms of carcinogenesis. However, none of these processes has been experimentally linked to the induction of tumors, either in animals or in humans by EM field exposure.

Finally, other key information was omitted. Such information, which further explained the current state of knowledge and scientific consensus, is summarized in the report as

> In evaluating the potential for carcinogenicity of chemical agents, the U.S. Environmental Protection Agency has developed an approach that attempts to integrate all of the available information into a summary classification of the weight-of-evidence that the agent is carcinogenic in humans. At this time,

such a characterization regarding the link between cancer and exposure to EM fields is not appropriate because the basic nature of the interaction between EM fields and biological processes leading to cancer is not understood. For example, a real possibility exists that exposure to higher field strengths is actually less hazardous than exposure to low field strengths. Because of this uncertainty, it is inappropriate to make generalizations about the carcinogenicity of EM fields.

But what the public is not told, the public cannot understand. Thus, the fear of developing cancer from the nearby power transmission lines was given the fuel it needed to stay alive.

The Evidence

In a word, the jury is still out on the charge that ELFs cause cancer and other health problems. M. Granger Morgan, Ph.D., and Indira Nair, Ph.D., head and associate head, respectively, of Carnegie Mellon University's department of engineering and public policy in Pittsburgh, and recognized experts on the topic of ELF, write in one of their reviews:

> In fact, it is by no means certain that exposure to fields will pose health risks. If it does, those risks will probably be small compared to the many other hazards of normal life.

Highlights from their extensive summary of the health studies on ELF[18] include:

1. ELF and childhood cancer: Six studies attempted to find a childhood cancer/ELF link, comparing children from homes with higher ELF to those of children whose homes had much lower ELF levels. One found no increased risk of cancer; five found a risk ratio from 1.4 for all types of cancer to 3.7 for central nervous system tumors. According to Morgan and Nair, the most carefully conducted study (by Savitz and co-workers in Denver) concluded that while there *was* a higher incidence of cancers in higher ELF homes, there may have been some other factor present when the ELF also was. Savitz found, for example, that traffic density was always higher in cases with the ELF/cancer connection.

2. Occupational exposure to ELF and leukemia: In the United States, twelve studies have been undertaken to investigate this claim. All have been positive, with risk ranging from 1.4 to 3.2 for all leukemias considered together.

One of these studies, by Matanoski and colleagues at Johns Hopkins University in Baltimore, also revealed a higher incidence for several other cancers, including those of the gastrointestinal system, prostate, and brain. Of eight studies conducted in other countries, two showed no association between leukemia and field exposure. Six did uncover a positive association, with risk ratios varying between 1.3 and 3.8.

3. ELF and brain cancer: A total of sixteen studies have investigated this association. Six studies, already discussed above, which examined the ELF and brain cancer link as part of other research, did find a link. Five separate studies focused on this question exclusively, and in the occupational setting. All were positive, with relative risks between 1.5 and 8. Nair and Morgan point out that while the brain tumor–electrical worker link seems real, the cause may not be ELFs, but some other factor. Electrical workers are simultaneously exposed to other agents, such as chemicals, which may be the culprit. Indeed, five occupational studies conducted in Sweden failed to find an excess risk for cancer of the brain in electrical workers.

4. ELF and birth defects: Most information about the effect of ELF on reproduction, growth, and development comes from animal studies. Results are inconsistent from species to species, revealing no pattern. The only human research was conducted by Wertheimer and Leeper, who used birth announcements to link the use of electric blankets or electrically heated waterbeds to irregularities in pregnancy outcomes. Although they did report a higher rate of spontaneous abortion, longer gestation periods, and lower birth weights in babies of people who used these electrical items, results must be considered cautiously, as the study was small and had uncontrolled variables. Researchers at Yale University School of Medicine are currently conducting a large study of human pregnancy outcome and field exposure.

Similarly, Leonard Sagan, M.D., summarized the state of knowledge in his 1992 *Journal of the American Medical Association* article, concluding that, due to poor and inconsistent exposure assessment in EMF studies, as well as the absence of any supporting laboratory evidence, it is premature to conclude that EMF poses a risk to humans.[19] Specifically, he made the following conclusions:

1. Childhood cancer: while there appears to be some association, especially with leukemia, the results are conflicting and studies suffer from bias.

2. Occupational studies: studies are conflicting and inconclusive. Job title alone, for example, was taken as the sole evidence of exposure in some studies.

Science agreed in their 1992 article on EMF, confirming that the central problem with studies is inconsistent exposure assessment, as job title alone cannot be taken as evidence of exposure and other risks associated with occupation, such as hazardous chemicals not controlled for in studies.[20]

3. Adult cancer (non-occupational exposures): there has been no association found.

4. Reproductive and neurological effects: no conclusive evidence.

It is revealing to note that while there has been a tremendous increase in our use of electrical power over the last thirty years, there has not been an increase in the occurrence of childhood leukemias during that same time period. Total per capita electrical power generation, in fact, has increased tenfold since 1940 and per capita residential consumption twentyfold. At the same time, the age-adjusted cancer rate for the whole population has actually been declining (when one removes tobacco-associated cancer deaths).[21]

As John Boice, Jr., Sc.D., chief of the National Cancer Institute's Radiation Epidemiology Branch, points out: "[This is] not what one would expect to see if increasing EMF exposure were having a major effect."[22]

Yale University physicist Robert Adair, Ph.D., is an outspoken critic of ELF research. He says,[23]

> Anyone who would believe that ELFs could promote cancer would believe in perpetual motion or cold fusion. In my mind, this falls into the realm of aberrant science—very difficult experience, very marginal data that are never quite reproducible, and results that don't increase proportionally when the factor increases.

Dr. Adair also points out that "the effects people are seeing are at ELF levels many times smaller than the natural field already present in cells."[24]

In June 1990, some fifty engineers, biologists, psychologists, academics, and military personnel gathered to discuss a difficult topic: How to set standards for exposure to power-frequency electromagnetic fields when science does not yet understand what, if any levels, are dangerous. Discussion centered largely on whether such standards should indeed be set at all, given the current lack of definitive evidence for health effects. Dr. Eleanor Adair, wife of Robert Adair and a fellow at the John B. Pierce Laboratories in New Haven, Connecticut, said that "We shouldn't let emotions generated by nonscientists or media determine standards."

During politically charged hearings sponsored by the EPA in January 1991, experts again testified that the weak ELF fields could not affect cells because the naturally occurring fields on cell surfaces are more powerful. Many criticized the weak studies that have produced positive results, urging that such studies be disregarded. Dr. Eleanor Adair said that she was so overwhelmed by the very poor science in the field that she would rather see the big money go somewhere else. Dr. M. Granger Morgan asked, "In public policy, should standards be the same as in basic research?" The hearings produced no answer in regard to what direction the EPA should venture in ELF policy making. A final EPA document on the topic is not expected until early to mid-1992.[25]

Should We Cut the Power?

Given the current state of uncertainty, what, then, is prudent? The best advice is given by expert Dr. M. Granger Morgan:

> In the face of possible risk and incomplete evidence the wise strategy is to exercise prudence. Search for low cost steps that could get people out of fields, especially new fields, and then take them. At the same time, don't go off the deep end. Don't spend large amounts of money or incur great inconvenience until the evidence is clearer. . . . Given the uncertain nature of the evidence, and the fact that even if fields do pose risks the incremental risk to any exposed individual is probably small, when a change cannot be made without significant cost or inconvenience, it is probably not worth worrying about.[26]

With these important caveats, Dr. Morgan offers examples of how one can easily reduce exposure to ELF:

1. Many people sleep eight hours every night with their head a few inches from their motor-driven bedside clock. Pushing the clock to the back of the bedside table or replacing it with an old-fashioned "wind-up" or battery-operated clock easily reduces such exposure.

2. Many people spend several hours each day in front of their computer. Pushing the machine back a few inches on the desk is simple and causes no inconvenience. Also, some companies now make low frequency terminals, and you can purchase screen covers to block exposure.

Dr. Morgan also summarizes the prudent stance that regulators should assume as we all await better scientific understanding of ELF:

1. "Work to avoid exposing many more people to fields *when this can be done at modest cost and with little inconvenience* [emphasis added]."

2. "Work to preserve future options and avoid setting precedents that will cause serious problems in the future if fields do, or do not, turn out not to present significant risks to public health."

3. "Work to keep a sense of perspective, and help the public keep a sense of perspective about this issue. Even if fields do turn out to pose significant health risks, they are likely to be modest for most exposed individuals, and small compared with many other risks in modern life. *We should be prudent, not paranoid* [emphasis added]."

What Is All This Concern Costing Us?

According to *Science* magazine[27] the concern about EMF health risks is resulting in significant—and unnecessary—economic costs, including:

1. Delays and cancellations and moratoria on new transmission projects limiting economic benefits projects could provide.

2. Negative effect on property values along existing transmission routes.

3. Court cases.

4. To avoid litigation, avoid future problems, or because of public outcry, power companies are placing new transmission and distribution circuits underground, more compact, on higher poles. This costs, however, 30 percent more.

5. Moving current utility lines.

6. New equipment that is "low field" costs more than "high field" equipment.

Conclusion

There are as yet no conclusions to be drawn about the relationship between electromagnetic forces and the development of cancer or other ill health in the general population. There does appear to be some convincing, although not consistent, occupational data that definitely merit continued research. But exposure in occupations at highest risk cannot be compared to the much smaller exposures of the general population. Imre Gyuk, Ph.D, program manager for Electromagnetic Research at the U.S. Department of Energy, capsulizes the issue:

> There are most definitely biological effects of EMF exposure; few scientists would dispute that. The compelling question is: Do these biological effects translate into health effects? We still don't know.[28]

NOTES

1. *Discover,* December 1989, p. 62.

2. P. Brodeur, "Annals of Radiation," *New Yorker,* June, 19, 1989.

3. J. Naar, *Design for a Livable Planet* (New York: Harper and Row, 1990), p. 177.

4. M. E. Newman, "The Search for the Missing Link—Electromagnetic Fields and Cancer," *Journal of the National Cancer Institute* 81 (1989): pp. 1686–89.

5. S. Shulman, "Cancer Risks Seen in Electro-Magnetic Fields," *Nature* 345 (June 7, 1990).

6. C. Glendinning, *When Technology Wounds* (New York: William Morrow and Co., 1990), p. 57.

7. National Cancer Institute, *Questions and Answers: Collaborative Study of EMF Exposure and Childhood Leukemia,* March 1990.

8. Ibid.

9. U.S. Environmental Protection Agency, EPA Draft Report, "Evaluation of the Potential Carcinogenicity of Electromagnetic Fields," June 1990.

10. Ibid.

11. Ibid.

12. USEPA, "Potential Carcinogenicity"; I. Gyuk, *Mitigation of Potential Health Hazards of Transmission Line Fields,* U.S. Department of Energy, 1990; M. G. Morgan, *Electric and Magnetic Fields from 60 Hertz Electric Power: What Do We Know About Possible Health Risks?* Department of Engineering and Public Policy, Carnegie Mellon University, 1989.

13. L. Sagan, *Journal of the American Medical Association* 268(5): pp. 625-29, 1992.

14. American Cancer Society, "Cancer Response System #2681," July 12, 1991.

15. M. G. Morgan, "Power-Frequency Electric and Magnetic Fields: Issues of Public Perception and Public Policy," *Radiation Protection in Australia* 9 (1991): pp. 124–33.

16. Newman, "Search for Missing Link," p. 1686.

17. Morgan, "Electric and Magnetic Fields," p. 7.

18. M. G. Morgan and I. Nair, "Part I: Biological Effects," *IEEE Spectrum* (August 1990): pp. 23–27.

19. Sagan, 1992.

20. H. K. Florig, *Science* 257 (1992): pp. 468-92.

21. J. W. Jackson, *Proceedings of the National Academy of Science* 89 (1992): pp. 3508-10.

22. Newman, "Search for Missing Link," p. 1687.

23. Ibid.

24. Ibid., p. 1688.

25. T. Bearsley, "Guessing Game: The EPA Tries to Decide If There's Harm from ELF," *Scientific American,* March 1991, pp. 30-33.

26. Morgan, "Power-Frequency Electric and Magnetic Fields."

27. Florig, 1992.

28. Dr. Imre Gyuk, personal communication, U.S. Department of Energy, October 20, 1990.

14

How Healthy Is America?

The optimist proclaims that we live in the best of all possible worlds; and the pessimist fears this is true.
—James Branch Cabell, *The Silver Stallion*, 1926

Twixt the optimist and the pessimist
    The difference is droll:
The optimist sees the doughnut
    But the pessimist sees the hole.
—McLandburgh Wilson, *Optimist and Pessimist*, 1915

A membership solicitation letter from Ralph Nader's Public Citizen organization began its pitch thus: "Earlier generations lived in fear of polio and smallpox. Nowadays the most deadly epidemics are man-made."[1]

Obviously the intent of that statement, plus the current dismal reports about America's health, suggests that modern technology is responsible for an amount of death and disease equivalent to past epidemics of polio and smallpox, or perhaps even greater.

Yet, according to available health statistics, nothing could be further from the truth. *Americans today are healthier than ever before.* Modern technology has succeeded in drastically reducing the health risks to which we are exposed and preventing the deaths of many of those who become ill or injured.

In 1900, about a hundred of every thousand infants born in the United States died before their first birthday; today only ten of every thousand infants fail to survive their first year. An American born today can expect to live twenty-eight years longer than someone born in 1900.[2] The age-adjusted death rate declined by a phenomenal 53 percent from 1900 to 1950; by an additional

393

43 percent from 1950 to 1980, and by another 6 percent from 1980 to 1988.[3]

The death rates for infectious disease have plummeted to record lows in this century. With the reduction of infectious disease mortality, many more people are now living to an age where chronic diseases may become a problem. Consequently, chronic diseases now account for a much larger proportion of deaths then they did at the turn of the century.

Even the death rate for heart disease, the leading cause of death in the United States, has declined dramatically in the past thirty years or so. The death rates for cerebrovascular disease (stroke) have declined even more precipitously. Age-adjusted death rates for most cancers, with the exception of lung and skin cancer, have gradually declined since the 1930s for those under sixty-five years of age.

The leading cause of death for individuals aged one to the early forties is attributable less to our modern technology than to our own carelessness. Accidents are the largest single cause of death for young Americans.

The toll taken by the four leading causes of disease-related death could be substantially reduced by changes in lifestyle and control of risk factors such as hypertension and obesity.

The bottom line is that there is no evidence that the United States is in the grip of a "technological epidemic." On the contrary, the evidence indicates that the only epidemic Americans currently face is an epidemic of good health.

This is not to say that there is no room for improvement in Americans' health status, or that modern technology has not produced health hazards that must be dealt with. But, on the whole, the health benefits of modern technology have far exceeded the costs, despite what the poisoned press tells us.

How Health Is Measured

The health status of a population can be measured in several ways. The most commonly used measurements are those relating to mortality, such as life expectancy and death rates. Information on mortality is fairly accurate and is easy to obtain from death records, and comparable historical and international information is often available.

Information about the incidence or prevalence of illness (morbidity) is more difficult to obtain. Although physicians are required to report some diseases (mainly those that are infectious) to the Centers for Disease Control, most illnesses are not recorded in any central registry.

The morbidity information available from research studies, medical reports, and national surveys is often difficult to interpret, especially when comparisons are made over time or between countries. For example, an increase in the prevalence of a disease may only mean that diagnosis has improved over the years. Similarly, a high rate of reported illness in one country may simply reflect the fact that diagnosis is more accurate there than in other nations.

Life Expectancy

Life expectancy is the average number of years of life remaining to individuals of a given age. The most common measure of life expectancy is the number of years that the average newborn is expected to live.

During this century, there have been dramatic gains in this important health index (table 1). In 1900 the average newborn could be expected to live only forty-seven years,[4] whereas a child born today can be expected to live seventy-five years.[5] The gains in life expectancy were especially evident in the first half of the century and were largely attributable to the control of infectious and parasitic diseases, which were major killers of the young.[6]

It is not just the young who have benefited from an increased life expectancy. Within the past thirty years, adults have realized greater gains in life expectancy than have infants. From 1900 to 1950 life expectancy at birth increased 38 percent, while the life expectancy of a forty-five-year-old person rose only 15 percent. From 1950 to 1980, however, life expectancy at birth increased 8 percent, whereas life expectancy at age forty-five increased 13 per-

Table 1. Changes in Life Expectancy in the United States

Year*	Life expectancy at birth	Decade's gain (%)	Life expectancy at age 45	Decade's gain (%)
1900	49.2	—	24.8	—
1910	51.5	4.7	24.5	-1.2
1920	56.4	9.5	26.3	7.3
1930	59.2	5.0	25.8	-1.9
1940	63.6	7.4	26.9	4.3
1950	68.1	7.1	28.5	5.9
1960	69.9	2.6	29.5	3.5
1970	70.8	1.3	30.1	2.0
1980	73.7	4.0	32.1	6.6
1987	75.0			

Source: J. M. McGinnis, "Recent Health Gains for Adults," *New England Journal of Medicine* 306 (1982): p. 671; National Center for Health Statistics, Prevention Profile, *Health United States, 1987* (Hyattsville, Md.: Public Health Service, 1990).

*Except for 1910 and 1980, the numbers given are three-year composites. For example, the 1970 data reflect changes occurring from 1969 to 1971.

cent.[7] Adults experienced continued health gains through 1988. Such gains, in fact, are measured by remaining life expectancy at age sixty-five, rather than at age forty-five. In 1988, the average sixty-five-year-old could expect to live an additional 16.9 years, compared to just 13.9 additional years in 1950.[8] This appears to be a major reversal of an historical trend which may trace, in large part, to the recent drop in deaths from cardiovascular disease.

In spite of the increases in life expectancy, the maximum lifespan of Americans has not increased, probably because there is a biological limit to lifespan. Population statistics suggest that under ideal societal conditions, the average age of death would be approximately eighty-five years.[9] During this century, Americans have rapidly approached that ideal. The average person died thirty-eight years "prematurely" in 1900, seventeen years "prematurely" in 1950, and only twelve years "prematurely" in 1980. Moreover, violent death accounts for three of the years by which we fall short of the ideal.

Death Rate

Perhaps most indicative of Americans' improved health is the declining death rate. The age-adjusted death rate decreased 53 percent between 1900 and 1950, from 18 deaths to 8 deaths per 1,000 people per year. From 1950 to 1977 the death rate fell 27 percent more, to approximately 6 deaths per 1,000 people per year. The age-adjusted death rate has stayed fairly constant since 1984, at slightly under 6 per 1,000.[10] These decreases are especially remarkable when one considers that a 100 percent decline in the death rate would mean that we had achieved immortality.[11]

Major reductions in the death rate have occurred in all age, sex, and race groups although some groups have benefited more than others.

Americans Assess Their Health

While self-assessment of health may be subjective, it has been found to correlate well with utilization of health-care services and a physician's judgment of health status.

When asked to rate their own health status in comparison with that of others within their age group, the vast majority (88 percent) of Americans say that their health is excellent or good. Only 12 percent of more than 100,000 individuals questioned in the 1978 National Health Interview Survey reported that their health was fair or poor.[12] A response of perceived poor health was given by only 9.6 percent of nearly 250,000 questioned in 1989.[13]

People tend to perceive their health status as declining with age. In the

1989 survey, only 10.6 percent of young adults (seventeen to forty-four years old) said that their health was fair or poor, whereas 28.5 percent of those sixty-five and over rated their health as fair or poor. Those with low incomes are more likely to report fair or poor health than are those with higher incomes.[14]

Infectious Diseases

Many infectious diseases that once claimed the lives of thousands of Americans annually have decreased remarkably in incidence and lethality because of improved sanitary conditions, effective immunization, and antimicrobial therapy.

Deaths from influenza and pneumonia declined from 200 per 100,000 people in 1900 to 22.1 per 100,000 in 1970; in 1988, the figure had dropped to 14.2.[15] In 1900, 194 of every 100,000 people died from tuberculosis, compared to fewer than 3 in 1970. Similarly, deaths from enteric (intestinal) diseases dropped from 143 per 100,000 in 1900 to less than 1 in 1970.[16]

Perhaps the most noteworthy example of the impact that immunization has had on health is poliomyelitis. When a vaccine first became available in 1955, there were about 29,000 reported polio cases. Five years later the incidence had dropped to 3,190 and by 1989 only 5 cases were reported.[17]

As indicated in figure 1, many infectious diseases that were once common among children have become increasingly rare because of widespread immunization. As the number of cases of these diseases has decreased, so has the number of deaths caused by their complications. Unfortunately, these dramatic reductions in morbidity and mortality have increased the visibility of the rare adverse effects of immunization, resulting in unwarranted reluctance of some parents to have their children immunized. Since these childhood diseases have not been eliminated, but merely controlled, by immunization, this could pose a serious threat to public health.

Between 1979 and 1988 the number of reported measles cases fluctuated, ranging from a high of 13,597 cases in 1979 to a low of 1,497 cases in 1983. In 1989, 18,193 cases were reported, which is twelve times the 1983 low.[18] Outbreaks have occurred among both preschool-aged children, many of whom were unvaccinated, and high school- and college-aged persons, many of whom had been vaccinated. It has become apparent from recent outbreaks that persons who had received measles vaccine at age twelve to fourteen months are at higher risk for measles than those vaccinated at age fifteen months and over.[19]

From 1980 to 1985 the reported cases of mumps declined from 8,576 to 2,982. In 1987, however, there were 12,848 cases, an increase of 331 percent over the 1985 low. These increases largely reflected outbreaks in high schools and colleges and probably resulted from the absence or lack of enforcement of school immunization requirements in some states.[20] Fortunately, the number

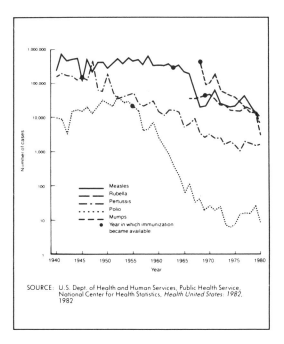

Fig. 1. Reported cases of selected diseases before and after availability of immunization, United States, 1950–80

of cases in 1989 fell to 5,712, which hopefully represents better enforcement of school immunization.[21]

The incidence of one class of infectious disease—sexually transmitted infections—increased from the mid-1960s to 1980 and then began to decrease. The number of reported gonorrhea cases rose about 12 percent from 1966 to 1973.[22] Fortunately the rate of gonorrhea began to drop after its peak of 445 per 100,000 population in 1980; by 1989 it was down to 297 per 100,000.[23] However, concomitant with the AIDS epidemic, rates of other sexually transmitted diseases, including gonorrhea and syphilis, are on the rise.

Reported cases of syphilis have increased since 1977. The rate for all syphilis infections was 30.5 per 100,000 population in 1980 and had risen to 45 in 1989.[24] Genital herpes infections have become increasingly common. It is estimated that 500,000 to 1 million Americans are infected each year.[25]

More recently there has been an outbreak of a relatively new disease, acquired immunodeficiency syndrome (AIDS), that is caused by the human immunodeficiency virus (HIV). As of June 31, 1991, 182,834 cases of AIDS have been reported in the United States, where over 115,000 AIDS deaths have occurred since 1981.[26]

The human immunodeficiency virus gradually incapacitates the immune system by infecting at least two types of white blood cells, the macrophage and a specific type of lymphocyte called a T4 cell. Depletion of the white blood cells leaves the infected person vulnerable to a multitude of infections and certain types of cancer. These infections and cancers rarely occur, or produce only mild illness in people with normally functioning immune systems.

Transmission of HIV occurs through sexual contact, piercing of the skin by HIV-contaminated instruments, transfusion of contaminated blood products, and the transplantation of contaminated tissue. An infected mother can transmit the virus to her child before, during, or shortly after birth. There is no evidence that HIV is transmitted by casual contact.[27]

Leading Causes of Death

At the turn of the century, most deaths resulted from infectious diseases. The age-adjusted death rate from influenza and pneumonia in 1900 was equal to the present heart disease death rate, and the death rates for tuberculosis and diarrheal diseases exceeded the present cancer death rate.[28]

The turn-of-the-century population was subject to a much greater variety of potentially lethal illnesses than are today's citizens. Although the four leading causes of death accounted for only 40 percent of all deaths in 1900, in 1988 they accounted for 71 percent of all deaths.[29]

The leading cause of death in the United States today is heart disease. Cancer ranks second, stroke third, accidents fourth, and chronic obstructive pulmonary disease fifth.[30]

Today's leading causes of death partially reflect the fact that more people in the United States are living longer. A quarter of a century ago, only 8 percent of the population was sixty-five years of age or older. Today, over 12 percent of the population is in this age group, which is more prone to develop and die from chronic disease.[31]

HEART DISEASE AND STROKE (CARDIOVASCULAR DISEASE)

Heart disease, stroke, and related disorders kill more Americans than all other causes of death combined. In 1988 nearly one million deaths—42 percent of all deaths for that year—were attributable to these diseases.[32] Information obtained from the 1989 National Health Interview Survey indicated that 2.8 percent of those under age forty-five suffered from cardiovascular disease, whereas 11.9 percent of those aged forty-five to sixty-four and 27.8 percent of those sixty-five and older were affected.[33]

Despite the high proportion of deaths from cardiovascular disease, the outlook is encouraging. Age-adjusted death rates from heart disease fell 18 percent in the twenty years from 1950 to 1970—an average annual decrease of 1 percent. From 1970 through 1977, the heart disease death rate dropped 2.6 percent per year; from 1980 through 1988, there was an additional 1.9 percent decline per year.[34] The reductions in age-adjusted heart disease mortality rates have been much greater for females than for males, particularly between 1950 and 1970.[35]

Mortality rates from cerebrovascular disease (stroke) declined about 25 percent from 1950 to 1970. In recent years, they have continued to decrease more rapidly than have heart disease death rates, dropping by 55 percent from 1970 to 1988.[36]

The improvement in cardiovascular disease death rates may be partially explained by improvements in medical treatment and care, but it is likely that other factors also contributed. Some possible explanations for the decline in heart disease and stroke mortality include decreased cigarette smoking, improved detection and control of hypertension, decreased dietary intake of total calories and calories from fats, and increased emphasis on physical activity. It is difficult, however, to quantify the effect that any one or a combination of these factors may have had.

CANCER

The American Cancer Society estimated that some 510,000 Americans died of cancer in 1990. Of these, about 142,000 or 28 percent died from lung cancer. There is no need to repeat the "good news" about cancer in the United States here. A simple summary will do.

- With the exception of lung and skin cancer (which are caused almost entirely by our own behavior), the age-adjusted death rates for cancer among those under sixty-five have declined slightly from 1933 to 1988 (see figure 2).

- Although it is widely believed that the United States has an unusually high cancer death rate compared with other countries, the data do not support this. In a comparison of age-adjusted cancer death rates for forty-two countries, the United States ranked seventeenth for male and nineteenth for female cancer death rates (see figure 3).

- From 1947 to 1971 the age-adjusted overall cancer incidence rate appeared to have declined slightly.[37]

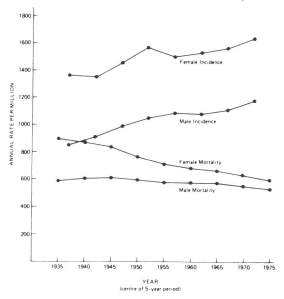

Fig. 2. Age-standardized certified death rates for entire U.S. population 1933–77, contrasted with Connecticut registered incidence rates 1935–74; all cancers except lung and skin. Rates per million, standardized to the age distribution of all respondents under 65 years to the U.S. 1970 census, as described in appendix.

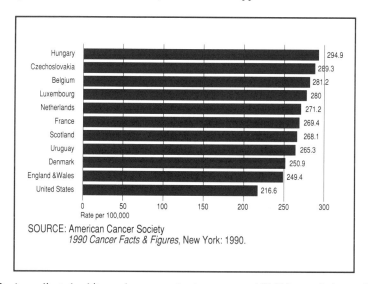

Fig. 3. Age-adjusted white male cancer death rates per 100,000 population, selected countries, 1990.

- The two most recent cancer incidence surveys, conducted in 1969–71 and from 1974 to the present, show no increase in cancer incidence when viewed separately. Although the cancer rates from these two studies are often compared to support contentions of an increase in cancer incidence during the 1970s, it is statistically inappropriate to make such a comparison.[38] Therefore, the prophets of gloom and doom have no factual basis for telling us that we are in the midst of a cancer epidemic.

ACCIDENTS

Accidents are the leading cause of death of Americans from the age of one through thirty-four.[39] In 1988, over 97,000 people died as a result of accidents.[40] The age-adjusted death rate among males was about three times the rate among females.

Although there has been a slight upward trend in the death rate from motor vehicle accidents since 1975 (with an unexplained drop in 1982), the death rate from all other accidents and adverse effects has been decreasing gradually since 1950.

CHRONIC OBSTRUCTIVE PULMONARY DISEASE

This category includes deaths from chronic bronchitis, emphysema, and asthma. It accounted for over 82,000 deaths in the United States in 1988.[41] Approximately 85 percent of emphysema and chronic bronchitis deaths are attributable to smoking.[42]

Health Status of Americans in Different Age Groups

It is a little misleading to examine only the health statistics for the population as a whole. There are significant differences in the death rate, leading causes of death, and general health status of different age groups.

HEALTH OF AMERICAN INFANTS

At the turn of the century about a hundred of every thousand infants born in the United States died before their first birthday. In 1959 fewer than thirty of every thousand infants failed to survive their first year.[43]

Progress in reducing infant mortality has not been quite so dramatic in recent years, although important gains have been made (figure 4). The infant mortality rate remained fairly stable between 1950 and the mid-1960s, but it has again begun to decline rapidly in recent years. Between 1960 and 1980,

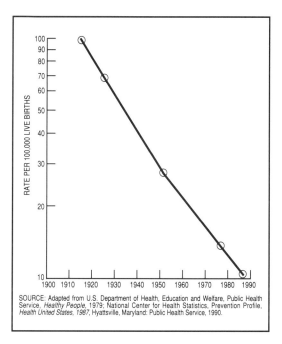

Fig. 4. Infant mortality rates: United States, selected years 1915–1987

the infant mortality rate fell over 50 percent.[44] In 1988 the infant mortality rate had fallen to ten infant deaths per thousand live births.[45]

There are marked differences in the infant mortality rates for different groups within the United States. The infant mortality rate for blacks is over double that for whites.[46]

The U.S. infant mortality rate is higher than that reported in certain other industrialized nations (figure 5). There are, however, significant differences in the manner in which infant mortality statistics are gathered in the various countries. Thus, international comparisons of infant mortality rates may not accurately reflect survival differences among infants in different countries. For example, Sweden and the Netherlands have consistently been ranked as having the lowest infant mortality rates. In Sweden, infants that do not breathe, but that display other signs of life at birth, are registered as being stillborn and are excluded from infant mortality statistics. In the United States, on the other hand, such infants are declared as "live at birth" and their deaths are included in the infant mortality statistics. In the Netherlands all infants who die before registration are excluded from birth or death statistics. Since it sometimes takes as long as a week to register an infant, many deaths may be omitted from the infant mortality statistics. In addition, all fetal deaths that occur after twenty

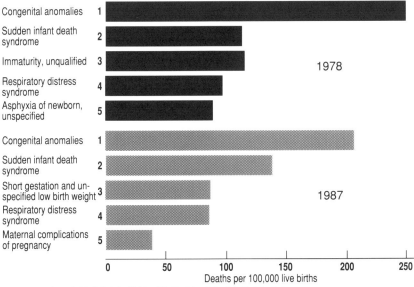

Source: National Center for Health Statistics, Division of Vital Statistics, National Vital Statistics System.

Fig. 5. Leading causes of death for infants: United States, 1978 and 1987

weeks of gestation are recorded in the United States, whereas in many European countries, only those fetuses that die after twenty-eight weeks of gestation are registered. Nevertheless, the United States still has a higher infant mortality rate than some other countries, even when such factors are taken into consideration.[47]

There is some evidence that the higher incidence of low birth weight infants in the United States may be largely responsible for the higher rate of infant death here. When U.S. mortality rates in specific weight groups were compared with those of corresponding weight groups of Swedish infants, the U.S. rates were consistently lower, even though Sweden has a lower overall infant mortality rate.[48]

Factors contributing to low birth weight include poor maternal nutrition, maternal cigarette smoking, alcohol abuse, lack of prenatal care, poor physical condition and several specific diseases that are not related to pregnancy.

The chances of an American infant being born alive have increased rapidly in recent years. Between 1970 and 1988, fetal death rates declined 48 percent in whites and 45 percent in all races.[49] Other races still have much higher fetal death rates than do whites, however, caused at least in part by differences in medical care, nutrition, etc.

Recently there appeared a widely publicized report indicating that the incidence of birth defects in the United States had doubled during the past twenty-five years. This report was based upon research done at the University of California, utilizing data obtained from the National Health Interview Survey.

In that survey, parents were asked to describe any congenital physical, mental, or behavioral disabilities that their children had. There was no attempt to verify the presence of the alleged birth defects from medical records. In addition, the diagnosis of "birth defects," when applied to learning and behavioral disabilities, is influenced by the publicity that such disorders receive—and by the absence of other, more overriding health concerns, such as the complications of poliomyelitis or measles. Changes in such factors could account for an increase in *diagnosis* of these disorders in the absence of an increase in incidence.

Researchers at the Centers for Disease Control (CDC), whose data collection methods are more controlled and reliable than those used in surveys, have found no such generalized increase in physical deformities or chromosomal abnormalities in recent years.[50] The CDC information is based upon hospital discharge records of several hundred thousand births from nearly a thousand hospitals around the country.

According to the CDC, in 1980 the number of children born with major defects, such as anencephaly and spina bifida, was *less* than expected based upon 1970–73 rates. The incidence rates of some birth defects, such as those affecting the cardiovascular system, were higher than expected, but the rates of most defects remained essentially unchanged.[51]

It is also of interest to note that the University of California researchers found no increase in the number of children born that were so severely impaired that they required institutionalization. If there actually were a major increase in the incidence of birth defects, one would expect that the rate of major, as well as less serious, birth defects would have risen.

HEALTH OF AMERICAN CHILDREN

In 1900, 870 of every 100,000 children aged one through fourteen died. By 1925 the death rate had fallen to 330; by 1977, to 43 per 100,000 children per year; and by 1987 to 33.3 (figure 6). Most of this improvement was due to a marked reduction in deaths from natural causes. Deaths from pneumonia and influenza declined 89 percent in preschool children from 1950 to 1979, with most of the decline occurring since 1960. Mortality from cancer dropped 68 percent from 1950 to 1988.[52]

Other highlights from the 1990 *Health United States* survey include:[53]

- Unintentional injuries were the leading cause of death for each group of children, accounting for about 40 percent of the deaths among black, Asian, Hispanic, and white children and for about 55 percent of deaths among native American children.

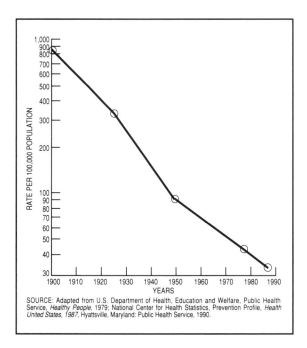

Fig. 6. Death rates for ages 1–14: United States, selected years 1900–1987

- In 1988, homicide was the second leading cause of death among black children, who had a death rate three to four times the rate for any other group.

- Malignant neoplasms ranked second for all others, with minimal racial variation.

HEALTH OF ADOLESCENTS AND YOUNG ADULTS

The death rate of adolescents and young adults fell until 1960, but since then it has risen. This is the only age group that now has a higher death rate than it did twenty years ago (figure 7).

Highlights from the 1990 *Health United States* survey include:

- Unintentional injuries were the leading cause of death for all except black youth, for whom it was the second leading cause. Between 74 and 79 percent of injury deaths in this age group were motor vehicle fatalities, except among black youth, where they accounted for 66 percent.

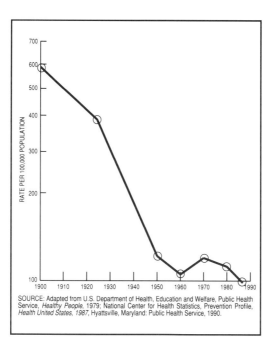

Fig. 7. Death rates for ages 15-24 years: United States, selected years 1900–1987

- Homicide was the leading cause of death among black youth, with the black homicide rate more than seven times the homicide rate for white youth.

- Suicide remains an important cause of death for young people in this age category.

HEALTH OF AMERICAN ADULTS

The death rate of American adults decreased more than 2 percent annually from 1970 through 1977, and continued to decrease by approximately 3 percent annually from 1980 to 1987 (see figure 8).[54]

American adults have experienced a significant decline in deaths due to heart disease since the turn of the century, with the largest drop in heart disease deaths since 1965. In 1978 the leading cause of death for adults 25 to 64 years of age was diseases of the heart. However, since 1983 cancer has ranked number one for this age group. This shift represents not so much a change in the death rates for cancer, but more notably a decline in the death rates for heart disease among persons 55 to 64 years of age.[55]

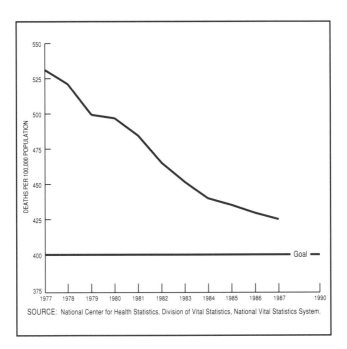

Fig. 8. Death rates for persons 25–64 years of age: United States, 1977–87 and 1990 goal

In 1978 the death rate for heart disease for persons aged 55 to 64 years was 530.8 per 100,000 population. This rate fell to 400.9 in 1988.[56] In contrast, the death rate for cancer among persons 55 to 64 years of age was slightly higher in 1987 than in 1978. In 1978 the death rate for cancer among persons 55 to 64 years of age was 440.5; although the rate was down to 434.8 in 1981, it had risen to 448.4 by 1984. Little decrease has occurred since, and in 1988 the rate was 447.3.[57] Throughout the period 1978–87, stroke was the third leading cause of death among this age group, with the death rate charting a decline from 79.5 to 52.2.[58]

HEALTH OF OLDER AMERICANS

From 1950 to 1979, the age-adjusted death rate among those 65 and older fell 17 percent (figure 9). (It is necessary to age-adjust because the proportion of elderly people over 85 has grown more rapidly than the proportion of those 65 to 84 years old.) The decline has continued through 1987.

Between 1978 and 1987 the ranking of the five leading causes of death among persons 65 years of age and over shifted very little. However, the magnitude of their toll in this population has changed significantly (figures

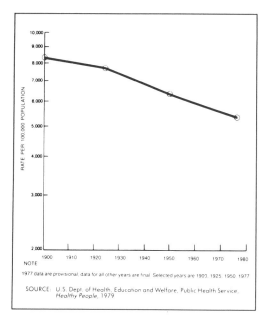

Fig. 9. Death rates for ages 65 and over: United States, selected years 1900–1977

10 and 11). Although heart disease remained the predominant cause of death, the death rate for heart disease fell 11 percent during this period. Cancer remained the second leading cause of death from 1978 through 1987, but the rates for cancer increased 6 percent during the period. Of the three leading causes of death as of 1987, the rates for the third, stroke, showed the greatest change between 1978 and 1987. The death rates for stroke declined from 662.0 per 100,000 population in this age group in 1978 to 435.0 in 1987—a 34 percent decrease. Chronic obstructive lung disease, which was not added to the cause-of-death list until 1979, ranked fourth in 1987. In 1978 pneumonia and influenza was the fourth leading cause of death among persons aged 65 years and over; in 1987 this cause ranked fifth.[59]

The proportion of the population aged 65 years and over is increasing rapidly. Moreover, persons reaching age 65 can look forward to a greater number of years of life. In 1978 life expectancy at age 65 was 16.3. By 1988 life expectancy at age 65 was 16.9 for a total of 81.9 years. In other words, people who attained age 65 in 1988 could expect to live, on average, about another 17 years. Life expectancy at age 65 varies by race and by sex.[60]

Not only are Americans living longer, but older Americans are enjoying better health. People over 65 years of age have enjoyed more unrestricted activity days in 1987 than in the past.[61]

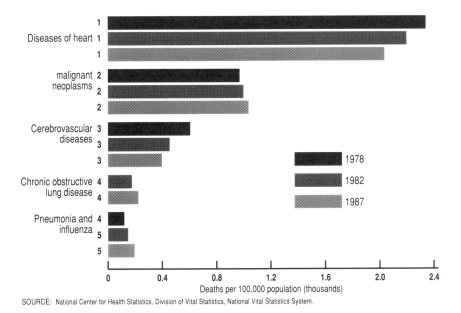

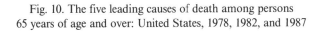

SOURCE: National Center for Health Statistics, Division of Vital Statistics, National Vital Statistics System.

Fig. 10. The five leading causes of death among persons
65 years of age and over: United States, 1978, 1982, and 1987

Preventing Preventable Deaths

Everyone has to die of something, but we prefer that it happens at a ripe old age. The best one can hope for is not to escape death, but to prevent premature death. Public health programs should, therefore, focus on preventable causes of untimely death.

The five leading causes of death—heart disease, cancer, cerebrovascular disease, accidents, and chronic obstructive pulmonary disease—claimed the lives of over 1.5 million Americans in 1988.[62] Almost one-third of these deaths could have been prevented by modifying just three risk factors: smoking, hypertension, and alcohol abuse.

Four of the five leading causes of death are directly related to cigarette smoking. It is estimated that smoking is responsible for 30 percent of all cancer deaths, or 143,000 deaths in 1987.[63] Thirty percent of all heart disease fatalities, or 228,000 deaths in 1987, are also attributable to smoking.[64] It is a major, but unquantifiable, risk factor for cerebrovascular disease and is responsible for 85 percent of chronic bronchitis and emphysema deaths—66,600 in 1987.[65]

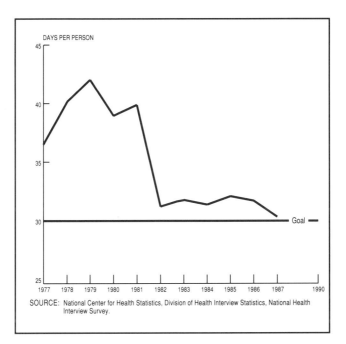

DAYS PER PERSON

SOURCE: National Center for Health Statistics, Division of Health Interview Statistics, National Health Interview Survey.

Fig. 11. Restricted-activity days for persons 65 years of age and over:
United States, 1977–87 and 1990 Goal

Infant and fetal mortality could also be substantially reduced by decreased cigarette smoking. Smoking is responsible for elevated rates of spontaneous abortion and stillbirth and accounts for up to 14 percent of all premature births in the United States.[66]

It is obvious that if Americans really want to prevent premature deaths and improve their health, giving up smoking is the place to start. As the World Health Organization has stated, "The control of cigarette smoking could do more to improve health and prolong life in [developed] countries than any other single action in the whole field of preventive medicine."[67]

Hypertension, or high blood pressure, is responsible for approximately 3 percent of heart disease deaths, or 22,810 deaths in 1987.[68] Thus, further improvements in public awareness, detection, and control of hypertension could significantly reduce cardiovascular disease mortality.

Accidents are the leading cause of death for Americans from the age of one through thirty-four.[69] Any reduction in accidents would thus have a sizable impact on the rate of premature death in the United States.

Alcohol-related accidents are the leading cause of death of adolescents and young adults. Some 49 percent of motor vehicle fatalities (22,415 deaths in 1989) involved an intoxicated driver.[70] Curtailing the use of alcoholic beverages by teenagers, and more cautious use by all age groups, would diminish America's highway death toll.

Cigarette smoking, alcohol abuse, and hypertension are known to have contributed to more than 500,000 deaths in 1990. In contrast, there is little evidence that most of the recently introduced chemicals in our food, air, and water play a significant role in premature death. They may, in fact, promote good health.

To prevent early death, the choices are clear. With limited resources, money should be allocated where it will do the most good. A comparison of the number of premature deaths known to be caused by allegedly toxic agents and the number of premature deaths known to result from the effects of cigarette smoking, alcohol, and hypertension indicates that our resources are better spent on the latter. By keeping our priorities straight, we can have some control over the time and cause of death—even if we all must succumb eventually.

Conclusion

One conclusion should emerge clearly from a perusal of the health statistics presented here: America is not in the midst of a "technological epidemic" caused by environmental contaminants, food additives, or anything else for that matter. On the contrary, the health of Americans has never been better and continues to improve.

Even though a time bomb has supposedly been ticking away for years, no evidence exists of the "explosion" of death and disease cited by the environmentalists. Those "seeping," "oozing," and "brewing" chemicals about which the nation is all shaken up seem not to have affected our health in any measurable way. Indeed, the technological society that produced these chemicals has improved our health far more than harmed it.

All one has to do is look at the substantial increase in life expectancy and decrease in the death rate that Americans have enjoyed during this century to realize that the sum of all the health hazards to which we are exposed must be less than it was in the past.

Certainly our current good health should not lull us into a sense of false security that we will be forever safe from our environment, no matter what we put into it. Modern technology has produced, and will no doubt continue to produce, substances that are *proven* dangers to our health. These must be dealt with expediently and effectively.

The important thing to remember, however, is that technology's benefits to our health have far exceeded the risks. It is no coincidence that the dramatic health gains experienced in the United States have paralleled dramatic innovations and growth in technology. It is thus apparent that if we follow the call of the environmentalists to ban pesticides, eliminate nuclear power, and make air- and water-pollution standards even stricter, demonstrable health benefits will very likely not accrue. Instead, we will face food shortages, higher taxes, fewer jobs, slower economic growth, greater dependence upon foreign energy sources, a reduction in our standard of living, and, probably, a decline in health, all for naught.

NOTES

1. Joan Claybrook, Public Citizen membership and fundraising appeal, undated.

2. U.S. Department of Health and Human Services, Public Health Service, National Center for Health Statistics, *Health United States 1990,* DHHS Pub. No. (PHS) 91-1232, March 1991, p. 67.

3. *Health United States 1990,* p. 77.

4. J. F. Fries, "Aging, Natural Death and the Compression of Morbidity," *New England Journal of Medicine* 306 (1982): p. 131.

5. *Health United States 1990,* p. 67.

6. L. A. Fingerhut, K. W. Wilson, and J. J. Feldman, "Health and Disease in the United States," *Annual Review of Public Health* 1 (1980): p. 8.

7. J. M. McGinnis, "Recent Health Gains for Adults," *New England Journal of Medicine* 306 (1982): p. 672.

8. *Health United States 1990,* p. 67.

9. Fries, "Aging, Natural Death and Morbidity," p. 131.

10. *Health United States 1990,* p. 77.

11. J. Enstron, *New York Times,* September 9, 1980.

12. U.S. Department of Health and Human Services, Public Health Service, Center for Health Statistics, "Americans Assess Their Health," *Data from the National Health Survey,* series 10, no. 142, DHHS pub. no. (HS) 83-1470, 1983, p. 21.

13. P. F. Adams and V. Benson, *Current Estimates From the National Health Interview Survey* (Hyattsville, Md.: National Center for Health Statistics, 1989), p. 8.

14. *Data from the National Health Survey,* p. 21; Adams and Benson, "Current Estimates from Interview Survey," pp. 113–14.

15. *Health United States 1990,* p. 78.

16. M. Eisenbud, "The Environment, Technology and Health: A Century of Progress but a Time of Despair," *American Journal of Medicine* 68 (1980): p. 476.

17. U.S. Department of Health and Human Services, Public Health Service, National Center for Health Statistics, *Health United States 1982,* DHHS Pub. no. (PHS) 83-1232, p. 14; *Health United States 1990,* p. 108.

18. *Health United States 1990,* p. 108.

19. *Health United States 1989,* p. 15.

20. Ibid.

21. *Health United States 1990,* p. 108.

22. U.S. Department of Health and Human Services, Public Health Services, Centers for Disease Control, *MMWR Annual Summary: 1981*, DHHS pub. no. (CDC) 82-8241, 1982, p. 38.

23. *Health United States 1990*, p. 108.

24. Ibid.

25. *Health United States 1989*, p. 149.

26. Centers for Disease Control, *HIV/AIDS Surveillance Report*, July 1991, pp. 1–18.

27. P. T. Cohen et al., eds., *The AIDS Knowledge Base* (Waltham: The Medical Publishing Group, 1990).

28. U.S. Department of Health and Human Services, Public Health Service, Office of Health Research, Statistics and Technology, *Health United States 1979*, DHHS Pub. no. (PHS) 81-1232, 1980, p. 272.

29. *Health United States 1979*, p. 272; *Health United States 1990*, p. 79.

30. *Health United States 1990*, p. 79.

31. Ibid., p. 51.

32. Ibid., p. 80.

33. *Health United States 1989*, p. 127.

34. *Health United States 1990*, p. 79.

35. Fingerhut, Wilson, and Feldman, "Health and Disease in the United States," p. 9.

36. *Health United States 1990*, p. 79.

37. Data from the 1947–48 Second National Cancer Survey and the 1966–71 Third National Cancer Survey.

38. N. F. Knowlden, W. R. Burach, and T. S. Burack, "Cancer: 1. Analysis of Recent New Case Incidence Reports," *Fundamental and Applied Toxicology* 1 (1981): pp. 458–68.

39. *Health United States 1990*, pp. 13–14.

40. Ibid., p. 80.

41. Ibid.

42. National Cancer Institute and National Heart, Lung and Blood Institute, *Smoking and Health: A Program to Reduce the Risk of Disease in Smokers, Status Report*, December 1978.

43. *Health United States 1979*, p. 8.

44. *Health United States 1990*, p. 68.

45. Ibid.

46. Ibid.

47. J. R. Evrard and C. Evrard, "How Disgraceful Are the Facts About Infant Deaths in the United States?" *Today's Health* 44 (1966): p. 72.

48. *Health United States 1989*, p. 12.

49. *Health United States 1990*, p. 68.

50. U.S. Department of Health and Human Services, Public Health Services, Centers for Disease Control, *Congenital Malformations Surveillance Report, January-December, 1980*, 1982, pp. 1–22.

51. Ibid.

52. *Health United States 1990,* p. 89.

53. Ibid., p. 13.

54. *Health United States 1989,* pp. 21–22.

55. *Health United States 1990,* p. 80.

56. Ibid., p. 85.

57. Ibid., p. 89.

58. *Health United States 1989,* pp. 21–22.

59. Ibid.

60. *Health United States 1990,* p. 67.

61. Ibid., p. 121.

62. Ibid., p. 80.

63. *Health United States 1989,* p. 123.

64. Ibid.; National Cancer Institute and National Heart, Lung and Blood Institute, *Smoking and Health.*

65. *Health United States 1989,* p. 123; National Cancer Institute and National Heart, Lung and Blood Institute, *Smoking and Health.*

66. U.S. Department of Health and Human Services, Public Health Service, Office on Smoking and Health, *Health Consequences of Smoking for Women: A Report of the Surgeon General,* 1980, pp. 10–11.

67. *Healthy People,* p. 124.

68. *Health United States 1989,* p. 123.

69. *Promoting Health,* p. 45.

70. U.S. Department of Transportation, National Highway Traffic Safety Administration, *Drunk Driving Facts,* September 1990.

15

The Environmental "Bad-News Syndrome" and Some Unanswered Questions

This book has emphasized that we are the victims of toxic terrorism because the overwhelming majority of the news we get from radio, television, and the print media about health and the environment is bad news—generally, very bad news, despite the fact that national health statistics indicate we have never been healthier. We are swindled because this bad news means that we pay more in taxes and in goods and services to eradicate alleged health risks that may not exist at all, or could be handled in simpler, less costly ways.

We have become almost numb to reports of our "cancer epidemic," industry's uncontrolled release of toxic chemicals and life-threatening radioactivity, polluted air and water, and the possibility of even worse things to come—for example, the type of near-meltdown we watched in horror in the fictional movie *The China Syndrome.* And what scientific evidence do the media present to back up these prophecies of imminent disaster? As I've mentioned before, they have their clique of "experts" on whom they call repeatedly.

What does the environmental movement tell us about the changing world in which we live? What are the real environmental concerns? Although published eight years ago in the April 1984 *Reader's Digest,* an excerpt of Ben Wattenberg's book *The Good News Is the Bad News Is Wrong* still offers valuable insight about the popular environmental movement:

> In terms of specifics the environmental viewpoint is often valuable. As a comprehensive vision of our time, however, it is in my judgment, typically both wrong and damaging. . . . No sane people are antienvironmental; we are all for improving the quality of life. No one proposes to swim in polluted

417

waters; no one gobbles carcinogens just for the hell of it. And surely some of the alarm bells that have sounded point to real problems.

But that is not the point. The point is that the environmental movement has argued that the overall quality of our lives is poor and getting worse. Such a view is incorrect.

In light of the fact that there is so much *good* news about America's health, the quality of our environment, and the contribution American technological know-how has made to this happy state of affairs, we are, in the end, left face to face with three very difficult questions:

1. Why are the media (with rare but notable exceptions, such as the *Washington Times,* the editorial page of the *Wall Street Journal,* and sometimes the *Chicago Tribune*) so eager to give us bad news? Although there is no solid evidence to back this impression up, it *seems* as if reporters *relish* bad news. Why do they demonstrate such gullibility— or willingness—to accept the views of that small cadre of scientists who sing the refrain of gloom and doom for a living? Why hasn't the investigative-reporting instinct of the media turned its skill to an exposé of the doomsdayers, calling their bluff and allowing us a welcome gust of airwaves filled with good news?

2. Why do the same scientists, whether the focus is Love Canal or Three Mile Island, show up in reports to confirm the bad news? Why don't scientists from the mainstream of academic thought contact the media, or, alternatively, why don't the media seek them out? Why aren't American scientists outraged that science is being distorted, and their whole profession discredited and abused?

3. Who are these self-styled environmentalists, those bearers of all this bad news? What motivates alarmists like Samuel Epstein, Ralph Nader, and Lewis Regenstein, and groups like the Environmental Defense Fund, the Natural Resources Defense Council, and the Sierra Club? Why do they constantly overlook the good news, never crediting technology for improving our standard of living, never choosing to pursue areas of investigation that may place the blame for accidents, disease, and poor health on, not industry, but our own negligent behavior? For whom are these individuals speaking: that is, who is their constituency? And since they so frequently dismiss those who disagree with their anti-technology views as "hired guns for industry," it seems appropriate to ask, Who funds *them?* What do they *really* want for social and economic change?

Question 1: Gloom and Doom and the Media

There is no simple answer to why we get such large helpings of pessimism mixed with our daily diet of news from the American media. But there are some observations and clues that give us at least an incomplete understanding of why the news is not presented in a more evenhanded way.

First, we are faced with what appears to be, for better or worse, an inherent quality of the definition of the word *news*. North, east, west and south, news seems to be, by definition, bad news characterized by sensationalism, because that is apparently what the public wants, or what the media think the public wants. R. M. Campbell, president of the Massachusetts Voice of Energy, once observed that "the dark side of human nature seems to enjoy horror movies, auto racing when there is a good chance of fiery death, and electronic pictures of the latest disaster."[1] And George Will, *Newsweek* columnist, said much the same thing: "Only man is perverse enough to feel most alive when the news is most lurid. . . . If some great catastrophe is not announced every morning, we feel a certain void. Nothing in the paper today, we sigh."[2]

Some say that the public is getting what it wants, that it somehow inwardly craves bad news. Ben Wattenberg expands on this phenomenon by breaking down news judgments into three categories:

1. Bad news is big news.
2. Good news is no news.
3. Good news is bad news.[3]

Throughout this book, examples of categories one and two have been presented. The sensational Alar and apple scare, Love Canal, and Three Mile Island—these kinds of events consistently captivate the nation's media. Bad news is big news. The health statistics that show that America's health has never been better are rarely, if ever, picked up by the press—good news is no news. The third category, that good news is bad news, provides an illuminating example of the media's skewed approach to environmental and public health issues.

Remember the threat to our resources and to our ability to maintain our high standards of living because of the population explosion? Well the good news is that population growth has stabilized in America. And how do the media deal with this positive development? They report the school closings, teacher layoffs, and declining college enrollments—all bad news caused by the good news of declining fertility.[4]

Here we are interested in whether or not the media report environmental bad news accurately. Has bad-news reporting gone too far, beyond the realm of what science tells us is the truth? Theodore White, distinguished author, historian, and career journalist, alludes to the "bad-news phenomenon" in what amounts to a reporter's credo:

> You don't make your reputation as a reporter, and I did not make my reputation as a reporter, by praising anybody. You make your reputation as a reporter by gouging a chunk of raw and bleeding flesh from the system. And I did that, all young reporters do that. You gotta be able to prove you can snap your jaws for the kill. But maybe we've gone too far and there should be someone to call us to account for this.[5]

Obviously, the press feels it can serve its own best interest and give its audience the entertainment (we usually call it news) it is looking for by seeking out the darker side of human life. The *Washington Post* even made such an admission, similar to the one made by White, describing its interest in the Three Mile Island story:

> The press, no matter its nationality, thrives on red meat. Red meat is disaster, tragedy, conflict-wars, assassinations, Jonestown massacre, exploding coal mines. The Three Mile Island nuclear accident was red meat, of a sort never before experienced by the press: all the fine fiber of Delmonico. It was a story of technology run amok, man forced from his home by the peaceful atom, the prospect of a stretch of the eastern seaboard being turned into an irradiated wasteland.[6]

Psychiatrist Robert DuPont offers some deeper insight into why bad news sells. He says that what makes news is fear, and "fear is news because fear is interesting."[7] He stresses, however, that the media are selective in using the powerful element of fear to attract attention to themselves, focusing the fear-induced methods on technology and "big business," *not* on everyday risks around us. He writes:

> You can understand how absurd this position is if you think about water instead of nuclear energy. I can see the television picture closing in on a swimming pool, and the voice-over saying, "Do you realize that there is enough water in this pool to drown 100,000 people?"[8]

Thus, in some cases, there is a desire to make environmental news dramatic and anxiety-producing to ensure our attention. It often seems as if reporters are reluctant to present a balanced perspective; that is, for example, to relate the alleged hazards of technology to other common risks, like the risk of drowning in a pool. Perhaps the reason they are presumably reluctant is that it would weaken the impact of their story. Thus in discussing dioxin traces found in Times Beach, Missouri, we are rarely reminded that no one has ever died from dioxin—but five hundred thousand people will die this year from cigarettes. Nor have very many news stories, in discussing the "risks" of nuclear power, ever told us that the risks to the average American of an all-nuclear electric power system would be equivalent to smoking one cigarette every ten years, an overweight person increasing his weight by .03 ounces, crossing a street one extra time every twenty weeks, or increasing the national speed limit from 55 miles per hour to 55.02.[9] Bad news is exciting. Balance and perspective, when not created by a clever reporter, are blah.

But, encouragingly, the public has gotten its fill of bad news. A 1989 survey by the Times Mirror Center for the People and the Press of Washington, D.C., revealed that 60 percent of the respondents think that news organizations pay too much attention to bad news. Let's hope the press responds to this charge appropriately.[10]

Second, the news media thrive on conflict. Anyone who has appeared on a television and radio program to defend food additives, pesticides, nuclear energy, or any other aspect of technology knows that it is *de rigueur* for the media to concoct a debate format, even though the protechnology guest represents 99.9 percent of the scientific community's views. (The reverse is not necessarily true. The alarmists frequently are not presented with an opponent because they are generally regarded as sincere in their views, unencumbered by a tie to industry, selfless in their motivation, and thus not requiring a balanced force; and apparently their views are considered so frightening and newsworthy that debate is not necessary.)

A debate—more appropriately, a fight—is in the mind of the producer, and perhaps the audience, entertaining. "We of the media like conflict, tension and suspense. . . . We like all those things because they make good copy. Our banner might well carry the motto "Let's you and him fight. . . . We desperately need a contest," says Charles Seib, editor of the *Washington Post*.[11] Never mind if the debate is between a Nobel laureate in geophysics and the Flat Earth Society, or between the president of the American Cancer Society and a spokesperson for the Tobacco Institute. Equal weight in credentials means little to the media. A fight is a fight.

Third, and related to the bad-news-sells phenomenon, is the much overlooked reality that news itself is a product. Indeed, news is a heavily marketed commodity in a highly competitive, carefully monitored marketplace.

Controversy and sensationalism draw viewers. Unfortunately, science and common sense, in the forms most often presented, do not. Television and radio stations want to attract an audience; that's their business, and that's how they stay in business.

One could decry this emphasis on audience size and insist that high-quality programming be presented no matter the ratings, but this view ignores an important consideration—ratings mean people. If the environmental alarmist on channel 1 is reaching 30 percent of the viewing audience, while the scientist on channel 2 is reaching his best friend, his neighbor, and his mother, it's clear who's having the greater impact on the public, and at the same time who is keeping which channel's ratings high.

If CBS can raise its ratings for its evening news by making its stories more sensational, then it will. The more the CBS ratings rise, the more advertising revenues come in, and if sensationalism or anything else works, you can be sure that ABC and NBC will follow in style. It appears that members of the media are frequently influenced by what has been successful—and the all-important ratings—not by what might be factual. So bad news is good for business. As John Madigan, the seasoned commentator for WBBM in Chicago put it, the media are "only interested in the guy who kicks his mother down the stairs."[12] One gets the distinct impression that the bystander who comes to a poor mother's rescue gets slighted in the coverage. Perhaps Dr. Ralph E. Lapp best makes the point about the marketability of environmental horror stories; in his book *The Radiation Controversy* he writes that "the scientist with the deepest voice of gloom and the direst prophecy wins the precious air seconds of prime time."[13]

And, according to that Times Mirror poll, even the press believes they have sensationalized too far. Seventy-four percent of the press who were interviewed believe that the use of video re-enactments in news broadcasts is adversely affecting journalism. Fifty-seven percent believe network television news is going too far to entertain its audience.[14]

For those who feel that the honor of the media is being unfairly maligned here, with the clear implication that those writing material for radio, television, and print are willing to give only one side of the story, all for the sake of the almighty dollars that pursue good ratings, consider two points. First, the media almost never report the good-news stories that follow the bad-news ones; for example, when in the early 1980s a study from the Harvard School of Public Health indicated that coffee consumption could increase the risk of pancreatic cancer, the headlines were spectacular. One could not even swallow a sip of the habitual morning brew before "Today" informed us of the risks. But when subsequent studies showed no causal relationship between coffee consumption and cancer, the silence in the press was deafening. Second, one tends to become skeptical about the media's willingness to put the best interest of their audience ahead of their quest for advertising revenues. Recall, if you will, the bitter fight the broadcasters put up in 1969 when it was proposed that cigarette advertisements be banned from the electronic media, and the fact that the current presence of tobacco ads in magazines seems to have such chilling effect on the coverage of health hazards of smoking.

Third, and following up on the point just made, it is clear that advertising dollars can influence the nature of the news and commentary. A detailed survey by the American Council on Science and Health confirmed that magazines that carried cigarette advertisements (which accounted for 15 to 30 percent of their total ad revenues) failed miserably in reporting about the contribution of cigarettes to environmentally induced disease.[15] Candid reports by journalists have revealed that magazines carefully discouraged pejorative comments about their advertisers, particularly those of tobacco products. Interestingly, then, when a magazine editor covering issues related to health and the environment feels inhibited in writing about cigarettes, the main cause of environmental disease, he or she by definition must *overstate* the contribution of other factors—dioxin, Love Canal, radioactivity—to fill the void left by the silence on tobacco. But, you might argue, this type of pressure could not apply to radio and television, because they do not now carry cigarette advertisements (banned in 1970). That radio and television, like their counterparts in print, rarely report on the hazards of cigarettes, and frequently report on how "pollution," occupational chemicals, and PCBs are a potential cause of cancer could not possibly be related to advertising pressure. Maybe yes. Maybe no. What is important to keep in mind is that many big television advertisers are owned by cigarette companies. For example, Del Monte products like Hawaiian Punch are owned by R. J. Reynolds (RJR/Nabisco), and Velveeta and Jello from Kraft-General Foods are ultimately owned by Philip Morris. It is not inconceivable, then, that advertising pressure through the parent companies plays a role in minimizing the coverage of cigarettes on radio and television, thus, as a secondary result, leaving more room for discussion of the other, more hypothetical hazards in the environment.

Radio and television producers might defend their relative silence on cigarettes by saying that it is "old news," that everyone knows cigarettes are harmful, and that because so many people are helplessly addicted to them the subject is depressing. That may well be. But if the electronic media, unlike the print media, were unencumbered by tobacco advertising pressure, one would think they would at least occasionally conjoin the hypothetical risks of nuclear energy, dioxin, and other topics they cover with regularity with the reality of the devastation wrought by cigarettes.

Fourth and again related to the general underlying bad-news theme, the media representatives who cover environmental issues, like their colleagues in other specialties, are in a hurry. Their deadline is always yesterday, and they have no time to listen to the pros and cons of an issue. Even when more moderate scientists attempt to dissuade them from yet again citing one of the handful of fringe, antiestablishment scientists, encouraging reporters to call a few of the local universities to check out this person's reputation among fellow scientists, the answer is that there is too little time. One scientist-bird in the hand is better than none, even if he or she is representing a fringe point of view.

What the journalist under pressure is looking for is the scientist who can give him the one-liner he wants to make his news pitch. Most writers and reporters do not have the time or expertise to put, for example, the results of a new animal study on the health effects of chemical X in perspective. To attempt to do so would mean coming up with a dreadfully boring and evenhanded story that communicates the accurate but ho-hum message that "a laboratory study today revealed that chemical X can increase the risk of liver tumors in mice, but scientists cautioned against rash regulatory actions against this chemical because dozens of other animal studies and many observations on humans have shown no ill effects." Now, where is the story line there? What would that do for ratings? The intense thirst of the media for titillating news in the context of their inevitable deadlines is a major discouraging factor in whatever quest they may have for balanced coverage.

At the Business Journalism Awards banquet of the Interstate National Gas Association held on 28 October 1983, Dow Chemical chairman of the board Robert W. Lundeen said,

> TV and some print journalists demand snappy answers to snappy questions. The reality is that more often than not, especially in matters relating to science and technology there simply are no snappy answers. To get it right, you must check . . . double check . . . and check once again.

Many reporters seem to have an aversion to checking back with their sources to check facts and the accuracy of quotes. They mumble words like "censorship" or worse. But checks for factual and technical accuracy need not have overtones of censorship if the reporter stays in charge.[16]

Apparently, the public is beginning to perceive that the press isn't careful. The 1989 Times Mirror survey found that public confidence in the press has dropped sharply since the mid-1980s survey. In 1985, 83 percent of the public thought the press was believable; by 1989 that figure had dropped to 74 percent. Other results of that survey include:

- Seventy-six percent of the public felt there is a great deal or fair amount of political bias in news coverage, and 75 percent of the politicians who were polled agreed, as did 88 percent of business leaders;
- Daily newspapers suffered a greater decline in believability than their electronic news rivals;
- Fifty-four percent of the public thinks news organizations get the facts straight, but 44 percent think news stories are often inaccurate; what is most revealing is that 14 percent of the press themselves felt their stories and reports were inaccurate.

Fifth, for whatever reason, whether it is a thirst for bad news, or a quest for something sensational, shocking, or frightening, the U.S. media are willing to accept, almost uncritically, preliminary scientific evidence no matter how tenuous and preliminary it is. Whether it is because of time pressure, the search for sensationalism, simple lack of expertise, or fear that their competition will get the story first, peer review does not exist in television, radio, and print media circles.

The process of peer review is the tried-and-true method that has evolved in the scientific community and is the sole method of applying the self-imposed standards that scientists use to separate good science from bad. When a scientist completes the research for a project, he or she interprets the results, writes them up, and submits them to a scientific journal in his or her field for publication. Scientific journals then submit the information they receive to peer review and meticulous editing before publication. However, unreviewed studies slip out into the public through the media before their results or scientific validity are confirmed. For example, as William R. Barclay wrote in the *Journal of the American Medical Association,* "Many of the reports on carcinogenesis that have been made public have been flawed both in design and interpretation but have been accepted by [government] agencies that funded them, by the news media, and, finally, by the public."[17] Dr. Barclay goes on to say:

> Although ignorance of the existence of a hazard can be dangerous, false information can be even more dangerous, and while one cannot quarrel with the concept of a fully informed public or defend science's cloaking itself in secrecy, one can demand responsible evaluation and reporting of scientific data.

In short, stories that go straight to the press without benefit of scientific peer review often end up causing unneeded concern and even panic. And, of course, when follow-up studies discredit earlier alarming reports, well—that's just not news.

IS THE "MEDIA BIAS DISEASE" CURABLE?

An immediate obvious antidote for the media bias syndrome might be the influx into journalism of a substantial number of establishment-supported, protechnology young writers and reporters who might be able to detect and present the good news and put the bad news in proper perspective. But realistically, this is not the answer. Journalists have their own club atmosphere, and dissenters find it exceedingly difficult to gain admittance, unless they openly identify themselves clearly as being "different," representing the politically conservative point of view.

With the great majority of the scientists mute on these raging controversies, understandably the public is left with the opinion that the four or five physicians and scientists who are repeatedly quoted by the media in their tirades against anything that makes this country great represent the majority opinion, or, at least, represent half of that opinion.

A number of explanations, some of which are at least partially correctable, come to mind.

First, it could be argued that American scientists are simply too busy to get into public, and sometimes controversial, dialogues on chemicals, the environment, and health. They are busy in laboratories, teaching, or, if physicians, in private medical practice. But, "too busy" is relative. If something is important—if, for example, your reputation is at stake—you are never too busy to defend it.

Second, perhaps scientists and physicians feel incompetent and uncomfortable appearing in public with glib, well-rehearsed "environmental performers." The trained scientist may never have been on TV and he or she might fear handling it badly. He doesn't want to make a fool of himself; she's afraid that professional colleagues might question the propriety of her presence on a program that also features a quack, two unemployed actresses, and a male stripper.

Not only are most Ph.D.s and M.D.s trained to use highly technical terms, but those true experts in the fields of epidemiology, toxicology, and the related disciplines feel obliged to speak with constant qualifications, clarifications, and exceptions to the rule. When one is on the offensive, for example, claiming that Love Canal residents were dropping dead like flies, giving birth to deformed children, and suffering from nervous breakdowns because of seeping chemicals, it is far easier to present your case than it is to be on the defensive, stating that no such problem exists, but in all honesty having to admit that since you cannot prove a negative, the possibility of disaster always exists. Legitimate scientists are at an immediate disadvantage in interviews with the media because they, unlike their pseudoscientific counterparts, are morally and emotionally confined to sticking to the facts.

Another reason pertains to time and money. Ralph Nader, on the other side of the fence, is paid well to do what he's doing—it is his full-time job to make waves over nothing. Most scientists have competing interests—industrial problem solving, research, or teaching—which claims higher priority than debunking pseudoscience. Most creators of pseudoscience—like Ralph Nader—have little else to do.

Perhaps of most importance is that the legitimate scientist rejects the attractive yet fatally flawed practice known as "intuitive science." Intuitive science is the easy way to reach conclusions without subjecting a hypothesis to a rigorous set of tests as part of a carefully planned methodology. In a recent public issues publication of the Dow Chemical Company, the intuitive approach was discussed:

> The intuitive approach draws its strength from appealingly reasonable conclusions about the nature of things. It's the kind of thinking, for example, that says if you tie a string to a stone and twirl it around your head, and suddenly let go of the string—the stone will continue to follow a curved path. This kind of "self-evident" reasoning has charm for many people today, including college students whose background and education should equip them for more thoughtful inquiry. Indeed, when a group of them was questioned about the string-and-stone example, three out of ten saw no need for any factual confirmation. They knew "intuitively" that this would happen. Of course, that isn't what happens. The stone actually flies off on a tangent, a straight line, in keeping with the laws of Newtonian physics.[18]

This kind of "science" makes clear to the parent of a child with leukemia that the nearby high-voltage line caused that malady and proves to the former resident of Love Canal that his or her cancer was caused by leaking chemicals there. This is also the kind of science that the Ralph Naders and Samuel Epsteins of the world can generate rapidly, to the delight of a voracious media. This kind of "science" in fact, should really be called science policy analysis. In this arena, political skills are more important than scientific credentials.

The only answer here seems to be the traditional one, whereby a commodity loses favor because consumers become dissatisfied with it. When "manufacturers," in this case the network or local news producer, know of that dissatisfaction, either by letters to the editor and other critical correspondence, or by learning that consumers are simply not purchasing the product (turning off the network news if it is not up to standards; not buying the *New York Times,* but trying an alternative source), then perhaps there is hope—economic incentive—for change. Similarly, advertisers could show their dissatisfaction with biased media coverage by pulling out their accounts when there is obvious evidence of distrust and an attempt to misinform the public.

Question 2: The Case of the Missing Scientists

Drs. Claus and Bolander, in *Ecological Sanity,* observe, with regard to the missing scientist, "One of the most obvious questions that may come to the reader's mind is: if the authors alleged that a considerable number of the scientific claims of the environmentalists are false and some of the papers which support these claims are worthless or filled with errors, how does it happen that out of more than 200,000 scientists in the United States so few have spoken up in a similar vein of protest?"[19]

Dealing with the media is, like everything else, an acquired skill. One does not automatically get a Ph.D. in biology from Yale, become a professor at the University of Michigan, and overnight become a qualified and at-ease guest for a debate on the "Today" program opposite a rabid environmentalist. Scientists and physicians are not trained to debate in public. They are not educated to be advocates or to be available for instant response to "new findings." Scientists are committed to the philosophy that the search for truth takes time and effort, and that one set of data does not necessarily make a conclusion. Certainly they do not feel comfortable evaluating for a reporter the results of a report they have never seen.

Environmental alarmists like Dr. Samuel Epstein, and his counterparts in the journalism world like Lewis Regenstein, Ralph Nader, and Karl Grossman, are self-appointed experts on everything. They are "generalists," quite willing, without other professional backup, to pontificate on subjects ranging from dioxin to Love Canal to aldrin and dieldrin and nuclear energy. On the other hand, most scientists and physicians are successful because they have become specialists and would not think of speaking authoritatively outside their field unless they were presenting the conclusion of a peer-reviewed group effort. Since the media much prefer roundup-type topics to specific ones (that is, they might want to talk about the safety of pesticides, herbicides, food additives, and food processing in the same breath rather than, as academics would in a seminar, focus exclusively on the toxicology of saccharin), the true expert remains stymied, while the alarmist, short on useful information but long on unfounded opinion, is willing to step forward to condemn a variety of technologies with one sweeping stroke.

Too, many mainstream scientists and physicians may simply be afraid of the media, and what they might do to them. The fear goes way beyond the anxiety of the lights and the countdown in an NBC studio. More important, it is the fear of public humiliation. As was mentioned before, members of the U.S. media, though quick to accept unchallenged the frightening and pessimistic reports of the environmentalists, are skeptical of scientists who defend technology. "Who funds you?" is the common, aggressively asked question for the scientist who brings good news. Many scientists in the United States have *some* connection with U.S. industry, either because they have offered consultant services or been a speaker at a corporate convention, or because their university department has a grant from one or more members of the food, chemical, or pharmaceutical industries. Thus they deem themselves vulnerable to the probes of the press representatives who want to reinforce the proconsumer versus proindustry dichotomy by using introductions like, "Dr. Smith, a professor at Harvard University, admits that his department has received a grant from the Dow Chemical Company."*

Beyond the funding phenomenon, some scientists fear the media because they don't trust them and have no control on how the material they give them will be used. Dr. Merril Eisenbud explains this reluctance:

> Many of us complain that we are expected to take the time to be taped for TV or radio interviews, but have no control over what finally appears. All too often, the most useful things we say end up on the cutting-room floor. Over the years I have grown camera-shy because all too often a single brief sentence, totally out of context, is all that is aired after an interview that involved many minutes of taping. I believe that unless the interview is going to be published in its entirety, it is proper that the scientist be given an opportunity to approve the edited version.[20]

This reluctance to submit to editorial whim is growing not only among scientists like Eisenbud but also among the corporate community, where a sentence out of context can help to develop a serious case against industry.

In addition, another funding question, one *never* raised by the media but an important roadblock to some scientists who might otherwise "go public," is the fear of losing government money. If a scientist's research program is being funded by the Environmental Protection Agency, the Occupational Safety and Health Administration, or other federal agencies, he might think twice before he steps forward to criticize a government study, or to defend the safety of a product that falls in the jurisdiction of his funder.

Moreover, the reluctance of the scientific community, particularly environmental and public health specialists, to come to the defense of pesticides and offer perspective to relieve public anxiety about dioxin, air and water pollution, and various Love Canals may be rooted in professional self-interest, or survival, or what is sometimes called the "medical student phenomenon."

What one finds from reviewing scientific journals committed to public health or environmental sciences is that they are very much one-sided, very much feeding the anxiety about environmental contamination and industry irresponsibility. Nowhere within publications such as the *Archives of Environmental Health* does one find a critique of environmentalism. In that sense, the profession of environmentalism is very different from, for example, the profession of the microbiologist. Microbiologists will be needed, and their profession will thrive, no matter the events in the news. Microbiology is a

---

*What is perplexing about the media is that while they are quick to dismiss the views of any scientist with even the remotest connection with industry, they never reflect on who funds the *media*. Every network and local radio and television station and almost every newspaper and magazine are funded by none other than the food, chemical, pharmaceutical, and other industries through their substantial advertising revenues.

basic science that stands by itself.

On the other hand, environmental science thrives on bad news. The more bad news we have about pesticide residues on food, dioxin, Love Canal, and general pollution, the more we will need environmental scientists. There seems to be an inherent, self-serving bias here, with public health advocates and environmentalists looking for problems that may not exist, but finding almost every one they look for, just as the medical student is sure he has every disease he reads about.

Individuals training in epidemiology, public health, or a particular environmental science are likely to be a self-selected group, having chosen their profession because of their feeling that the end of the world was near and their services were needed to postpone that inevitability. After receiving their professional training, they are understandably defensive of their own vocation and the educational commitment they have made to it and seek to ensure that the problems they built their careers on don't go away. One might want to dismiss this explanation by saying this is as ridiculous as saying that some dentists are against fluoridation so they can keep their customers coming in. But it is different. Dentists are health professionals who deal with a full spectrum of dental problems. The environmentalist, without environmental problems, does not have a job. So again, in the words of Ben Wattenberg, "Bad news is good news."

GETTING THE SCIENTIFIC COMMUNITY TO PARTICIPATE

Although there are a number of serious roadblocks in the way of scientists who want to, or should want to, become part of the public dialogue on health and the environment, the problem is solvable if scientists become more aggressive in defense of their profession and more active in challenging misinformation when it is served up. As the late Dr. Philip Handler, former president of the National Academy of Science, once observed,

> Scientists best serve public policy by living within the ethics of science, not those of politics. If the scientific community will not unfrock the charlatans, the public will not discern the differences—science and the nation will suffer.[21]

First, scientists must come to appreciate how irresponsible the mass media are in disseminating information, or misinformation, about the relationship of health and the environment. People tend to believe what they hear on radio or TV. After all, if something weren't true, that man on the program wouldn't be allowed to say it, would he? Especially on *national television?*

Of course, people are allowed to say almost anything they want to on the air as long as it doesn't libel someone. They are protected by the First

Amendment. Most of us wouldn't want it any other way. However, this freedom, combined with our tendency to trust TV and radio, makes misinformation from these sources especially potent.

If a scientist reads about a "startling medical discovery" or "new deadly toxin found in Kalamazoo" in a supermarket tabloid, or if he hears about it from the guy sitting next to him on the plane, his skepticism is going to be operating at full steam. Unfortunately, most consumers don't retain this high level of suspicion when listening to radio or TV. They need an opposing scientist, with better credentials, to challenge the alarmists, and make the viewer think twice before accepting the grim news.

Second, health professionals should convince the media, by example, that scientifically sound medicine and science aren't intrinsically dull; prime-time and daytime medical dramas are relatively accurate, and many of them have earned high ratings. Those ratings might plummet, however, if the actors were replaced by real doctors. A haughty, multi-syllabic presentation from high in the ivory tower does little to hold an audience. Unfortunately, many real-life health professionals (unlike their fictional counterparts) cannot communicate their messages well, and they're anything but entertaining. If the health professions are to utilize the media effectively for communications, their spokespersons must learn to be believable and appealing.

It would also help if both the media and health professionals devoted some thought to reevaluating their priorities and responsibilities.

Third, scientists whenever possible—through personal contacts, letters to the editor, or a call to a TV producer—should announce their availability to answer questions on specific topics well in advance of a breaking story. If each station had a continuing relationship with a few medical and scientific consultants (from the local university faculty, perhaps), it would not be difficult to verify the accuracy of a purported health fact, or to determine whether a controversial talk-show guest would best appear together with a spokesperson for the opposite viewpoint.

Obviously, *all* scientists and health professionals can't be expected to ditch their careers in favor of media tours, but it seems reasonable to ask *some* of them, particularly academic physicians, to make themselves available to the media from time to time, and to learn to present their messages with a proficiency at least comparable to that of the average quack.

All health professionals should make a point of keeping track of the current fads and frauds being promoted via the media. Even if they never go on the air, health professionals can exert some social and economic pressure by praising those stations that are fair and responsible in their coverage of health topics.

The health professions must also stop ignoring the America-the-poisoned authors and the like, and the media appearances they make. These people have a powerful impact on the public and gain credibility with each broadcast.

Physicians and scientists should not deny or fight the power of the media; they should join it. If a charlatan is in town, a qualified professional should be demanding a debate. To stand back is to permit facts to be distorted— a dangerous error of omission. Says Gary Flamm, a former Food and Drug Administration staffer, about scientists who didn't come forward to clarify the Alar-and-apple issue:

> My own feeling is that scientists who sit by and watch [such] things happen without protesting are no different from scientists who fudge data.[22]

Question 3: The Environmentalists and Health Pessimists: Who Are They and What Do They Want?

The term *environmentalist* encompasses many different people. Presumably there are sincere, well-meaning individuals who worry about the disappearance of natural resources and the quality of this country's lakes, rivers, streams, oceans, and beaches, and are understandably concerned about the threat to wilderness lands. There *is* sound reason to take steps to ensure that our air and water remain acceptably free of pollutants, and that irresponsible industries do not dump toxic material into our environment. *Environmentalist* is not synonymous with *alarmist*.

But in this section, as throughout this book, we are focusing on the extreme end of the environmentalist spectrum. We are referring to those who so frequently make claims and suggest regulations that have no basis in science, that serve to interrupt the growth of the American economy, and that have no perceivable positive impact on the public's health.

Environmental groups, and authors of books like *The Toxic Cloud* and *America the Poisoned*, often style themselves as defenders of the "public interest," crusaders who protect the American public from the greed and callousness of American industry. The term *public interest* sounds good, and it would initially seem that it is such a neutral humanistic goal that there would be something in it for everyone. After all, Walter Lippmann, writing in 1955, before the label public interest assumed its current connotations, wrote:

> The public interest may be presumed to be what men would choose if they saw clearly, thought rationally, acted disinterestedly and benevolently.[23]

Indeed, the names of many of these public-interest groups do seem to suggest they are speaking for all of us: Common Cause, Public Citizen, Consumer Federation of America. They sound about as American as 100 percent naturally, purely organic apple pie and about as free from vested interest as possible.

Why would those speaking in the public interest constantly want to sound the chimes of doom, predict the end of the world through environmental, technology-induced disaster? One might begin with an "optimistic" explanation for their pessimism, namely, that it is a natural phenomenon to experience feelings of terminability as we approach the close of another millennium. As Rene Dubos wrote in *So Human An Animal,* "As the year 2000 approaches, an epidemic of sinister predictions is spreading all over the world, as happened among Christians during the period preceding the year 1000.[24]

But this explanation in itself is not satisfying. If it were simply a natural reaction to the turning of centuries, why wouldn't the environmentalists be focusing on natural as well as man-made sources of disaster? Why would they not be predicting earthquakes, flood, collision of the earth with a comet, or simply the falling of the skies, as in Chicken Little?

Another charitable explanation, as presented by Maddox, is that the first landing on the moon by the crew of Apollo 11 provided those left on earth with a vivid impression of our precarious foothold in an otherwise inhospitable solar system. But then, in rejecting that, Maddox reminds us that the landing on the moon took place when the environmental movement was well established, so it could hardly be a cause.[25]

But indeed, a close look at the public-interest leaders clearly suggests that they are *not* worried about the turn of the century or our precariousness in the solar system, and are *not* representing the interests of the vast majority of Americans. Further, they are *not* mainstream in their political orientation. And perhaps they are *not* as selfless as they would like us to believe.

The purpose in stressing the politically liberal views of the public-interest leaders is not necessarily to be critical of liberal political philosophy. The point here is that public-interest leaders do not represent a cross-section of political views. They represent a homogeneous political philosophy, one that makes their pronouncements on scientific subjects suspect, because if science and health were their primary goals, it seems logical that their political attitudes would be as diverse as they are in the rest of the nation's population.

So public-interest leaders, including those who espouse environmentalism, have their own unique profile: they are politically liberal, highly educated at the best schools, and the offspring of relatively affluent, educated parents. Indeed, it is this profile that has led a few analysts to conclude that environmentalism is an elitist movement consciously or unconsciously designed to preserve its members' own high standard of living.

Herbert Meyer, for example, in his book *The War Against Progress* actually defines the environmental movement as just that, a war against progress. This war, he writes, "is being fought by people who themselves enjoy a high standard of living and who believe that to protect their own comfort they must prevent others from becoming equally comfortable. . . ." In other words, Meyer sees the environmental movement as a self-interest–motivated protest by a small group of "haves" against all of those "have nots."[26] Thus, with this interpretation, the resistance to the development of land and the construction of more apartments in urban areas is based not on "preserving the quality of the environment," but on a threat to their own lifestyle through the mechanism of overcrowding and disappearance of properties that they enjoy for leisure purposes.

William Tucker in his book *Progress and Privilege,* in articles for *Harper's* magazine, and in interviews expresses a similar philosophical basis for the environmental movement:

> Environmentalists today are not saying anything different than what most aristocracies have been saying all along. Invariably, there's a strong conservatism, a strong cautiousness and a tendency to downgrade industrial society and industrial accomplishments. Environmentalism is a kind of elitist expression of a group which is already well off, and doesn't welcome new upstarts or technologies. It's the old "we can do without it" sort of attitude that aristocracies have always had toward progress and innovation.[27]

Thus Tucker believes basically that environmentalism is a selfish enterprise run by people who are able to make sacrifices by giving up "material production,"[28] which they personally don't need anyway, to make marginal gains in health and safety.

The findings in a Lichter and Rothman survey of public-interest leaders that there is a "general dissatisfaction with the American social and economic order" suggest yet another thread of motivation, one that does not conflict with, but parallels, that presented by Meyer and Tucker.[29] Any careful reading of environmentalist rhetoric and a close analysis of the targets that the health alarmists choose for manipulating to "improve health" clearly indicate that these individuals are bitterly antagonistic toward American industry. If there were ever a way of solving a problem *without* economically penalizing an industry, they show no interest in that alternative. If there are zero known deaths caused by routine use of agricultural pesticides in this country, and hundreds of deaths among children who accidentally ingest household pesticides that their parents have imprudently left in their reach, the environmentalists would still choose the route of attempting to restrict the sale of agricultural pesticides made by the "agribusiness" complex they seem so suspicious of. Ron Arnold, author of *At the Eye of the Storm: James Watt and the Environmentalists,* minces no words when he characterizes the goals of environmentalists as the desire to "drastically reduce or dismantle industrial civilization" and to "impose a fundamentally coercive form of government on America" through the implementation of a wide range of environmental laws and controls.[30]

The motives of the environmentalists in claiming death and destruction through exposure to the chemicals at Love Canal, air and water pollution, pesticides, low-level radiation, and other potential environmental contaminants are clearly suspect primarily because they will fully disregard the scientific facts that do not support their case. They skillfully avoid the topic of the costs of their suggestions while pleading a utopian, pollution-free existence. They criticize, they condemn. But they appear to have no workable solutions that do not entail greater political coercion and control.

In the end we are left with the possibility that, for some environmental agitators, although certainly not all, environmentalism is a means to an end, rather than the end itself. Perhaps their primary interest is not in preserving health and ecological quality, but in changing the political and economic system by dwarfing the power of corporation, replacing the free-enterprise system with public agencies, and redistributing the country's wealth. Perhaps the extreme environmentalists simply are rejecting the traditional goals and philosophy of American society and are out to dismantle it and replace it with some poorly defined alternative structure.

WHO FUNDS THE ENVIRONMENTALISTS?

These days if you picket a nuclear power plant, hold a national news conference to condemn a pesticide, make charges that the chemical industry is polluting our air and water, or deplore the sale of infant formula overseas, the chances are your view will be accepted by the media and the public as an honest expression of your feeling on the subject.

But if, after examining the facts, you conclude that nuclear power plants are safe, that food additives and pesticides are not only safe but necessary, or that bottle feeding is a fully acceptable form of infant nutrition, then you are in big trouble, inevitably confronted with the question, Who funds you? The implication of the question is always clear: what the asker really wants to know is, Can you be trusted or are you bought off to say what you say?

Why, then, haven't the media been equally skeptical in evaluating the environmentalists? Who *does* fund them?

The answer is far from clear. The funding sources for a tax-exempt group need not be publicly revealed. Such groups are required to disclose funding sources to the Internal Revenue Service, but even the Freedom of Information Act has not allowed access to this information. The limited information available by means of "backward searches" to examine which groups foundations (which are required to disclose) are funding triggers a number of fascinating observations. First, the budgets of the large environmental groups are significant. For example, the budget of the Natural Resources Defense Council in 1984 was in excess of $7 million. (It's now about double that or more.) Second, most all the environmental groups receive substantial contributions from a small group of foundations, including the Rockefeller Brothers Fund, the Charles Stewart Mott and Ruth Mott Foundation, and the George Gund Foundation. Third, many of the environmental groups, including the Natural Resources Defense Council, receive moneys from tobacco family foundations, including the Mary Reynolds Babcock Foundation.

The last observation—the support from tobacco family money (another Reynolds family foundation that frequently shows up on funding lists is the Arca Foundation)—tantalizes. It is of course possible that, in addition, the environmentalists receive money directly from the tobacco companies, although this is not easy to verify because corporations need not publicly disclose to whom they are giving money. Philip Morris, among other tobacco manufacturers, has a contribution committee that proclaims a special interest in funding environmentalism. In any case, the environmentalists are silent on the health devastation caused by cigarettes, and surely, whether or not the tobacco companies are funding them, the cigarette manufacturers are pleased when the country is in a state of hysteria about Alar on apples instead of focusing attention on the more than five hundred thousand deaths each year from smoking. Are tobacco interests fueling the environmental movement? All the answers are not in, but this surely would be a likely area for an aggressive investigative reporter to pursue.

What Is the Cost of Environmentalism?

According to a 1992 report "Why Is the Cost of Environmental Regulations So High" by the Center for the Study of American Business at Washington University, the cost of environmental policies has risen steadily while their effectiveness has not.[31]

Writes one of the report's authors, Robert Crandall, a senior fellow at the Brookings Institute:

> Given nearly 20 years of experience with the environmental policies that were launched in the 1970s, one would hope that Congress and the administration would not repeat the errors of the past that resulted in a federal government policy that is absurdly inefficient.

Crandall cites studies that showed compliance with environmental legislation has reduced economic growth by 0.2 percentage points per year from 1974 through 1985, totaling $150 billion. That figure may even be too low, says Crandall, since these studies did not include the effects of regulatory policies deliberately biased against new investments and "It is very difficult to measure the effects of investments not made."

Looking to the Future

What kind of an impact ought environmentalism to have on America in the coming years? How should the quest for a "cleaner" environment be incorporated into the policies and regulations that will guide us into the third millennium?

A healthy environment is synonymous with healthy standards of living for all people. To the environmental extremists of the 1990s the ultimate goal is the widescale restriction of man-made chemicals in all facets of society. But to the truly concerned public health specialist, the better world that we work to build is a world void of preventable illnesses and deaths. Drug abuse, suicide, highway fatalities, and tobacco-induced mortality are some of the grim agents of human misery that affect our daily lives. These, and not parts per billion of pesticide residues, are the real causes of human pain and suffering. Sanitary housing and abundant food supplies for all segments of the population are the kinds of goals that, when reached, will genuinely improve our society.

Americans and citizens all over the Western world can be proud of the strides we've taken to improve our environment. The innovative technological breakthroughs of the twentieth century have resulted in the healthiest population ever to live on this planet. While the advances have not come without risks, the ultimate benefits have in fact vastly outweighed the costs, despite what the scaremonger lobby would have us believe.

It is time for scientists to speak out on environmentalism and public health. The public has a right to receive credible scientific information concerning important environmental issues. And it's also time for knowledgeable consumers to scrutinize and protest the steady diet of misinformation supplied by the holier-than-thou activists and lobbyists who would have us believe that technology-run-amok is the enemy that is successfully destroying our health and well-being.

Environmental health problems do exist. Many have been addressed, and many warrant strong commitments for the future. But the toxic terrorists have egregiously overreacted to a frightening extent. Their spread of chemophobia threatens our ability to create the new technologies that can continue to benefit our environment and our standard of living. Understanding that we must respect the potential hazards inherent in new technologies, we will see our public health continue to improve. For when used responsibly, technology provides us with our most valuable tools as we strive to build a safer, healthier world.

NOTES

1. R. M. Campbell, "Plutonium—A Precious Fuel," *Patriot Ledger,* September 15, 1982.

2. R. Arnold, *At the Eye of the Storm: James Watt and the Environmentalists* (Chicago: Regnery Gateway, 1982), p. 210.

3. B. Wattenberg, "The Good News Is the Bad News Is Wrong," *Reader's Digest,* April 1984, pp. 103–5.

4. Ibid., p. 202.

5. Arnold, *Eye of the Storm,* p. 210.

6. *Washington Post,* April 9, 1979.

7. Media Institute, *Nuclear Phobia: Public Thinking About Nuclear Power: A Discussion with Robert L. DuPont, M.D.* (Washington, D.C., March 1980).

8. Ibid.

9. B. L. Cohen and I. S. Lee, in *Health Physics* 36 (1979): p. 707.

10. Center for the People and the Press, "Times Mirror Study Finds 'Erosion' in Public Confidence in News Media," press release, November 15, 1989.

11. Arnold, *Eye of the Storm,* p. 210.

12. Personal communication, August 4, 1983.

13. R. E. Lapp, *The Radiation Controversy* (Greenwich: Reddy Communications, 1979), p. 140.

14. Center for the People and the Press, "Times Mirror Study."

15. American Council on Science and Health, *ACSH News and Views,* January/ February 1982.

16. R. W. Lundeen, *The Media and Industry: Two Different Worlds* (Dow Communications Department, Dow Chemical Company, 1983), pp. 12–13.

17. W. R. Barclay, "Science Reporting to Alarm the Public," *Journal of the American Medical Association* (August 24–31, 1979): p. 754.

18. Dow Chemical Company, *Rush to Judgment,* no. 67, December 5, 1983.

19. G. Claus and K. Bolander, *Ecological Sanity* (New York: David McKay, 1977), p. 49.

20. M. Eisenbud, "Statement Before the Public Information and Public Relations Panel," New York Academy of Medicine Symposium on the Health Aspects of Nuclear Power Plant Incidents, April 7–8, 1983.

21. P. Handler, "Science and the American Future," speech at Duke University, March 6, 1980.

22. E. Marshall, "A Is for Apple, Alar and . . . Alarmist?" *Science* 254 (1991): pp. 20–22.

23. S. R. Lichter and S. Rothman, "What Interests the Public and What Interest the Public Interests," *Public Opinion* (April/May 1983): pp. 44–48.

24. R. Dubos, *So Human an Animal* (New York: Charles Scribner's Sons, 1968), p. 10.

25. J. Maddox, *The Doomsday Syndrome* (New York: McGraw Hill, 1972), p. 24.

26. H. E. Meyer, *The War Against Progress* (New York: Storm King, 1979), p. 83.

27. American Council on Science and Health, William Tucker interview, *ACSH News and Views* (September/October 1983): pp. 4–5.

28. W. Tucker, *Progress and Privilege* (New York: Doubleday, 1982), p. 5.

29. Lichter and Rothman, "What Interests the Public," pp. 44–48.

30. "Behind the Campaign Against Watt," *Nation's Business,* March 1983, p. 56.

31. "Environment Policies Costlier But Less Effective, Report Says." *Journal of Commerce,* (March 9, 1992).

Appendix

The Myth of a Cancer Epidemic*

Cancer Statistics: Terminology

A thorough discussion of cancer statistics must begin with definitions of cancer incidence and cancer mortality.

Cancer incidence refers to the number of new cases of cancer diagnosed during a given year. Cancer incidence rates are the number of new cases per year for a fixed population. These rates are usually expressed as the annual number of new cases per hundred thousand population. For most of the United States, it is not required that each new case of cancer be reported to a government agency. Thus, exact figures on the total number of new cancer cases are not available. Instead, cancer incidence is estimated from an ongoing survey in several states and urban areas which represent the nation as a whole.

Cancer mortality refers to the number of cancer deaths reported for a given year. Cancer death rates are expressed as the annual number of cancer deaths per hundred thousand population. Most deaths in the United States are reported and the primary cause of death is usually specified. Because of this broader reporting system, there is more accurate information on cancer mortality than on cancer incidence.

A comparison of cancer mortality and incidence time trends is found in figure 1. Certified death rates, age-standardized for the total U.S. population, show a moderate decline for both sexes, 1933–77, whereas opposite trends are observable for Connecticut-registered, age-standardized incidence rates, 1935–74.

Age standardization is an averaging method of calculating mortality and/

---

*Reprinted with permission from the American Council on Science and Health publication, *Cancer in the United States: Is There an Epidemic?*

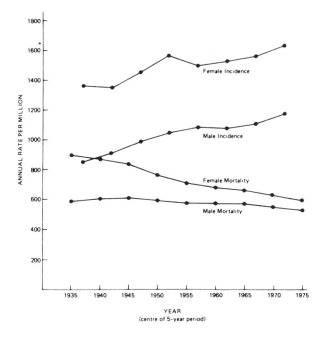

Fig. 1. Age-standardized certified death rates for entire U.S. population 1933–77, con-trasted with Connecticut registered incidence rates 1935–74; all cancers except lung and skin. Rates per million, standardized to the age distribution of all respondents under 65 years to the U.S. 1970 census, as described in appendix.

or incidence rates to remove the confounding effect tracing to the age distribution in a given population. Such procedures are required to compare cancer inci-dence and mortality rates for population groups whose age makeup may differ in time or geographic place.

Cancer Statistics: Sources

The National Cancer Institute (NCI), American Cancer Society (ACS), and the National Center for Health Statistics (NCHS) regularly publish national cancer information. However, because each agency uses different methods of analysis and presentation their cancer statistics are often not comparable.

In the past, the National Cancer Institute estimated cancer incidence on the basis of periodic surveys. More recently, the NCI has developed an ongoing program that continually reports new cases of cancer in several states and cities. The information collected from the Surveillance, Epidemiology and End

Results (SEER) program is then used to estimate national cancer patterns.

The SEER program is currently based on cancer data from eleven geographic locations. These include five entire states (Connecticut, Iowa, New Mexico, Utah, and Hawaii), five large metropolitan areas (Atlanta, New Orleans, Detroit, San Francisco, and Seattle) and the entire commonwealth of Puerto Rico. New Jersey and New York have also established cancer registries to monitor new cases and cancer deaths, but these data are not included in the SEER reporting system.

The American Cancer Society also publishes annual information on cancer incidence. Using data from the SEER program, the ACS estimates the number of new cancer cases that will occur in each state. These estimates can be misleading, however, because they are not related to a fixed population.

Cancer death rates are published by the National Center for Health Statistics, the American Cancer Society, and the National Cancer Institute. Each of these agencies uses a different standard population for presenting mortality data.

The National Center for Health Statistics collects crude cancer mortality information and adjusts it to the age distribution of the 1940 census population. Because cancer occurs primarily among older persons, it is important to take into account the proportion of each age group in computing a single death or incidence rate. Age adjusting permits comparisons of rates from different years without the influences of a continuously aging population.

The American Cancer Society uses the information collected by the NCHS and prepares its own analysis of cancer death rates. The ACS also uses these data to estimate the number of cancer deaths that will occur during the following year. But because these cancer death rates are not age-adjusted, they are not comparable with the NCHS cancer death rates.

In 1975 the National Cancer Institute published a report, *U.S. Cancer Mortality by County: 1950–1969*. This study calculated cancer death rates for each county in the continental United States according to sex and race. These rates were age-adjusted to the 1960 census population, a different standard than that used by the NCHS. These NCI data also give the death rate for the entire twenty-year period for each type of cancer as a single composite figure. Although these rates permit intercounty comparisons, they cannot be compared with either ACS or NCHS annual cancer statistics.

U.S. Cancer Incidence*

The American Cancer Society estimates that 1,100,000 new cases of cancer will be diagnosed in 1991. If current rates prevail, one in three to four Americans

---

*Incidence rates in this section are taken from the 1947–48 Second National Cancer Survey (SNCS), the 1969-71 Third National Cancer Survey (TNCS), and the 1973–87 data of the SEER program.

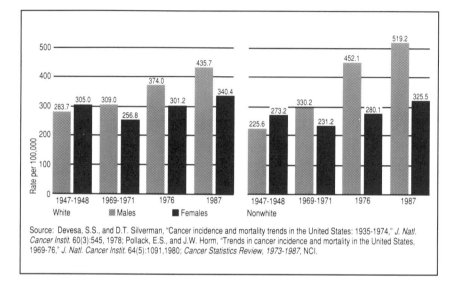

Source: Devesa, S.S., and D.T. Silverman, "Cancer incidence and mortality trends in the United States: 1935-1974," *J. Natl. Cancer Instit.* 60(3):545, 1978; Pollack, E.S., and J.W. Horm, "Trends in cancer incidence and mortality in the United States, 1969-76," *J. Natl. Cancer Instit.* 64(5):1091,1980; *Cancer Statistics Review, 1973-1987*, NCI.

Fig. 2. Estimated cancer incidence rates per 100,000 population by race and sex, SNCS (1947–48), TNCS (1969–71), SEER (1976), SEER (1987)

now living will eventually develop cancer, although many will die of other causes. For the twenty-four-year period 1947–71, the composite age-adjusted cancer incidence rate *declined* slightly, even though the total number of new cases increased. However, between 1973 and 1987, the most recent period for which data are available, age-adjusted incidence rates have increased about 1.0 percent annually.

In general, cancer incidence has decreased among women under the age of forty-five. Incidence has increased since 1947 among men and among persons forty-five and older. Figure 2 shows how the combined cancer incidence rates have changed for men and women during the period 1947–87. Again, the differences in age-adjusted standards for each survey period require caution in drawing any firm conclusions from this information.

Some types of cancer occur more frequently than others. Among men, prostate cancer is now the most common form followed by lung and colon-rectum cancer. Among women, breast cancer is the leader followed by colon-rectum and lung cancers. Figure 3 shows estimates of the proportion of all cancers that occur at each major body site. Table 1 shows the changes in cancer incidence for selected body sites for the period 1947–76.

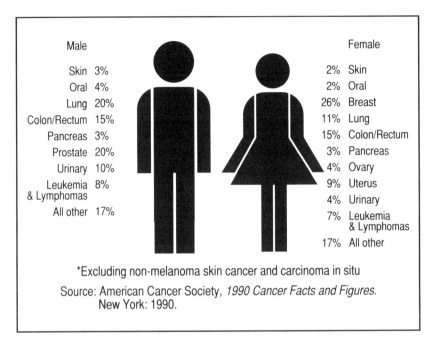

Male

Skin	3%
Oral	4%
Lung	20%
Colon/Rectum	15%
Pancreas	3%
Prostate	20%
Urinary	10%
Leukemia & Lymphomas	8%
All other	17%

Female

2%	Skin
2%	Oral
26%	Breast
11%	Lung
15%	Colon/Rectum
3%	Pancreas
4%	Ovary
9%	Uterus
4%	Urinary
7%	Leukemia & Lymphomas
17%	All other

*Excluding non-melanoma skin cancer and carcinoma in situ

Source: American Cancer Society, *1990 Cancer Facts and Figures.* New York: 1990.

Fig. 3. 1983 estimated cancer incidence by site and sex

As with all statistical data, several factors will influence the interpretation of these estimates. First, as knowledge about cancer increases, changes occur in medical diagnosis. (There are currently more than one hundred known types of human cancer.) Past incidence surveys may have either under- or over-reported certain kinds of cancer because of these diagnostic changes.

Second, the survey areas from which data are collected also change with time. For example, two southern cities with large black populations (Atlanta and New Orleans) were added to the SEER network in 1974 and 1976. As a result, the estimates of cancer incidence among blacks from the past surveys cannot properly be compared with the newer data. And as noted earlier, the SEER program adjusts its data to a different standard population than the earlier National Cancer Surveys. These and other methodological differences suggest that the incidence data for 1971–87 may be somewhat higher than they would be if the pre-1971 techniques were used. Therefore any small increases or decreases should be interpreted cautiously.

Table 1. Estimated Cancer Incidence Rates per 100,000 Population
by Race and Sex, Selected Body Sites SNCS (1947–48),*
TNCS (1969–71),** SEER (1976),*** SEER (1987)****

		White		Nonwhite†	
Cancer site	Total	Males	Females	Males	Females
All Sites Combined					
SNCS	288.9	283.7	305.0	225.6	273.2
TNCS	277.7	309.0	256.8	330.2	231.5
SEER (1976)		374.0	301.2	452.1	280.1
SEER (1987)		441.3	344.0	520.1	321.8
Lung					
SNCS	17.6	29.5	6.7	23.3	4.9
TNCS	39.2	68.0	14.9	77.9	13.5
SEER (1976)		77.8	23.7	112.8	25.6
SEER (1987)		82.3	38.7	118.9	37.5
Colon					
SNCS	23.8	23.8	26.0	13.7	11.9
TNCS	26.4	29.0	24.8	22.9	23.6
SEER (1976)		36.9	31.4	37.8	32.4
SEER (1987)		41.6	29.7	44.7	36.1
Rectum					
SNCS	16.6	20.7	13.9 ₁	11.4	12.3
TNCS	12.2	16.0	9.6 '	13.0	7.6
SEER (1976)		19.4	11.4	12.6	8.6
SEER (1987)		18.9	10.9	13.8	10.5
Breast					
SNCS		0.9	73.6	0.2	50.4
TNCS		0.8	73.3	0.7	53.7
SEER (1976)			83.5		66.7
SEER (1987)		0.8	115.9	1.0	90.9
Prostate					
SNCS		37.4		43.8	
TNCS		45.2		68.6	
SEER (1976)		68.6		107.9	
SEER (1987)		99.2		136.1	
Bladder					
SNCS	11.3	17.2	7.1	4.8	5.6
TNCS	11.7	21.3	5.6	9.8	3.5
SEER (1976)		26.4	7.3	13.2	6.1
SEER (1987)		33.0	7.3	16.7	5.9
Uterus Corpus and Uterus NOS‡					
SNCS			22.9		25.0
TNCS			23.2		13.1
SEER (1976)			31.2		15.2
SEER (1987)			22.5		13.0

Cancer site	Total	White		Nonwhite†	
		Males	Females	Males	Females
Melanoma					
SNCS	2.7	2.6	3.3	0.6	0.4
TNCS	4.3	4.8	4.7	0.8	0.6
SEER (1976)		6.8	6.1	1.3	1.1
SEER (1987)		12.8	10.1	1.4	0.8
Pancreas					
SNCS	7.1	8.9	5.6	9.9	4.1
TNCS	8.7	10.7	6.5	14.1	8.2
SEER (1976)		11.5	8.0	17.7	11.1
SEER (1987)		10.3	7.3	15.2	14.5
Kidney					
SNCS	4.0	5.2	2.9	4.8	2.5
TNCS	5.7	8.2	3.8	6.9	3.3
SEER (1976)		9.6	4.8	9.0	3.8
SEER (1987)		11.9	5.8	13.4	6.2
Leukemia					
SNCS	7.6	9.0	6.9	9.2	3.0
TNCS	8.4	11.0	6.7	8.7	5.3
SEER (1976)		13.1	7.1	9.2	6.1
SEER (1987)		12.5	7.4	12.0	6.8
Uterine Cervix					
SNCS			38.3		74.6
TNCS			15.1		31.3
SEER (1976)			10.6		26.4
SEER (1987)			7.3		15.1
Stomach					
SNCS	25.2	32.4	17.8	38.6	18.9
TNCS	9.1	12.1	5.8	18.6	7.9
SEER (1976)		12.6	5.6	20.3	9.2
SEER (1987)		10.4	4.5	19.8	7.7

SOURCE: S. S. Devesa and D. T. Silverman, "Cancer Incidence and Mortality Trends in the United States: 1935–74," *Journal of the National Cancer Institute* 60, no. 3 (1978): p. 545; E. S. Pollack and J. W. Horm, "Trends in Cancer Incidence and Mortality in the United States, 1969–76," *Journal of the National Cancer Institute* 64, no. 5 (1980): p. 1091.

*SNCS: Second National Cancer Survey, 1947–48, rates adjusted to age distribution of 1950 census population.

**TNCS: Third National Cancer Survey, 1969–71, rates adjusted to age distribution of 1950 census population.

***SEER: Surveillance, Epidemiology and End Results, 1976, rates adjusted to age distribution of 1970 Census population.

****SEER: Surveillance, Epidemiology and End Results, 1987, rates adjusted to 1970 Census population.

†Nonwhite rates for SEER program are for black population only.

‡Not otherwise specified.

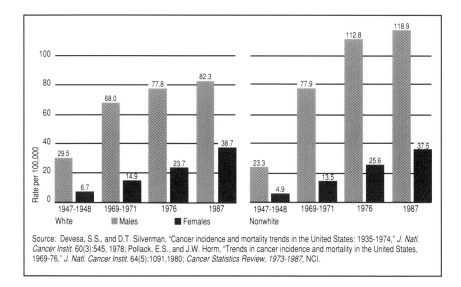

Fig. 4. Estimated lung cancer incidence rates per 100,000 population by race and sex, SNCS (1947–48), TNCS (1969–71), SEER (1976), SEER (1987)

LUNG

Since 1947 the greatest increase in cancer incidence has been for lung cancer. In 1947, white male incidence was estimated at 30 per 100,000 population. By 1987 this rate had risen to 82.3, an increase of more than 174 percent (figure 4).

An even greater increase has been noted among nonwhite males. In 1947, nonwhite male incidence was estimated at 23 per 100,000; by 1987 it had increased to 119 per 100,000 or more than 500 percent. These large increases are believed to be from the effects of cigarette smoking, although some of the increase for nonwhites may be explained by a lack of medical care in the past. Nonwhites had fewer contacts with the health-care system in 1947 than they did after legislation of Medicaid in 1965. This suggests that the number of new cases identified in 1947 was lower than it should have been.

The incidence of lung cancer among women has also steadily increased since 1947. Lung cancer incidence among white females increased from 7 in 1947 to 38.7 per 100,000 in 1987; from 5 to 37.5 per 100,000 among nonwhites.

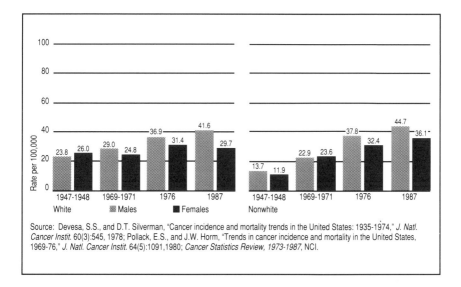

Fig. 5. Estimated colon cancer incidence rates per 100,000 population by race and sex, SNCS (1947–48), TNCS (1969–71), SEER (1976), SEER (1987)

The American Cancer Society, in fact, estimates that deaths due to lung cancer in 1990 will surpass those due to breast cancer (50,000 vs. 44,000).

At present, lung cancer incidence is increasing at a faster rate for females than for males. Indeed, a substantial proportion of the overall increase in cancer incidence during the 1970s can be explained by the dramatic surge in female lung cancer cases. This increase is also believed to trace to the increase in female cigarette smoking following World War II.

COLON

Colon cancer incidence among white males increased from 24 per 100,000 in 1947 to 41.6 in 1987 (figure 5). Among nonwhite males, incidence increased from 14 in 1947 to 44.7 per 100,000 in 1987. Nonwhite female incidence also increased during this period from 12 to 36.1 per 100,000.

Colon cancer incidence among white females decreased slightly during the period 1947–71 from 26 to 25 per 100,000. By 1987 this incidence had increased to 29.7 per 100,000.

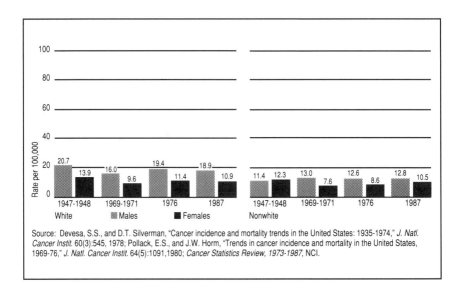

Source: Devesa, S.S., and D.T. Silverman, "Cancer incidence and mortality trends in the United States: 1935-1974," *J. Natl. Cancer Instit.* 60(3):545, 1978; Pollack, E.S., and J.W. Horm, "Trends in cancer incidence and mortality in the United States, 1969-76," *J. Natl. Cancer Instit.* 64(5):1091,1980; *Cancer Statistics Review, 1973-1987,* NCI.

Fig. 6. Estimated rectal cancer incidence rates per 100,000 population by race and sex, SNCS (1947–48), TNCS (1969–71), SEER (1976), SEER (1987)

RECTUM

The incidence of cancer of the rectum among white males and females and nonwhite females decreased from 1947 to 1971, then increased between 1971 and 1976 (figure 6). White males and females once again showed a decrease from 1976 to 1987, but nonwhite females continued to increase during this latter period. The incidence has fluctuated for nonwhite males.

BREAST

The breast is the leading site of cancer incidence among women. In whites, breast cancer incidence increased from 74 to 115.9 per 100,000 during 1947–87 (figure 7). Among nonwhites, it increased from 50 to 90.9 cases per 100,000 population during the same time period.

One report has suggested that there may be two distinct forms of breast tumors in women. One form is a malignant type that can be fatal if not detected early, while the other is a benign tumor that does not develop into malignancy. During the 1970s, many women became more aware of breast cancer because

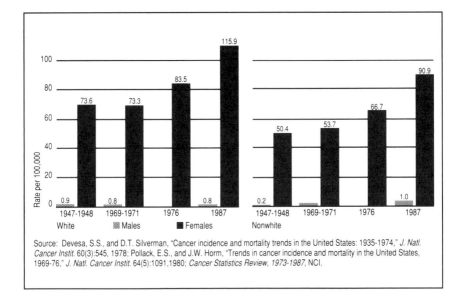

Source: Devesa, S.S., and D.T. Silverman, "Cancer incidence and mortality trends in the United States: 1935-1974," *J. Natl. Cancer Instit.* 60(3):545, 1978; Pollack, E.S., and J.W. Horm, "Trends in cancer incidence and mortality in the United States, 1969-76," *J. Natl. Cancer Instit.* 64(5):1091,1980; *Cancer Statistics Review, 1973-1987,* NCI.

Fig. 7. Estimated breast cancer incidence rates per 100,000 population by race and sex, SNCS (1947–48), TNCS (1969–71), SEER (1976), SEER (1987)

of the publicity over the breast cancer diagnoses of Betty Ford, Marvella Bayh, and Happy Rockefeller. The increase in self-examination and other early-detection methods may therefore have led to a diagnosis of more benign tumor types. This suggests that there may have been no real increase in the incidence of malignant breast cancer in recent years.

PROSTATE

Prostate cancer incidence has increased substantially among white and non-white males (figure 8), making it the most common type of male cancer. Among whites, it increased from 37 to 99.2 per 100,000 during 1947–87. Among nonwhites, prostate cancer incidence increased from 44 to 136.1 cases per 100,000 population during the same period. These increases may again reflect better diagnosis of prostate cancer in its early stages and, for nonwhites, better access to medical care. Since prostate cancer occurs more in older males, longer male life expectancy will also allow for the discovery of new cancer cases although another illness or disease may actually cause death.

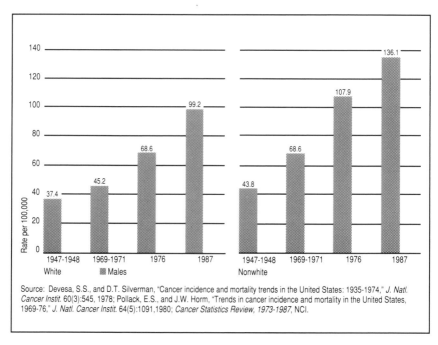

Fig. 8. Estimated prostate cancer incidence rates per 100,000 population by race, SNCS (1947–48), TNCS (1969–71), SEER (1976), SEER (1987)

BLADDER

For males, bladder cancer incidence increased from 1947 to 1987 (figure 9). Among white males it increased from 17 to 33 per 100,000. Among nonwhite males bladder cancer increased from 5 in 1947 to 16.7 per 100,000 in 1976. Female bladder cancer incidence decreased slightly from 7 in whites and 6 in nonwhites in 1947 to 6 and 4 per 100,000, respectively, in 1971. Since 1971, female bladder cancer has increased to 7 per 100,000 in whites and 6 per 100,000 in nonwhites.

The increases in male bladder cancer are likely due to cigarette smoking and occupational exposures to certain toxic chemicals. Among females the recent increases are probably from smoking alone. In general, bladder cancer is far more likely to occur in males than females.

UTERUS OTHER THAN CERVIX

The incidence of cancer of the uterine corpus increased among whites from 23 in 1947 to 31 per 100,000 in 1976 (figure 10). Among nonwhites, incidence

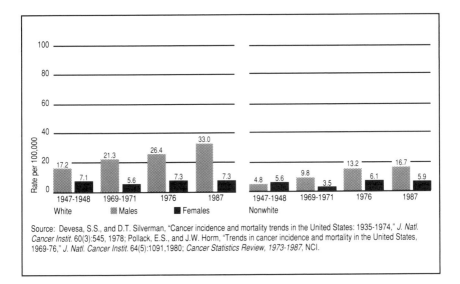

Fig. 9. Estimated bladder cancer incidence rates per 100,000 population by race and sex, SNCS (1947–48), TNCS (1969–71), SEER (1976), SEER (1987)

substantially decreased during the period 1947–71, then increased slightly during 1971–76. Research has suggested that increases in that time period may have traced to the long-term use of estrogen compounds in treating menopausal symptoms. However, from 1976 to 1987 the incidence decreased for both races to 22.5 among white women and 13 in nonwhite women. This may represent improved knowledge of the use of estrogen in the management of menopausal symptoms.

MELANOMA

The incidence of melanoma, a malignant skin cancer, has increased in all groups since 1947 (figure 11). Among white males, it increased from 3 to 12.8 per 100,000 during the period 1947–87. Among white females melanoma incidence increased from 3 to 10.1 per 100,000 in 1987. Although slight increases in melanoma incidence have also been reported for nonwhites, this form of cancer is rare among dark-skinned individuals. Geographic variation in melanoma incidence suggests that it may trace in part to exposure to solar radiation, but this relationship is still uncertain.

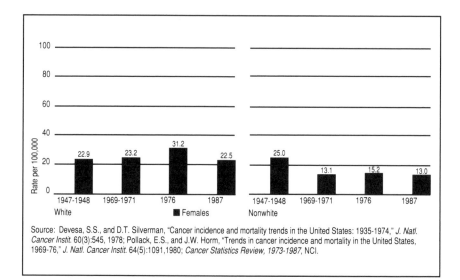

Fig. 10. Estimated cancer incidence rates per 100,000 population by race, uterus corpus and uterus not otherwise specified, SNCS (1947–48), TNCS (1969–71), SEER (1976), SEER (1987)

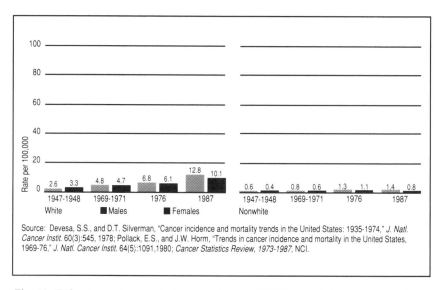

Fig. 11. Estimated melanoma incidence rates per 100,000 population by race and sex, SNCS (1947–48), TNCS (1969–71), SEER (1976), SEER (1987)

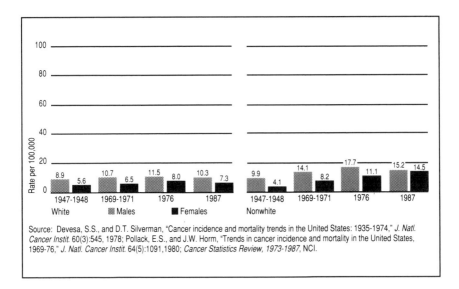

Fig. 12. Estimated pancreatic cancer incidence rates per 100,000 population by race and sex, SNCS (1947–48), TNCS (1969–71), SEER (1976), SEER (1987)

PANCREAS

The incidence of pancreatic cancer increased in all sex and race groups since 1947 (figure 12). The incidence of pancreatic cancer increased in all sex and race groups from 1947 to 1976, and then declined for all except nonwhite females from 1976 to 1987.

KIDNEY

The incidence of kidney cancer has increased among males and females in both race groups (figure 13). Among white males it rose from 5 to 11.9 cases per 100,000 during the period 1947–87. For nonwhite males incidence increased from 5 to 13.4 per 100,000 during this same period. Increases in female incidence during 1947–76 were substantially less than those for males, suggesting differential exposure to some carcinogenic agent. However, female increases from 1976 to 1987 more closely followed increases among males.

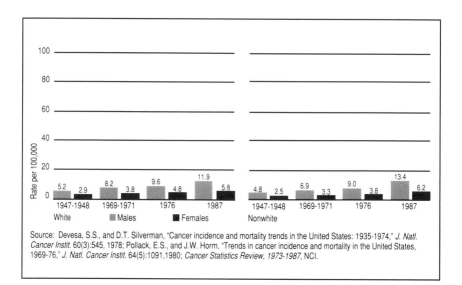

Fig. 13. Estimated kidney cancer incidents rates per 100,000 population by race and sex, SNCS (1947–48), TNCS (1969–71), SEER (1976), SEER (1987)

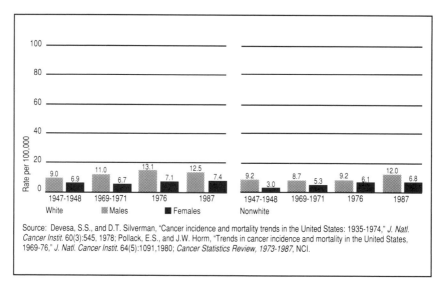

Fig. 14. Estimated leukemia incidence rates per 100,000 population by race and sex, SNCS (1947–48), TNCS (1969–71), SEER (1976), SEER (1987)

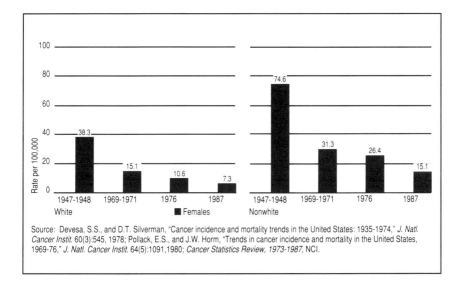

Source: Devesa, S.S., and D.T. Silverman, "Cancer incidence and mortality trends in the United States: 1935-1974," *J. Natl. Cancer Instit.* 60(3):545, 1978; Pollack, E.S., and J.W. Horm, "Trends in cancer incidence and mortality in the United States, 1969-76," *J. Natl. Cancer Instit.* 64(5):1091,1980; *Cancer Statistics Review, 1973-1987,* NCI.

Fig. 15. Estimated uterine cervix cancer incidence rates per 100,000 population by race and sex, SNCS (1947–48), TNCS (1969–71), SEER (1976), SEER (1987)

LEUKEMIA

Leukemia incidence increased among white males and nonwhite females during the period 1947–76 (figure 14). In nonwhite females the rate doubled from 3 to 6 per 100,000. During this same period, the incidence for white females and nonwhite males has remained relatively constant. From 1976 to 1987, the incidence dropped slightly for white males and increased most dramatically for nonwhite males.

CERVIX

The incidence of cervical cancer has decreased substantially since 1947 in both white and nonwhite females (figure 15). Among whites it declined from 38 in 1947 to 11 per 100,000 in 1976; in 1987 the incidence was down to 7.3. Among nonwhites cervical cancer incidence decreased from 75 to 15.1 during 1947–87. Most, if not all, of this decline can be explained by use of the Pap test, which can detect precancerous changes in uterine tissue before they become cancerous and thus allow for surgical treatment or other therapy.

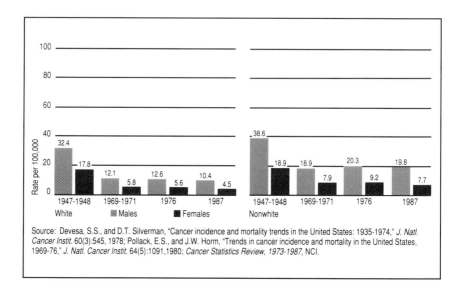

Source: Devesa, S.S., and D.T. Silverman, "Cancer incidence and mortality trends in the United States: 1935-1974," *J. Natl. Cancer Instit.* 60(3):545, 1978; Pollack, E.S., and J.W. Horm, "Trends in cancer incidence and mortality in the United States, 1969-76," *J. Natl. Cancer Instit.* 64(5):1091,1980; *Cancer Statistics Review, 1973-1987,* NCI.

Fig. 16. Estimated stomach cancer incidence rates per 100,000 population by race and sex, SNCS (1947–48), TNCS (1969–71), SEER (1976), SEER (1987)

STOMACH

Stomach cancer incidence also declined substantially for all sex and race groups during the period 1947–87 (figure 16). The combined rates for males and females dropped from 25 to 8 per 100,000. Between 1971 and 1976, U.S. stomach cancer incidence remained stable at the lowest level in the world. The cause of this decline is unknown, but many believe it is related to the widespread use of refrigeration and antioxidant food additives rather than salting to preserve food. In countries where salting and pickling are still the main forms of food preservation, stomach cancer rates are considerably higher than those in the United States.

U.S. Cancer Mortality

Cancer is the second leading cause of death in the United States after diseases of the heart and circulatory system.

The American Cancer Society estimates that about 514,000 Americans

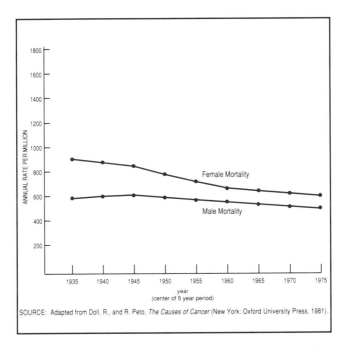

SOURCE: Adapted from Doll, R., and R. Peto, *The Causes of Cancer* (New York: Oxford University Press, 1981).

Fig. 17. Age-standardized certified death rates for entire U.S. Population, 1933–77. All cancers except lung and skin. Rates per million, standardized to the age distribution of all respondents under 65 years to the U.S. 1970 census.

will die of cancer in 1991. Of these, 142,000, or 28 percent, will die of lung cancer. Recent data (figure 17), however, indicate a gradual decline from 1933 to 1977 in the age-adjusted cancer death rates (except lung and skin cancer) for both sexes under the age of sixty-five; there was a continued decline from 1971 to 1987. These general declines in most cancer death rates among both men and women contrast sharply with the rapid increases in lung cancer death rates for males (figures 18 and 19). It is important to bear in mind that these sharp increases in mortality are due to lung cancer. Figures 18 and 19 summarize the long-term trends in cancer death rates for whites and nonwhites, males and females.

These declining trends in cancer death rates trace in part to the decrease in certain forms of cancer, especially stomach and cervical cancer. They are also the result of the increased use of screening methods that can detect cancers early, when therapy can be more successful. Some of the decrease can also be attributed to improved medical and surgical treatments for diagnosed cancers. These improvements have increased the survival rates for several forms of cancer, particularly leukemia, Hodgkin's disease, and breast cancer in young women. On the other hand, survival rates for lung and pancreatic cancers remain very low.

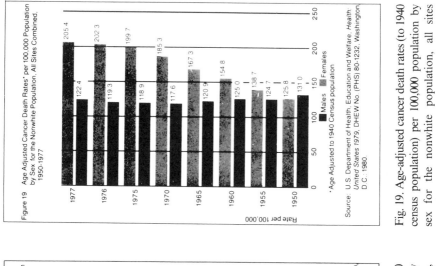

Fig. 19. Age-adjusted cancer death rates (to 1940 census population) per 100,000 population by sex for the nonwhite population, all sites combined, 1950–1977

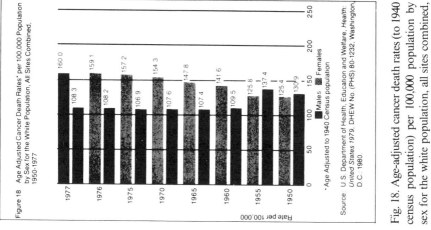

Fig. 18. Age-adjusted cancer death rates (to 1940 census population) per 100,000 population by sex for the white population, all sites combined, 1950–1977

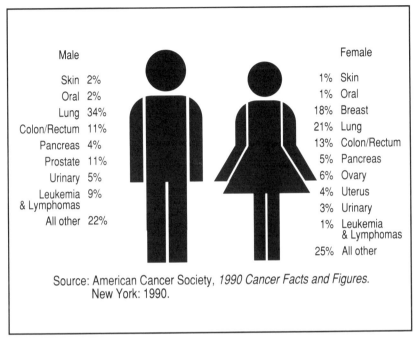

Source: American Cancer Society, *1990 Cancer Facts and Figures.*
New York: 1990.

Fig. 20. 1990 estimated cancer deaths by site and sex

Lung cancer is the most common cause of cancer deaths among men, followed by colon-rectum and prostate cancers. Lung cancer is also the leading cause of cancer deaths among women, followed by breast and colon-rectum cancers. Figure 20 shows the proportion of all cancer deaths for specific body sites of the disease.

As is evident in figures 21, 22, and 23, the only cancer deaths that qualify as "epidemic" are those from lung cancer. The rapid increase in lung cancer deaths is most evident for males, but has also become evident in recent years for women as well. This delayed increase in female lung cancer death rates is consistent with the rise in female cigarette smoking that followed World War II. In contrast, men began smoking in large numbers after World War I, almost thirty years earlier. The usual latency period for lung cancer is twenty to thirty years, which accounts for the delayed increase in lung cancer mortality rates among women, whose smoking patterns are known to lag twenty-five to thirty years behind those for males. Table 2 summarizes the recent trends in the site-specific cancer death rates for men and women.

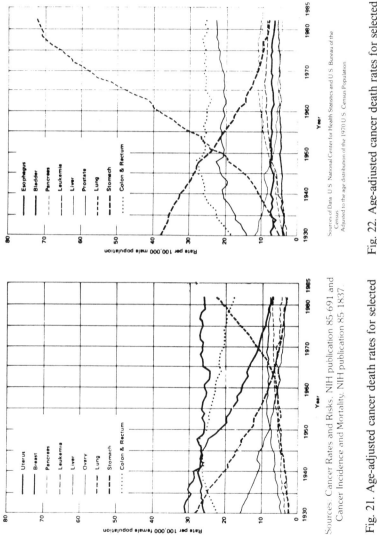

Sources: Cancer Rates and Risks. NIH publication 85 691 and
Cancer Incidence and Mortality. NIH publication 85 1837.

Fig. 21. Age-adjusted cancer death rates for selected
sites, females, United States, 1930–82

Sources of Data: U S. National Center for Health Statistics and U S. Bureau of the
Census.
Adjusted to the age distribution of the 1970 U.S. Census Population.

Fig. 22. Age-adjusted cancer death rates for selected
sites, males, United States, 1930–1982

An International Comparison

It is widely believed that the United States has a high cancer death rate compared with other countries. One network television program on cancer opened with the statement: "The news tonight is that the United States is number one in cancer. The National Cancer Institute estimates that if you're living in America your chances of getting cancer are higher than anywhere else in the world."

However, cancer mortality data gathered by the World Health Organization and analyzed by the American Cancer Society provide a much different view.

Table 2. Thirty-five-Year Trends in Age-adjusted Cancer Death Rates per 100,000 Population, 1949–51 to 1984–86

Sites	Sex	1949–51	1984–86	Percent Changes	Comments
All sites	Male	168.0	218.7	+ 30	Steady increase mainly due to lung cancer.
	Female	147.8	139.3	– 6	Early decrease, but recent increases due to lung cancer.
Bladder	Male	7.2	6.0	– 17	Slight decrease in recent years.
	Female	3.2	1.7	– 46	Some fluctuations; noticeable decrease.
Brain	Male	3.3	4.9	+ 47	Early increase in both sexes; later leveling off, reasons unknown.
	Female	2.2	3.3	+ 51	
Breast	Male	0.4	0.2	– 36	Steady decrease.
	Female	25.9	27.3	+ 5	Slight fluctuations; overall no change.
Colon & Rectum	Male	25.4	24.9	*	Slow steady increase; then leveling in recent years.
	Female	24.8	17.5	– 29	Slow, steady decrease.
Colon	Male	16.9	21.2	+ 26	Slow, steady increase; then leveling in recent years.
	Female	18.8	15.3	– 18	Slow, steady decrease.
Rectum	Male	9.3	3.8	– 59	Slow, steady decrease in both sexes.
	Female	6.5	2.2	+ 42	
Esophagus	Male	4.7	5.7	+ 20	Some fluctuations; small increase.
	Female	1.2	1.5	+ 19	Slight fluctuations; small increase.
Kidney	Male	3.3	4.7	+ 44	Steady increase.
	Female	2.0	2.2	*	Slight fluctuations; overall no change.
Larynx	Male	2.6	2.6	*	Slight fluctuations; overall no change.
	Female	0.3	0.5	+ 88	Steady increase in females.
Leukemia	Male	7.3	8.4	+ 15	Early increase; later leveling off and decrease.
	Female	5.0	5.0	*	Early slight increase; later leveling off and decrease.
Liver†	Male	6.9	4.8	– 31	Decreasing rapidly early; later leveling off.
	Female	8.0	3.3	– 59	Some fluctuations; steady decrease.
Lung	Male	22.0	73.9	+236	Steady increase in both sexes due to cigarette smoking.
	Female	4.8	26.2	+450	
Non-Hodgkin's Lymphoma	Male	3.6	6.9	+ 92	Steady increase in both sexes.
	Female	2.3	4.7	+103	
Hodgkin's Disease	Male	2.2	0.9	– 60	Steady decrease in both sexes.
	Female	1.3	0.5	– 61	
Multiple Myeloma	Male	1.1	3.5	+215	Steady increase in both sexes.
	Female	2.3	4.7	+103	
Oral	Male	6.4	5.0	– 21	Steady decrease.
	Female	1.6	1.8	+ 15	Slight fluctuations; overall no change.
Ovary	Female	7.9	7.7	*	Early increase; then leveling off and decrease.
Pancreas	Male	8.2	10.2	+ 24	Early increase; later leveling off.
	Female	5.5	7.2	+ 32	Steady increase.
Prostate	Male	20.6	23.7	+ 15	Slight increase in recent years.
Total Skin	Male	3.3	4.1	+ 23	Some fluctuations; slight increase.
	Female	2.1	1.8	– 14	Slight decrease.
Melanoma of Skin	Male	1.0	2.8	+183	Steady increase in both sexes.
	Female	0.8	1.5	+ 88	
Other Skin	Male	2.2	1.3	– 42	Steady decrease in both sexes.
	Female	1.3	0.3	– 74	
Stomach	Male	24.6	7.5	– 70	Steady decrease in both sexes; reasons unknown.
	Female	13.5	3.4	– 75	
Uterus	Female	21.6	6.9	– 68	Steady decrease.

*Percent changes not listed because they are not meaningful.
†Primary and non-specified.
Source: American Cancer Society, *1990 Cancer Facts & Figures.*

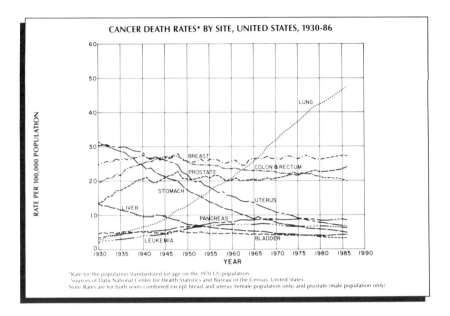

Fig. 23. Cancer death rates by site, United States, 1930–86

In a comparison of age-adjusted cancer death rates for fifty countries, the United States ranked twenty-sixth for male, and twentieth for female cancer death rates. Hungary experienced the highest age-adjusted cancer death rate, followed by Czechoslovakia, Luxembourg, the Netherlands, and Scotland (figure 24).

As with other statistical data on cancer, this comparison must be interpreted cautiously. There are many differences in the completeness and accuracy of cancer death reports among countries. So, too, the quality of medical care differs substantially and affects the diagnosis of specific types of cancer. For some countries, low cancer rates may also signify that the average life expectancy is too short to allow some kinds of cancer to occur; their citizens die of other causes well before the age when these cancers are diagnosed.

Cancer Clusters

Variations in the incidence of specific types of cancer in different time periods or geographic areas can provide valuable clues as to the causes of these cancers.

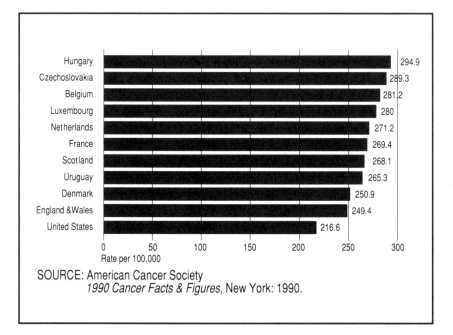

	Rate per 100,000
Hungary	294.9
Czechoslovakia	289.3
Belgium	281.2
Luxembourg	280
Netherlands	271.2
France	269.4
Scotland	268.1
Uruguay	265.3
Denmark	250.9
England &Wales	249.4
United States	216.6

Rate per 100,000

SOURCE: American Cancer Society
1990 Cancer Facts & Figures, New York: 1990.

Fig. 24. Age-adjusted white male cancer death rates per 100,000 population, selected countries, 1990.

The dramatic increase in lung cancer rates earlier in this century, for example, prompted research that incriminated cigarette smoking as the major cause of lung cancer. Differences in the rates of stomach and colon cancers between countries have suggested that dietary factors may influence the risk of developing these types of cancer.

From time to time there are reports of more localized variations in cancer incidence or "cancer clusters"—unusually high numbers of a specific type of cancer in a small area, such as a neighborhood or community, over a limited time period. Most of these reports have involved clusters of leukemia (malignancy of the blood-forming organs) or lymphomas (malignancies of the lymph glands). Because these cancers are relatively rare, the number of cases of these "outbreaks," although greater than expected, has usually been very small.

Clustering of a specific type of cancer may suggest that the disease is caused by a virus or some other infectious agent that can be transmitted from person to person. Clustering may also suggest that the victims have been exposed to a cancer-causing environmental substance. However, many apparent cancer clusters are merely the result of random fluctuations in the incidence of cancer.

Even if an event occurs totally at random, some clustering is bound to occur by chance. For example, if you thoroughly mix fifty red marbles into a tub of a thousand blue marbles, the red marbles should theoretically be evenly distributed among the blue ones. In practice, however, you might find one or two "clusters" of red marbles. There is no "reason" for the clustering, other than random fluctuation in the distribution of the marbles.

The same type of random fluctuations can account for clusters of cancer; and if enough people are looking for clusters, some will find them. For example, if twenty researchers look for unusual clustering among a small series of cases, on the average, one will identify a cluster even if there is no relationship between any of the cases. The one researcher with positive results will probably publish his findings, while the other nineteen probably will not publish their negative results.

Index